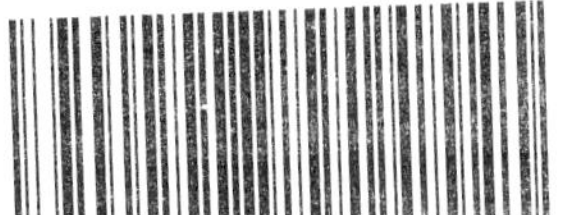
MW00780134

SCIENCE AND PRACTICE IN COGNITIVE THERAPY

Also from Robert L. Leahy

Cognitive Therapy Techniques, Second Edition: A Practitioner's Guide
Robert L. Leahy

Emotion Regulation in Psychotherapy: A Practitioner's Guide
Robert L. Leahy, Dennis Tirch, and Lisa A. Napolitano

Emotional Schema Therapy
Robert L. Leahy

Overcoming Resistance in Cognitive Therapy
Robert L. Leahy

Psychological Treatment of Bipolar Disorder
Edited by Sheri L. Johnson and Robert L. Leahy

Roadblocks in Cognitive-Behavioral Therapy: Transforming Challenges into Opportunities for Change
Edited by Robert L. Leahy

Treatment Plans and Interventions for Bulimia and Binge-Eating Disorder
Rene D. Zweig and Robert L. Leahy

Treatment Plans and Interventions for Depression and Anxiety Disorders, Second Edition
Robert L. Leahy, Stephen J. F. Holland, and Lata K. McGinn

SCIENCE AND PRACTICE IN COGNITIVE THERAPY

Foundations, Mechanisms, and Applications

edited by

ROBERT L. LEAHY

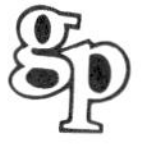

THE GUILFORD PRESS
New York London

A Division of Guilford Publications, Inc.
370 Seventh Avenue, Suite 1200, New York, NY 10001
www.guilford.com

Printed in the United States of America

This book is printed on acid-free paper.

Last digit is print number: 9 8 7 6 5 4 3 2 1

Library of Congress Cataloging-in-Publication Data

Names: Leahy, Robert L., editor.
Title: Science and practice in cognitive therapy : foundations, mechanisms, and applications / edited by Robert L. Leahy.
Description: New York : The Guilford Press, [2018] | Includes bibliographical references and index.
Identifiers: LCCN 2017050354 | ISBN 9781462533381 (hardback : alk. paper)
Subjects: | MESH: Cognitive Therapy
Classification: LCC RC489.C63 | NLM WM 425.5.C6 | DDC 616.89/1425—dc23
LC record available at *https://lccn.loc.gov/2017050354*

About the Editor

Robert L. Leahy, PhD, is Director of the American Institute for Cognitive Therapy in New York and Clinical Professor of Psychology in the Department of Psychiatry at Weill Cornell Medical College. His research focuses on individual differences in emotion regulation. Dr. Leahy is Associate Editor of the *International Journal of Cognitive Therapy* and is past president of the Association for Behavioral and Cognitive Therapies, the International Association for Cognitive Psychotherapy, and the Academy of Cognitive Therapy. He is a recipient of the Aaron T. Beck Award from the Academy of Cognitive Therapy. Dr. Leahy has published numerous books, including *Cognitive Therapy Techniques, Second Edition*; *Treatment Plans and Interventions for Depression and Anxiety Disorders, Second Edition*; and *Emotion Regulation in Psychotherapy*. He is Editor of Guilford's Treatment Plans and Interventions for Evidence-Based Psychotherapy series.

Contributors

Lyn Y. Abramson, PhD, Department of Psychology, University of Wisconsin–Madison, Madison, Wisconsin

Lauren B. Alloy, PhD, Department of Psychology, Temple University, Philadelphia, Pennsylvania

Arnoud Arntz, PhD, Department of Clinical Psychology, University of Amsterdam, Amsterdam, The Netherlands

Aaron T. Beck, MD, Beck Institute for Cognitive Therapy, Bala Cynwyd, Pennsylvania; Department of Psychiatry (Emeritus), University of Pennsylvania Perelman School of Medicine, Philadelphia, Pennsylvania

Judith S. Beck, PhD, Beck Institute for Cognitive Therapy, Bala Cynwyd, Pennsylvania

Taylor A. Burke, MA, Department of Psychology, Temple University, Philadelphia, Pennsylvania

Joseph K. Carpenter, MA, Department of Psychological and Brain Sciences, Boston University, Boston, Massachusetts

David A. Clark, PhD, Department of Psychology (Emeritus), University of New Brunswick, Fredericton, New Brunswick, Canada

Michelle Hanna Collins, MEd, Student Affairs Office, Moravian College, Bethlehem, Pennsylvania

Joshua Curtiss, MA, Department of Psychological and Brain Sciences, Boston University, Boston, Massachusetts

Frank M. Dattilio, PhD, ABPP, Department of Psychiatry, University of Pennsylvania Perelman School of Medicine, Philadelphia, Pennsylvania; Harvard Medical School, Boston, Massachusetts

Denise D. Davis, PhD, Department of Psychological Studies, Vanderbilt University, Nashville, Tennessee

Robert J. DeRubeis, PhD, Department of Psychology, University of Pennsylvania, Philadelphia, Pennsylvania

Keith S. Dobson, PhD, Department of Psychology, University of Calgary, Calgary, Alberta, Canada

Norman B. Epstein, PhD, Department of Family Science, School of Public Health, University of Maryland, College Park, College Park, Maryland

Amanda M. Ferguson, MA, Graduate Department of Psychological Clinical Science, University of Toronto Scarborough, Ontario, Canada

Nicole B. Gumport, BA, Department of Psychology, University of California, Berkeley, Berkeley, California

Allison G. Harvey, PhD, Department of Psychology, University of California, Berkeley, Berkeley, California

Stefan G. Hofmann, PhD, Department of Psychological and Brain Sciences, Boston University, Boston, Massachusetts

Steven D. Hollon, PhD, Department of Psychology, Vanderbilt University, Nashville, Tennessee

Emily A. Holmes, PhD, Department of Clinical Neuroscience, Karolinska Institute, Stockholm, Sweden

Sheri L. Johnson, PhD, Department of Psychology, University of California, Berkeley, Berkeley, California

Robert L. Leahy, PhD, American Institute for Cognitive Therapy, New York, New York

Bruce S. Liese, PhD, Department of Family Medicine, University of Kansas Medical Center, and Department of Psychology, The University of Kansas, Lawrence, Kansas

Anthony P. Morrison, PhD, Division of Psychology and Mental Health, University of Manchester, Manchester, United Kingdom

Elizabeth K. Murphy, Division of Psychology and Mental Health, University of Manchester, Manchester, United Kingdom

Cory F. Newman, PhD, Center for Cognitive Therapy and Department of Psychiatry, University of Pennsylvania Perelman School of Medicine, Philadelphia, Pennsylvania

Jared O'Garro-Moore, MA, Department of Psychology, Temple University, Philadelphia, Pennsylvania

Andrew D. Peckham, PhD, Behavioral Health Partial Hospital Program, McLean Hospital, Belmont, Massachusetts

Julia C. Poole, MSc, Department of Psychology, University of Calgary, Calgary, Alberta, Canada

Fritz Renner, PhD, Medical Research Council, Cognition and Brain Sciences Unit, Cambridge, United Kingdom

Patricia A. Resick, PhD, Department of Psychiatry and Behavioral Sciences, Duke University Medical Center, Durham, North Carolina

Rachael I. Rosner, PhD, Independent Scholar, Boston, Massachusetts

Zindel V. Segal, PhD, Graduate Department of Psychological Clinical Science, University of Toronto Scarborough, Scarborough, Ontario, Canada

Debbie Sookman, PhD, Obsessive Compulsive Disorder Clinic, Department of Psychology, McGill University Health Center, and Department of Psychiatry, McGill University, Montreal, Quebec, Canada

Jessica C. Tripp, MS, Department of Psychology, The University of Memphis, Memphis, Tennessee

Preface

When I was a young graduate student many years ago, the only model that interested me was the psychodynamic model. It appealed to me because it seemed to have depth, it promised to free people from the traumas and ghosts of the past, and it offered an approach to the bigger questions of love, war, and even the complexities of civilization. But as I began reading more about the lack of evidence of its effectiveness, I became disillusioned and turned away from what I thought was the magic key. Then I discovered the work of Aaron T. Beck, the visionary and pioneer whose work has influenced all of the contributors to this volume. That work has changed my life.

What Beck did was turn depression—and then anxiety, anger, and even personality disorder—on its head. Rather than digging for the buried treasures of the unconscious, Beck's cognitive model allowed us to access thoughts and images that were often right out in the open. It was as if the secret to treating depression and other disorders were hidden in plain sight. His work on depression provided both a model of what activated, maintained, and escalated negative moods and a treatment model that guided us in directly addressing each of the major symptoms of depression. Ever the objective scientist, he, together with colleagues, demonstrated the effectiveness of this approach and gave rise to a new field—cognitive therapy.

The contributors to this volume were all influenced by Beck's work, and it is a testimony to the cognitive model that it has expanded its conceptualization and treatment protocols for the past 45 years. It is not a doctrinaire model, and Beck himself has continued to expand it by integrating the cognitive model with contemporary neuroscience, evolutionary theory, and socialization research. In the chapters that follow, the reader will be taken on a journey from Beck's current work (on schizophrenia) to an overview of the emergence of this work in the early years when Beck broke away from the psychodynamic schools that were so dominant at the time. The cognitive model—or cognitive-behavioral therapy (CBT) model—is then described as it relates to a wide variety of disorders, the research supporting the various approaches is outlined, and the clinical implications are elucidated.

Not every application of the cognitive model is reflected in the current volume; that would require several books. But I hope the reader will share with me some of my fascination with the continuing impact of Beck's cognitive therapy model and will feel deep gratitude that we have come so far from those early days. Many of the "truisms" of CBT that we now take for granted were considered heresy—or even delusional—at one time. Though that is no longer the case, we must not rest on our laurels. No, we hope that new approaches will emerge, new techniques will be developed, and new hope will be given to those who suffer.

After all, we are really in the business of saving the world one person at a time.

Contents

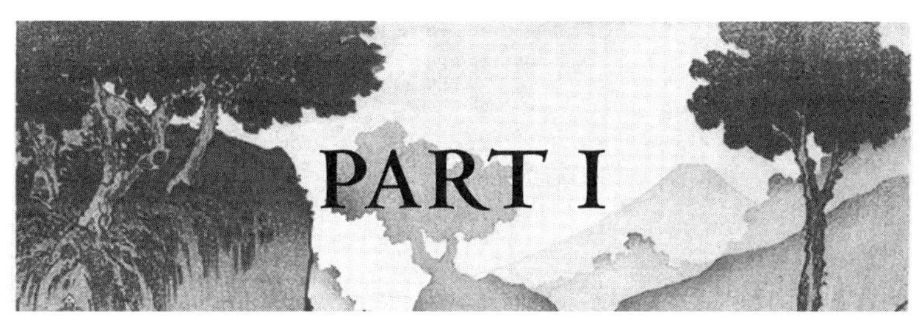

FOUNDATIONS OF THE COGNITIVE MODEL

CHAPTER 1

Recovery-Oriented Cognitive Therapy for Schizophrenia

A Personal Perspective

Aaron T. Beck

I have traveled a long road since my initial exposure to the images and descriptions of individuals with schizophrenia. My early exposure consisted of movies, such as *The Snake Pit*. In medical school, the exposure consisted of a kind of freak show, in which various individuals with schizophrenia were exhibited to show their bizarre behavior and to relate their fantastic delusions.

My first direct contact with these patients in my residency program was with individuals who were lying comatose as a result of insulin shock treatment, or were walking around with a shaven head with scars from their lobotomies, or sitting in straitjackets in seclusion rooms, or receiving hydrotherapy, in which they would lie in hot tubs covered with canvas up to their necks.

I had occasion to treat an individual with a delusion of being followed by government agents (Beck, 1952). At that time, I focused partly on the meaning of the delusion, but largely on supporting him to make an adjustment to civilian life.

For several decades after that, I had little contact with individuals with schizophrenia. In the 1990s, while attending a meeting at the Royal

College of Psychiatry in England, I came across a poster that described the application of cognitive therapy to a fairly large number of individuals[1] with schizophrenia. I finally located the authors, David Kingdon and Doug Turkington, and subsequently organized a meeting in Philadelphia attended by various groups from England who, to my surprise and pleasure, were also using cognitive therapy or cognitive-behavioral therapy in the treatment of individuals with schizophrenia (see also Morrison and Murphy, Chapter 16 of this volume, on CBT for schizophrenia).

At this point, I teamed up with Paul Grant, who was then a graduate student at the University of Pennsylvania and who was interested in schizophrenia. We realized that while the various English groups worked on the psychological aspects of the positive symptoms of schizophrenia (delusions and hallucinations), there was a large gap, specifically, the challenge of dealing with negative symptoms. At that time, it was believed that neurocognitive impairments (defects in executive function, attention, and memory) were responsible for the negative symptoms. Indeed, a positive correlation exists between these neurocognitive deficits and the negative symptoms. Yet Paul and I reasoned that it simply did not make sense that the deficits in behavior were directly due to deficits of neurocognitive functioning. We speculated that the individuals' dysfunctional beliefs mediated between these two processes. To test this hypothesis, we prepared a checklist of defeatist attitudes (see below), which we administered to individuals with schizophrenia. We found that defeatist beliefs correlated with negative symptoms and neurocognitive impairment; the missing link between neurocognitive impairments and deficits in behavior appears to be defeatist and asocial attitudes, as we suspected (Grant & Beck, 2009, 2010).

We inferred that the neurocognitive deficits probably led to substandard academic performance and social awkwardness during adolescence (for example, disappointment in oneself, disparagement, and even bullying by others). We proposed that individuals vulnerable to schizophrenia built a wall of protective attitudes to insulate themselves from being hurt (Grant, Beck, Stolar, & Rector, 2009). In addition to holding defeatist beliefs, we found that the individuals who had more negative symptoms scored higher on an asocial beliefs scale, demonstrating the importance of dysfunctional attitudes in the impoverished social lives of individuals with the deficit syndrome. The Asocial Belief Scale contained a number of isolating items such as "I prefer watching television to going out with others" (Beck, Grant, Huh, Perivoliotis, & Chang, 2013; Grant & Beck, 2010).

Having reached this point in our research and formulations, it seemed that the next step would be to conduct a clinical trial aimed at modifying these dysfunctional attitudes, with the hope that this would unlock the

[1]In this chapter, I refer to people with schizophrenia as "individuals" rather than as patients as a way of emphasizing personhood rather than patienthood.

individuals' proactive tendencies and facilitate their having a better quality of life, as well as greater independence, better social interactions, and vocational success. We conducted a clinical trial examining cognitive therapy as a treatment for low-functioning outpatients with schizophrenia (Grant, Huh, Perivoliotis, Stolar, & Beck, 2012). In this study, sixty individuals with prominent negative symptoms and neurocognitive impairments were randomly assigned to receive either standard treatment alone or standard treatment with cognitive therapy. Duration of treatment varied from six months to eighteen months. In addition to concentrating on negative symptoms in low-functioning individuals, therapists also used established cognitive therapy techniques to address the positive symptoms in the higher functioning individuals. Analyses of data from blind assessments revealed that participants who received cognitive therapy compared to standard treatment exhibited better global functioning, fewer negative symptoms (in particular, avolition and apathy), and fewer positive symptoms (hallucinations, delusions, and disorganization) by the end of treatment.

At the time we were conducting this study, we became aware of the increasing popularity in the mental health field of *Recovery*, and we endorsed the concepts underlying it: restoring the individual's self-respect, independence, and integration into the community. Of note, many individuals made an excellent social and vocational recovery without insight into the pathological nature of their voices and delusions (Grant, Reisweber, Luther, Brinen, & Beck, 2013; Perivoliotis, Grant, & Beck, 2009).

In order to fill the need for therapists trained in recovery-oriented cognitive therapy (CT-R), we embarked on a broad program of training clinicians in hospitals, assertive community therapy teams (ACT teams), community mental health centers, and outpatient clinics. We also established a recovery milieu in several hospitals and community mental health centers. The program enhanced activities of the individuals and greatly increased staff and individual participation. Our therapeutic approach (CT-R) is illustrated by the following case history.

Case History

A middle-aged Caucasian woman who was seen in a structured residence, had been hospitalized for twenty years. She believed she was the divine master of the universe and had created the planets and stars, as well as her fellow inhabitants of Earth. Some of the people she had created had turned against her, she believed. She stated that in order to protect herself, she withdrew from other people. In her isolated, regressed state, she spent time staring at a wall or, at times, smearing feces on it. She paid little attention to personal hygiene, was disheveled, and generally disorganized.

Her therapist began work with Jean by making a connection with her, developing a bond of trust and warmth. Once engaged, the next step was to ascertain her subjective needs: to belong, to be respected, to be independent, and to be productive. Jean revealed that her long-term goal was to return to teaching. Her therapist then collaborated with her to establish an activity that would appeal to her while she was still in the hospital. She expressed an interest in baking and then began to make cupcakes for herself and other individuals on the unit. Soon she began to teach others how to bake, not just cupcakes, but also soufflés and more complex dishes. Preparing food and teaching the other patients had a transformative effect on Jean. She began to take an interest again in her personal hygiene, to become more animated with others, and to talk in full sentences rather than in garbled speech.

Once Jean started baking and reestablished her role of teaching others, her "premorbid personality" reemerged, replacing her sullen, expressionless presentation. When Jean was in the regressive mode, she had a variety of fears and concerns, as well as a medley of beliefs designed to protect her from being hurt. Her fears centered on being exposed to ridicule by participating in group activities. She had a hypersensitivity to any actions of the staff that appeared controlling or rejecting, and she exhibited a strong impulse to retaliate verbally and sometimes physically when she felt threatened by the staff. Her image of herself at these times was that of being vulnerable, inadequate, and inept. Her aggressive behavior was a form of compensation for her sense of helplessness and inferiority to others. By cooking and ultimately providing for others, she shifted to a more adaptive mode. In this mode, she could see herself as adequate, competent, and commanding the respect of other people. Thus, her behavior changed to that of a tutor and teacher from that of a weak, threatened individual.

As can be suspected, however, the adaptive behaviors did not persist after she left the constructive situation in the kitchen. When she returned to her room, all of the maladaptive beliefs associated with the regressive mode became reactivated. Obviously, the matrix of regressive beliefs that had emerged and been reinforced on countless occasions were robust and nonamenable to radical change. Nonetheless, the more frequently the adaptive mode was activated (i.e., "I am competent" and "people respect me"), the more the positive beliefs associated with the adaptive mode became reinforced, and the negative and dysfunctional beliefs associated with the regressive mode gradually became weakened. Within three months of the initial contact with her therapist, she was discharged from the hospital. The interpersonal impact of her engagement with her therapist allowed her to feel safe, in what had seemed to be a hostile environment, and participating in meaningful activities with others restored her self-esteem and motivation to return to her previous life.

Jean had been dominated by a maladaptive, regressive mode, featuring negative views of herself, her world, and her future. Some of her beliefs included the following: "I have to protect myself. I'm better off being isolated from other people. If I interact with others, it only leads to trouble. I don't have the energy to do anything. There's no point in trying anything, because I would only fail." Grandiose delusions were a compensation for her negative concepts of herself and the outside world.

In working with a person with schizophrenia, we use the delusion as a source of information. Instead of challenging Jean's belief that she was God, we asked, "What is good about being God?" The therapist had expected her response to be something along the lines of: "If I'm God, I can create miracles, read people's minds and change the future." Jean's response was different. To her, being God meant: "I can help people." With this understanding—that she had a desire to help others, as well as information from her psychiatric record about her early career as a schoolteacher—we were able to create a context in which she could first nourish others and then help them learn the skills themselves.

THERAPEUTIC COMMUNITY

In our work in Jean's acute extended-care unit, we focused on instituting a therapeutic community in which such transformations could occur. We organized activities and projects to stimulate the individuals' motivation to interact with other people and to provide the staff with tools to help them. The program involved the integration of psychiatrists, nurses, and mental health workers, along with the individuals receiving care, in group projects that would benefit the entire hospital community, such as putting on an art exhibit, decorating the unit, and producing a play. The individuals with schizophrenia took the initiative in preparing a script for the play, memorizing lines, constructing sets, and designing costumes. An art therapist supervised their work. Staff members also had roles in the play. The most withdrawn individual played a role as usher giving out the programs. Interestingly, the members of the audience reported that they could not differentiate patients from staff in the play.

One week following the successful play on the unit, Jean, who had played a role preparing the script, said that her take-home message was: "I am capable, confident, and proud of myself. I feel hopeful, part of a group, and worthwhile." Similar responses were expressed by other participants in the play. Following the play and other similar successful experiences, the therapists regularly reinforced the positive conclusions invoked by the patients' successful performance.

INDIVIDUAL THERAPY

Engagement with the therapist plays an indispensable role in the psychotherapy of regressed individuals. Among the barriers to successful engagement are the individual's preoccupations with hallucinations, difficulty in deploying attentional resources to the therapeutic situation, and tendency to ward off intrusions from other individuals. Patients with paranoid delusions may find it difficult to engage if they perceive the therapist as an antagonist. For example, one individual was spending most of his time staring at the wall; the therapist was able to enlist the individual's attention by playing some music and asking the individual to name the song. The individual perked up at this point and was able to discuss the music and the musicians before regressing back into his torpor.

Over time, the therapist was able to extend the duration of contact. Not until they reach this point are the individual and therapist actually engaged. We have used a variety of methods, in addition to playing music, as a way to get the individuals involved with the therapist. For example, one of the female therapists on our team was able to penetrate the barrier of an individual who was essentially incommunicado by bringing a manicure set and informing her that she was going to do her nails. This experience evidently reminded the individual of talking to her manicurist, and she began a verbal exchange with the therapist. Other strategies that have helped to initiate meaningful contact with individuals were taking a walk together, bringing in food, and showing photographs of individuals' hometown. It was necessary for the therapist to cultivate the relationships to the point that the individual began to see the therapist as somebody she could relate to and trust.

ACTIVATING THE ADAPTIVE MODE

The therapeutic strategy is to provide as many corrective normalizing experiences as possible to activate and reinforce the positive adaptive mode and to reduce the strength of the negative mode, as illustrated in Jean's case. This is often a painstaking process, since the dysfunctional beliefs are very strong and require numerous corrective experiences to weaken them. It is possible to activate underlying abilities by promoting activity and social affiliation, increasing pleasure and mastery in individuals' daily lives, and improving communication skills. Once skills are enhanced, the negative symptoms become attenuated. Notably, we have seen most individuals begin to speak in a coherent and realistic way, make better decisions, and focus on long-term goals and aspirations.

The therapist and the individuals work collaboratively to formulate action plans. A main thrust of the action plan is to reactivate the latent skills and strategies that the individual had utilized, at an earlier time, prior to the onset of schizophrenia. In addition, we operated on the assumption that selecting a particular activity that was meaningful to the individuals would help to motivate—actually, energize—them to participate in the activity. The activation of the repertoire of related skills, such as reasoning or problem solving, occurred when a meaningful activity was carried out.

In the case of Jean, we found that her teaching the other individuals fulfilled the objective of a meaningful activity that mobilized her latent skills. Of course, utilizing this repertoire as part of a group activity had a greater impact than doing any activity solo.

In most instances, individuals are blocked by dysfunctional beliefs when they are engaging in a consensually agreed-upon activity. In some cases, the therapist has to work with the individuals to overcome these obstacles in individual therapy, before proposing the individual's participation in a group activity. As indicated previously, the therapist worked collaboratively with the individual in determining the action plan and dealing with the dysfunctional beliefs. Specific behavioral experiments that would contradict these deeply rooted attitudes are utilized. The behavioral experiment may consist of a simple activity, such as walking, which would contradict the individual's belief that he or she did not have enough energy to walk. The behavioral experiment, in Jean's case, consisted of testing her dysfunctional beliefs by baking and cooking for herself and the other individuals. This activity demonstrated conclusively to her that she did have the energy and that she was competent. It is essential after each activity to review what it demonstrated. She also learned that she had the energy to perform complicated tasks that seemed too demanding for her. She reported, "I do have the energy," "I can enjoy participating with other people," and "This shows that I am not inadequate."

OUTCOMES OF INDIVIDUAL THERAPY WITH LOW-FUNCTIONING INDIVIDUALS

A training project was conducted in the state of Georgia. Therapists were trained in cognitive therapy over a three-year period. The training consisted of workshops for all of the participants, followed by case supervision of each therapist for six months. Supervision included audioclips of sessions and ratings of audiotapes at the conclusion of supervision. Practically all of the therapists achieved competency in the treatment approach, using audiotapes rated by our team.

The therapist provided data regarding the individuals' progress over six months of supervised training. Out of a consecutive sample of the 376 individuals treated in the study, 69% showed improvement on at least one of the Recovery dimensions in the six-month period. On the Recovery dimension labeled "Purpose," 59% of the individuals showed improvement in at least one category, such as engaging in positive activity outside of sessions, participating in a hobby, and taking on a new role. Five percent became employed, and 2% returned to school/college. On the dimension "Community," which included the following—started dating, making new friends, or has joined an organization—20% of individuals showed an improvement. On the dimension "Health," at least 49% of individuals showed improvement in engaging in physical activity outside sessions and experienced improvement in obstacles to recovery. On the dimension "Home," which included environmental obstacles (legal, housing, support system), 10% of individuals showed improvement.

DISCUSSION: THEORETICAL CONSIDERATIONS

We have learned a great deal from our work with individuals with schizophrenia, especially those functioning at a very low level. We suggest that the positive symptoms of schizophrenia, such as delusions and hallucinations, can be conceptualized as the hyperactivation of imaginative and perceptual systems. A person with schizophrenia who is experiencing a hallucination or a delusion finds it as difficult to use reality-testing strategies as a sleeping person does when dreaming or a drug user does when high on LSD. Understandably, these powerful sensory and cognitive experiences can induce fear, which might lead to isolation and aggression.

We propose that negative symptoms represent an "idling" of the motivational, affective, and behavioral systems. In other words, systems that are operating at a minimum level of activation can be brought up to a more functional level of activation by appropriate stimulation. Jean's view of the world as overwhelmingly threatening led to extreme isolation and withdrawal. Behind the dysfunctional beliefs such as "I can't do it" are the basic self-images of Jean and like-minded individuals as being inferior, inadequate, and vulnerable.

To understand the transformation of Jean and other individuals more fully, it is important to review the structure and functions of personality. The personality organization consists of a number of suborganizations labeled "modes," designed to enable the individuals to adapt to changing conditions (Beck & Haigh, 2014). When individuals with schizophrenia withdraw from the social milieu, no longer attend to personal hygiene, and fend off approaches from other people, they fall into what we have previously described as "the regressive mode." This mode is complex in that it involves a global view centered on the cognitive triad—the self, the future, and the outside world. A matrix of specific beliefs forms the infrastructure of the triad. The regressive mode predominates over all other modes in the withdrawn individuals. While different modes prevail from time to time in normal people, the dominant mode in withdrawn individuals is the regressive mode. This mode can be changed temporarily by modifying the environmental input. We found, for example, that highly regressed individuals became animated when participating in a play, talent show, or other group activities. When the shift occurs to an adaptive mode, the beliefs take the form of "I am able to do things," "I can help other people," and "I have the energy to do things."

CONCLUSIONS

The cognitive approach to severe mental illness, with special attention to schizophrenia, is one of the first successful psychotherapies of this disorder. Moving from the effective British application of cognitive therapy for the positive symptoms, we first developed a cognitive model for the negative symptoms. We approached clinical symptomatology from the standpoint of asocial and defeatist beliefs blocking constructive motivation and activating avoidance. We found that the positive and negative symptoms of schizophrenia mask the latent adaptive personality.

When individuals are engaged in activity, such as acting in a play, they appear to be as normal as the staff. They are able to focus their attention on the demand of the situation and draw on their repertoire of cognitive skills, such as problem solving and reasoning.

The therapeutic challenge is to activate the adaptive mode and keep it activated through a progression of behavioral tasks directed toward the individual goals. As the individuals become more energized in the social world, their delusions and hallucinations become less prominent and disturbing. The therapist works collaboratively with the individuals to set the proximal and long-term goals. The goal setting helps to prime constructive motivation to overcome obstacles to these goals. Among the internal obstacles are the dysfunctional beliefs. Priming the latent adaptive beliefs and alleviating the negative beliefs energize mobilization of positive motivation to engage with the outside world.

The therapeutic regime consists of priming adaptive motivation through engagement with the therapist, collaboratively setting short-term and long-term goals, and promoting participation by the patient in the action plans to reach these goals. The medium for therapeutic change consists of alleviating the individual's loneliness, sense of helplessness, inadequacy, and inferiority. The alleviation of defeatist and asocial beliefs reduces the powerful motivation to avoid interactions and activities with other people.

We anticipate that emphasizing our goals and the strategies for achieving them will open up a new era in treating schizophrenia.

REFERENCES

Beck, A. T. (1952). Successful outpatient psychotherapy of a chronic schizophrenic with a delusion based on borrowed guilt. *Psychiatry, 15,* 305–332.

Beck, A. T., Grant, P. M., Huh, G. A., Perivoliotis, D., & Chang, N. A. (2013). Dysfunctional attitudes and expectancies in deficit syndrome schizophrenia. *Schizophrenia Bulletin, 39*(1), 43–51.

Beck, A. T., & Haigh, E. A. (2014). Advances in cognitive theory and therapy: The generic cognitive model. *Annual Review of Clinical Psychology, 10,* 1–24.

Beck, A. T., Rector, N., Stolar, N., & Grant, P. (2009). *Schizophrenia: Cognitive therapy, research, and therapy*. New York: Guilford Press.

Grant, P. M., & Beck, A. T. (2009). Defeatist beliefs as a mediator of cognitive impairment, negative symptoms and functioning in schizophrenia. *Schizophrenia Bulletin, 35,* 798–806.

Grant, P. M., & Beck, A. T. (2010). Asocial beliefs as predictors of asocial behavior in schizophrenia. *Psychiatry Research, 177,* 65–70.

Grant, P. M., Huh, G. A., Perivoliotis, D., Stolar, N. M., & Beck, A. T. (2012). Randomized trial to evaluate the efficacy of cognitive therapy for low-functioning patients with schizophrenia. *Archives of General Psychiatry, 69*(2), 121–127.

Grant, P. M., Reisweber, J., Luther, L., Brinen, A. P., & Beck, A. T. (2013). Successfully breaking a 20-year cycle of hospitalizations with recovery-oriented cognitive therapy for schizophrenia. *Psychological Services, 11*(2), 125–133.

Perivoliotis, D., Grant, P. M., & Beck, A. T. (2009). Advances in cognitive therapy for schizophrenia: Empowerment and recovery in the absence of insight. *Clinical Case Studies, 8*(6), 424–437.

CHAPTER 2

Three Myths and Truths about Beck's Early Years

Rachael I. Rosner

On September 29, 2006, Aaron Beck received the Albert Lasker Award for Clinical Medical Research, the U.S. equivalent of the Nobel Prize in Medicine. Sitting in the audience (and recognized in Beck's acceptance speech) was Dr. Marvin Stein of New York City. Stein was an old friend of Beck, from his early years in the psychiatry department at the University of Pennsylvania. Stein had been his best friend in those days. They were on the junior faculty at Penn together as well as candidates at the Institute of the Philadelphia Psychoanalytic Society. They lived within walking distance of each other, and their wives and children were friends. They played tennis and golf together. They spoke on the phone every day.

Stein was also the golden child of Penn psychiatry. Unlike anyone else in his cohort, Stein had begun his career as a scientist. Stein had come to Penn in 1953 just as he was catching the enormous wave of postwar government funding for medical science and with the promise to transform Penn's psychiatry department into a world-class scientific enterprise. With the blessing of his chairman, Kenneth E. Appel, in 1954 Stein built the university's first psychiatry laboratory, up in the turrets of the old Hare Building, where he studied the psychosomatics of induced asthma in guinea pigs. Stein was equally brilliant in inspiring his colleagues—all of whom were clinicians, like Beck, with no prior experience in the laboratory—to try science themselves. Stein encouraged Beck to undertake a large-scale experimental study of depression. Beck admired and emulated Stein so much that he described Stein to me as his "Steerforth," the streetwise older boy in Charles Dickens's *David Copperfield* who took the orphaned and naive David under his wing.[1]

One might imagine that Stein would play a role somewhere in our histories of cognitive therapy (CT). But Stein's name is unknown to cognitive therapists. Why? The answer is because in 1962 Stein suddenly dropped out of the picture. In fact, many of Beck's colleagues from his early years at Penn suddenly dropped out of the picture. Even the generation of clinicians and researchers with whom Beck collaborated in the 1960s—the formative decade of cognitive therapy—are not part of the CT origin story. They, too, remain unfamiliar names today.

This is a curious historical situation. Beck, at the age of 42, was not a young man when he published his first article on thinking and depression (Beck, 1963). And he was 55 when his first book on CT—*Cognitive Therapy and the Emotional Disorders)*—came out (Beck, 1976). Surely something must have happened, even larger than his discovery of the role of cognitions in depression, to cause such an astonishing "historical amnesia."[2] As a historian, I have spent almost two decades exploring both the known and the (vast) unknown territories of Beck's early years to try to paint a fuller and more nuanced picture of the origins and contours of the model.

The answer to the question "What happened in and around 1962 to generate this odd kind of amnesia?" lies in Beck's complicated break with psychoanalysis. The standard origin story of CT is that in the late 1950s Beck undertook a major study of the manifest dreams of depressed patients, funded by the National Institute of Mental Health (NIMH), to prove the psychoanalytic hypothesis that depression is a form of inverted hostility. As Beck has recounted many times, the results were sufficiently equivocal to cause him in the early 1960s to reconsider not only the psychoanalytic theory of depression but indeed all of the postulates of psychoanalysis. By 1963, he had completely dismantled psychoanalytic theory, was creating a new cognitive theory, and was refusing to look back. When Richard Suinn asked Beck in 1991 who his professional influences were, he answered: "I had a number of psychoanalytic advisors but none of them influenced my work as it eventually developed. I'm afraid I am a 'dead end.' "[3] Beck's

---

[1]Author interview with Aaron T. Beck, November 3, 2010; see also Beck's acceptance speech, Lasker Award Ceremony, September 26, 2006, Center for Cognitive Therapy, University of Pennsylvania.

[2]I am borrowing the phrase "historical amnesia" from historian Russell Jacoby, whose *Historical Amnesia: A Critique of Contemporary Psychology* (1975) focused on the rise of ego psychology.

[3]Letter from ATB to Richard Suinn, October 29, 1991. Personal Collection, Dr. Aaron T. Beck.

colleagues are familiar with this story. It is also completely in line with the historical record and even accounts for the fact that many of the people with whom he had previously been associated dropped off the map.

The problem with this story is not that it lacks truthfulness but rather that it is an incomplete telling of a larger story. Beck's break with psychoanalysis was actually one of the most protracted and convoluted in American history. From 1962 to 1976, he simultaneously broke from and sought an audience with psychoanalysts. A salient example of this phenomenon is the fact that even as he was training first-generation cognitive therapists—Jim Stinnette, Dean Schuyler, Martin Seligman, John Rush, Steve Hollon, Maria Kovacs, and others—he was simultaneously courting psychoanalysts and was even a fellow of a psychoanalytic organization. The tradition of dichotomous (dare I say black-and-white) thinking that has characterized most historical accounts of CT simply isn't adequate to the task of penetrating these complicated truths.

There are three aspects ("truths") to Beck's protracted break with psychoanalysis that challenge long-held assumptions about the origins of CT. Each has a corresponding "myth" which I have so named not because it is false but because it has had the effect of misdirecting the community's attention and unwittingly generating a false understanding of where the boundaries lie between the two schools.

MYTH #1: BECK'S DISCOVERY OF A COGNITIVE ASPECT OF DEPRESSION WAS *SUI GENERIS*

Beck has often told the story of an epiphany he experienced in 1956: while in session with a depressed patient, he suddenly intuited that there is a preconscious stream of thinking, accessible to awareness, in which we are constantly evaluating ourselves and our world. As he tells the story, he had been employing the standard psychoanalytic postulate that depression was a form of inverted hostility, and he had tried to convince his patient that she was really suffering from hostility. To his surprise, she rejected his interpretation and instead unloaded a complex of worries that he didn't like her, that he found her boring, and so on. This insight eventually led Beck to study experimentally the psychological correlates of depression (e.g., Bloch, 2004). While no hard data exist to confirm Beck's Martin Luther-like epiphany-in-a-thunderstorm, there is also no reason to doubt its truthfulness. Beck's memories nearly always map accurately onto facts I have found in the archival record.

There is more to this story, though, that helps cast light on the context of his early work. Beck's epiphany did not emerge fully formed out of nowhere. It was rather the result of having trained in the early 1950s with a Hungarian-born émigré and psychoanalytic psychologist named

David Rapaport. From 1950 to 1952, Beck was a psychiatry fellow at a small but influential private mental hospital in western Massachusetts called Austen Riggs. Rapaport was the dominant intellectual force there at that time. Rapaport and the other clinicians at Riggs were exemplars of a particular branch of psychoanalysis that flourished in America in the postwar years known as *ego psychology*. As a group, these Rapaport-affiliated ego psychologists were building on the work of Anna Freud, Heinz Hartmann, Ernst Kris, and others in studying what would now be called patients' metacognitions—how patients evaluate and make meaning out of their world.[4] Beck's mentors at Riggs conceptualized those beliefs as "the reality-testing capacities of the ego," or the patient's "ego strength." Beck learned to understand patients who were anxious, depressed, phobic, or overwhelmed as suffering from "defective ego-structures."

Rapaport was especially interested in systematizing the psychoanalytic theory of *thinking*. In 1950, the year Beck arrived, Rapaport had just completed a massive tome called *The Organization and Pathology of Thought* (Rapaport, 1951). This book was his life's work (he died prematurely in 1960). Rapaport argued that thinking—a category that included cognition, attention, perception, learning, and memory—was the bridge that connected psychoanalytic theory with experimental psychology. To be more specific, Rapaport was convinced that the *ego*, the hypothesized region of the mind that mediates between primitive urges and the demands of reality, was also the location in which the "conflict-free" mental functions of normal psychology operated. I have written elsewhere that Rapaport's passion for thinking and the ego dominated the Riggs conversations. Psychiatry fellows had frequent contact with him (Rosner, 2012, 2014).

Beck's epiphany occurred only four years after he had left Riggs (and two years after he completed a tour of duty as a psychiatrist in the Korean War). Given the close proximity between his 2 years with Rapaport and this insight into patients' metacognitions, it is highly likely that the influence of Rapaport and ego psychology were still strong. Indeed, we must assume this to have been so. The historical record is brimming with evidence that young clinicians who came under Rapaport's influence walked away with his cognitive stamp. Everyone who studied with him in the late 1940s and 1950s—ranging from those who hewed most closely to ego psychology (notably George Klein, Robert Holt, and Roy Schafer; see Friedman, 1991) to Nobel Prize-winning psychologist Daniel Kahneman (who studied with Rapaport in 1959) to master historian of American psychoanalysis John Burnham (who was also at Riggs in 1959)—has admitted Rapaport's influence.[5] Seen in this context, Beck surely would have been

[4]Author conversation with Dr. Jeremy Ridenour, Austen Riggs, October 5, 2015.

[5]For observations on Rapaport's influence on Kahneman, see "Daniel Kahneman—Biographical." *Nobelprize.org*. For influence on Burnham, see interview with author, November 22, 2013.

primed in the mid-1950s to be looking for how his patients evaluated themselves and their world. Beck himself has credited his "interest in cognition, which fitted under the umbrella term of ego psychology . . . (to) his contacts at that time with David Rapaport."[6]

What was *sui generis* about Beck's insights about thinking and depression, however—what set him apart from the ego psychologists—was that he eventually concluded that cognitions *were themselves* the psychopathology rather than the *sequelae* of the psychopathology. Rapaport had primed all of his students to look for cognitive patterns and even to postulate the existence of cognitive structures. But George Klein, Roy Schafer, and others who publicly followed Rapaport still believed that psychopathology was the result of a conflict between primitive wishes and the press of reality. For them, the locus of psychopathology was unresolved conflicts within the ego. Any changes in a patient's thinking were consequences of the ego's inability to manage those conflicts.

Beck flipped the situation around. He rejected the ideas of primitive wishes and conflict and held instead that *the structures themselves were cognitive in nature such that the psychopathology resided directly within them.* Now *faulty cognitive structures,* not defective ego structures in a motivational system, were the *locus of psychopathology.* In the early to mid-1960s, during a self-imposed five-year sabbatical from his department, Beck began fleshing out the contours of these cognitive structures (which he called "schemas"). He proposed that schemas develop in childhood and that in their primitive, childhood condition, they have the qualities of being fixed, rigid, dichotomous, and closely tied to emotions (good/bad, black/white, happy/sad etc.). As the child matures, the schemas take on the qualities of flexibility and distance from emotions such that the individual gains the capacity to evaluate situations rationally and resists the pull of strong emotions. Psychopathology results from a failure of primitive schemas to attain these mature qualities. Repeated exposures to situations that trigger a primitive schema can lead to a buildup of energy (Beck imagined a threshold–activation model) and a hyperactivation of the extreme ends of the structure. If enough energy builds up, the energy can then spill over into the extreme ends of neighboring schemas. In sum, these immature and poorly functioning schematic structures not only produce the primitive thinking typical of psychopathology but also create the cascade effect that leads people to generalize and extend their faulty thinking beyond the immediate situation (see Rosner, 2012, for a full exposition on this subject).

One of Beck's closest psychoanalytic collaborators at Penn in the late 1950s, Marvin Hurvich—who later became an ego psychologist himself—read a draft of one of Beck's papers in which he made public parts of this new theory and recognized immediately that

[6] Aaron T. Beck, draft of biographical sketch, extended version, Box 2 ff: Biographical write-ups—CV, 9/27/89. Personal Collection, Dr. Aaron T. Beck.

> the finding of consistent cognitive structures in depressives apparently has not been noticed by the psychological testers [ego psychologists like Roy Schafer], who are interested especially in cognitive structures. For example, Schafer maintains . . . that the diagnosis of depression is not based on any particular characterological picture . . . but rather on indications of speed, efficiency & variability of thought and action. Said another way, it appears that Schafer has only been impressed by the "speed," "efficiency," & "variability" aspects of the thinking of depressives as clues to differentiating the thought processes of depressives from the thought processes of other groups. Your work goes considerably beyond this.[7]

Seymour Feshbach, another psychoanalytically-oriented psychologist who was a consultant on Beck's depression study, agreed that "cognitive theorists will be very pleased by this paper. . . . My own view is that it will serve as an important and necessary corrective to certain motivational accounts of depression."[8]

In sum, one of Beck's earliest influences was ego psychology, particularly Rapaport's cognitive strain. Interestingly, Beck never divorced himself fully from ego psychology, even after he allied with behavior therapists in the 1970s. One could even make the case that his first book on CT, *Cognitive Therapy and the Emotional Disorders* (Beck, 1976), was actually an ego psychology text. The only publisher who took the manuscript was International Universities Press (IUP). For decades, IUP had been the main publishing house for ego psychology texts, including an edited volume from Austen Riggs (in which one of Beck's papers was included; Beck, 1952; Knight & Friedman, 1954), the ego psychology monograph series *Psychological Issues,* and George Klein's 1976 book on psychoanalysis (Klein, 1976).

Clearly, the editors at IUP put Beck in that camp. And so did Beck himself. In 1981, he wrote to John Bowlby that

> it might be a point of curiosity therefore for you to know that my psychiatric training was completely and exclusively psychoanalytic . . . I would consider my theoretical work as derivative from ego psychology rather than from cognitive psychology or learning theory. At the present time in fact I am trying to reformulate many of the basic psychoanalytic assumptions into cognitive terms.[9]

---

[7]Letter from Marvin Hurvich to ATB, February 25, 1963. Personal Collection, Dr. Aaron T. Beck.

[8]Letter from Seymour Feshbach to ATB, January 17, 1963. Personal Collection, Dr. Aaron T. Beck.

[9]Letter from ATB to JB, July 29, 1981. Personal Collection, Dr. Aaron T. Beck.

And he acknowledged to Paul Salkovskis in 1990 that "first I called [cognitive therapy] ego psychology, [and then I felt that this was] the psychoanalysis of the '60s, this is neo-analysis. What I am saying is that [cognitive therapy] is consistent to this day with Adler and Horney and so on."[10] And so the full truth about Beck's interest in cognitions is that it dates to 1950 when he came under the influence of David Rapaport and ego psychology. Rapaport's theory of thinking is the missing link between Beck's formative years as a psychiatrist, his expertise in cognitions, and his admission that CT is a derivative of ego psychology.

MYTH #2: COGNITIVE THERAPY IS BASED ON SCIENCE WHILE PSYCHOANALYSIS IS NOT

By the late 1960s, just as he was going public with CT, Beck set terms that would define the mission: CT would champion experimentalism in contradistinction to psychoanalysis, which relied on dogma and faith. It is true that Beck had felt enormous pressure to take what amounted to a loyalty oath to psychoanalytic theory. In 1968, he reflected on this pressure in a letter to Paul Meehl: "As time went on, I realized that support for [the psychoanalytic] postulate was ultimately derived from the declarative statements of the psychoanalytic authorities rather than from evidence; I began to quaver in my belief that '20,000 analysts can't be wrong.' "[11] He spoke more bluntly with his biographer, Marjorie Weishaar, in 1991:

> The personal element . . . that got me out of the whole psychoanalytic framework is the whole notion that authorities don't have to be taken at their face value and my own data seemed to contradict the authorities; that my own data can be trusted. . . . And there were no authorities that are more powerful in this world except maybe priests—the Pope—but no authority is more powerful than analysts because they know everything. They have the word.[12]

It might seem, therefore, that Myth #2 is really the whole truth. Indeed, it does convey the expectation of organized psychoanalysis—by which I mean the American Psychoanalytic Association and its local institutes—of loyalty to their interpretation of the model. For them, experimental science was anathema because to operationalize and standardize psychoanalytic

---

[10]Transcript of an interview with Aaron T. Beck/Interviewer Paul M. Salkovskis, November 3, 1990. Personal Collection, Dr. Aaron T. Beck.

[11]Letter from ATB to Paul Meehl, March 13, 1968. Personal Collection, Dr. Aaron T. Beck.

[12]Transcript of an interview with Aaron T. Beck/Interviewer Marjorie Weishaar, August 4, 1991, pp. 17–18. Personal Collection, Dr. Marjorie Weishaar; Weishaar, 1993.

constructs meant to observe and quantify them. And yet a creed of the psychoanalytic model was that the presence of any observing body in the therapy room would necessarily violate the mechanism of treatment, the transference. So from an epistemological point of view, they held, it was foolhardy to study psychoanalysis experimentally (see Rubenstein & Parloff, 1959; Rosner, 2005, for discussion of this particular epistemological position).

Regardless, Myth #2 is part of a more complicated story about the challenge of reconciling the epistemologies of psychoanalysis and experimentalism. Long before Beck trained as a psychoanalyst, a small but influential minority of psychoanalysts was exploring experimentalist approaches. Rapaport was one of them. So was Franz Alexander, yet another Hungarian-born émigré who had recently come to the U.S. from Berlin to lead the Chicago school of psychoanalysis. Alexander was in constant conflict with the American Psychoanalytic Association over his innovations with shorter treatments, behavioral exercises, psychological tests, and quantitative studies linking manifest dream themes with presumed psychosomatic illnesses such as hypertension, asthma, menstrual disorders, and others (Rosner, 1999).

One of Alexander's protégés was Leon J. Saul, who became Beck's training analyst in Philadelphia. Saul was even more of a renegade than Alexander. Saul regularly gave his patients homework assignments and conducted treatment over the telephone, in his back yard, and even in his car. Saul also championed experimentalism and assembled a team of scientists, even though he himself was not expert in the laboratory. In 1956 Saul offered a seminar on the quantification of hostility in manifest dreams. That seminar was Beck's introduction to scientific research. That same year Saul had published a "hostility scale" (for measuring the presence of hostility in manifest dreams) after which Beck modeled his own first scale (with the assistance of Marvin Hurvich), known as the "masochism scale." This was the beginning of what became Beck's NIMH-funded study of depression (Rosner, 1999).

As experimentalists, Saul and Beck joined the ranks of influential psychoanalytic psychologists like Lester Luborsky (first of the Menninger Clinic and later of the Department of Psychiatry at Penn), David Shakow (of the Intramural Psychology Laboratory at NIMH), and George Klein (Rapaport's protégé at New York University). They were also in the company of sympathetic psychoanalytic psychiatrists, especially Roy Grinker of Chicago who was editor of the *Archives of General Psychiatry*. Grinker's *Archives* published many of the papers that came out of Beck's first NIMH depression study, including the paper on the Depression Inventory (e.g., see Beck & Ward, 1961; Beck, Ward, Mendelson, Mock, & Erbaugh, 1961; Beck, Sethi, & Tuthill, 1963; Ward, Beck, & Rascoe, 1961, 1962). Beck modeled his first book, *Depression: Clinical, Experimental, and Theoretical Aspects* (Beck, 1967) on Grinker's 1961 monograph on depression

(Grinker, Miller, Sabshin, Nunn, & Nunnally, 1961). In 1972, Beck publicly acknowledged his debt to Grinker by contributing an essay to a *festschrift* in his honor (Beck, 1972). Finally, in 1968 Beck joined an organization that Grinker, Saul, and others had founded called the American Academy of Psychoanalysis. The mission of the Academy was to combat the "antiscientific" attitude of the American Psychoanalytic Association (Grinker, 1958). The Academy was actually the first organization Beck joined after he built CT. In other words, the very first national community to which Beck turned with CT was not behavior therapists but scientifically inclined psychoanalysts. Beck became a fellow in 1969, chaired sessions at meetings, and published articles in their journal. He stayed through 1976 (Rosner, 1999). So the truth is that a subgroup of American psychoanalysts was actively bridging psychoanalysis and experimental science, and Beck positioned the cognitive model in their camp, at least at first.

But why then was he simultaneously writing to Meehl disparaging comments about the antiscientific attitudes of psychoanalysts? Here a more sobering aspect of experimentalism and psychoanalysis becomes clear. The hard truth all of these analysts had to face was that to stay true to the epistemology of experimentalism they had to be willing to modify psychoanalytic theory should the data call for it—and few were willing to do so. I have described elsewhere the "epistemic frame" through which Saul and his cohort viewed scientific practice, which I have dubbed a "theory-trumps-data" mentality. For them, scientific data were valuable only as long as they supported psychoanalytic theories. Loyalty to the theory was paramount (Rosner, 2014).

They were therefore in an epistemological bind, and most of their efforts failed. Edith Sheppard, one of Saul's protégées and a close colleague of Beck in these early years, actually threw away data that didn't support her analytic hypotheses.[13] Rapaport's closest followers found his dizzying psychoanalytic constructs impossible to operationalize, but rather than question psychoanalysis, they revolted instead against Rapaport. David Shakow of the NIMH invested millions of government dollars in an effort to obtain objective knowledge about psychoanalysis through filming an entire course of treatment. But he abandoned the project with the sobering conclusion that it was simply too difficult to study psychoanalysis experimentally (Rosner, 2005). Even Roy Grinker lamented that the American Academy had failed in its mission to promote science in psychoanalysis.[14]

When viewed from the perspective of these failures and frustrations,

[13]Author Interview with Dr. Robert Daroff, Cleveland, Ohio, December 2012.

[14]Letter from Roy Grinker to Henry Laughlin, June 25, 1969. American College of Psychoanalysis Collection, Box 2, ff. 3. Courtesy of the New York Hospital and Cornell University Medical College, Oskar Diethelm Library, History of Psychiatry Section, Department of Psychiatry.

Beck's solution appears radical. His tactic was to switch out the "theory-trumps-data" mentality for "data-trumps-theory," and then to modify psychoanalytic theory with abandon (Rosner, 2014). Already in 1962, he had turned away from drive theory. This decision relieved him of the obligation to hold any other part of the theory sacrosanct. It freed him to design a study in the early 1960s that tested the hypothesis that depressed patients wish to suffer (he found they do not wish to suffer) (Loeb, Feshbach, Beck, & Wolf, 1964). In sum, in chucking drive theory Beck was free to forge ahead with the agenda of his early psychoanalytic mentors, namely, to explore the "conflict-free" cognitive aspects of the "ego"—which accounts for his comfort in identifying himself as an ego psychologist. It may sound heretical, but Beck's trajectory with CT was arguably the most successful adaptation of ego psychology to the demands of experimentalism. Still, the price Beck paid for doing so (abandoning drive theory) was too high for most psychoanalysts to pay.

MYTH #3: AARON BECK BROKE WITH PSYCHOANALYSIS

This myth seems so patently true that readers may be astonished I even question any aspect of its truthfulness. Didn't Beck admit that he broke with drive theory in 1962? Didn't he tell Paul Meehl, Marjorie Weishaar, and so many others over the course of decades that he rejected psychoanalysis?

The problem with this myth is not the actuality of a break but rather the assumptions that Beck was the one who did the breaking and that the break was clean. The truth is that Beck never actively sought to break with *organized* psychoanalysis. The opposite was true. Since 1950, he had diligently and thoroughly mastered the craft, jumped through the hoops, and become a fellow of the Philadelphia Psychoanalytic Society. He began formulating the cognitive model of depression while he was still an active member of the psychoanalytic community—and viewed the model as a reformulation of psychodynamic theory. He wrote to Leon Saul in 1961 that he believed the time had come to rethink the psychodynamics of depression because his data suggested that drives might not be involved.[15] Surely it was bold to suggest that drives were not involved anywhere in depression—but there was precedent. Karen Horney had made a similar argument, as had other neo-analysts who followed her. And still, Beck, as was true of them, did not originally plan to break with psychodynamics.

Instead, the psychoanalytic establishment broke with him. The establishment couldn't have done more than it actually did to kick him out. The

[15] ATB to Leon Saul, September 28, 1961. Personal Collection, Dr. Aaron T. Beck.

context of his break is the missing piece of the puzzle. Beck has never publicly spoken about the fact that in the early 1960s both he and his cohort became pawns in two different power plays, one by the American Psychoanalytic Association and the other by the senior faculty at Penn. These power plays occurred just as Beck was cresting with his new model. The crises took an enormous personal toll on him, and ultimately he had no choice but to walk away.

The first crisis was his failed attempt to join the American Psychoanalytic Association. Membership in the national organization was a given for any graduate of a local institute, and Beck followed the required procedures, including agreeing to a two-year waiting period after graduating from the Philadelphia Psychoanalytic Institute before applying. He finally applied in 1960. But the American Psychoanalytic Association nonetheless deferred his application, claiming Beck had insufficient training. Beck's patients had only needed two years of analysis, and the committee did not believe they could have been "symptom free" and "improve(d) . . . after such comparatively brief periods of analytic work." The committee advised him to undertake "additional supervisory work on the advanced or termination phases of a suitable analytic case, preferably a female, for about one year."[16] Although Beck did not undertake additional training, he did reapply in the fall of 1961 with a detailed description of his four control cases. The American Psychoanalytic Association again deferred his application: "I couldn't even get mad at something like that," he later told me. "It's like [when] a hallucinating schizophrenic starts calling you names. I was really quite disillusioned now. I can't say necessarily with psychoanalysis but with the people. They were so dumb, they really were dumb."[17] He did not reapply.[18]

What Beck couldn't have known was that his deferment was a warning from the American Psychoanalytic Association to Leon Saul that he was taking too many liberties with the orthodox model. Historian Nathan Hale has shown that the American Psychoanalytic Association used strategies like this—punishing the student as a slap on the wrist of the training analyst—to curb innovation and force loyalty (Hale, 1995). Beck was not Saul's only student to be deferred. Regardless, after 1961 Beck faced an uncertain future. He refused to undertake additional training, and yet without membership in the national organization his professional options

[16]Letter from Gerhart Piers to ATB, December 16, 1960. Personal Collection, Dr. Aaron T. Beck.

[17]Author interview with ATB, July 17, 1997.

[18]Undated, unsigned handwritten document, American Psychoanalytic Association Papers, RG11 Committees, Series 10, Subseries 1 (Committee on Membership 1961–1971), Folder: 1962–1964, Oskar Diethelm Library, Institute for the History of Psychiatry, Weill Cornell Medical College, New York.

were limited. An unfortunate truth about the American Psychoanalytic Association during this period in American history is that it had unchecked power and did not use that power wisely. It couldn't have done more to turn a creative psychoanalyst away.

The second crisis, which had been fulminating for 2 years, erupted in the summer of 1962, about six months after Beck learned of his second deferment. The crisis was a pitched battle between the psychiatry department and the university administration over who would succeed the retiring chairman of psychiatry, Kenneth E. Appel (Rosner, 2014). The battle became a referendum on the future of psychoanalysis. The senior faculty championed Marvin Stein, Beck's best friend and the brilliant scientist who promised to preserve old traditions like psychoanalysis and psychosomatics. The university administration, in contrast, wanted Eli Robins, a biological and experimental psychiatrist from Washington University who was vocally antagonistic toward psychoanalysis. The senior faculty, in their desperation to hold onto long-standing traditions, employed less-than-honorable tactics to secure Stein's nomination and pillory Robins.

Beck was caught in the crossfire. Appel (along with other senior faculty like Leon Saul) put tremendous pressure on Beck and other junior faculty to support Stein. Stein himself used pressure tactics to secure his nomination. Beck had originally supported Stein but eventually felt that the wisest political position was neutrality. He urged, indeed pleaded with, Stein to do the same—but the pressure was too much. Stein pushed hard for the chairmanship, Beck resisted being drawn into factions, and the result was a breech in their friendship and a split among the junior faculty in their loyalties. The crisis over Appel's successor nearly tore the department apart and irreparably damaged Beck's friendship with Stein. In the end, the administration chose someone else entirely, another junior faculty member named Albert J. (Mickey) Stunkard. But the damage was done. Stein grew enraged with Beck. Stein no longer saw a future for himself at Penn and within a year would leave for New York City.

Within weeks of Stunkard assuming the chairmanship, Beck requested a one-year sabbatical—which Stunkard granted. Stunkard's impression was that Beck needed time to heal from the break with Stein. One year turned to five. Between 1962 and 1967, Beck worked from his home-office (and saw patients in his office at the Girard Bank Building at 133 S. 36th Street at the corner of Walnut Street) in a self-imposed isolation from Penn psychiatry. It was during this "splendid isolation" that he composed the two foundational articles on thinking and depression, completed his first book (Figure 2.1 shows Beck ca. 1968 sitting in his home office looking at his new depression book), and built his new "cognitive" therapy. Other major events in Beck's life, by unfortunate coincidence, also dated to late 1961 and 1962, including the death of his mother, the NIMH's decision not to renew funding for his large depression project, and his family's move to a more affluent suburb. All of these major events converged to make 1962 a particularly difficult year and the prospect of a sabbatical even more appealing (Rosner, 2014).

One might imagine that by now Beck would have become allergic to organized psychoanalysis. So it is surprising that he immediately brought his cognitive model to the Philadelphia Psychoanalytic Society when he returned to active departmental life in 1967. In other words, he tried yet again to *find fellowship* with psychoanalysts. And yet again, psychoanalysts *broke with him.* In 1997, Beck reminisced about the moment he presented CT to the Philadelphia Psychoanalytic Society: "When I presented this material before the local analytic society, I said, 'this is really neo-analysis.' They said, 'Well, Beck, this is no longer analysis. You better stop calling yourself an analyst.'"[19] So Beck turned instead to the American Academy of Psychoanalysis. The Academy did not reject Beck, but, in failing to cultivate science in psychoanalysis, the Academy couldn't really take his ideas very far either. In 1970, Beck decided to court behavior therapists. But the behavior therapists didn't accept him either, at least initially:

> I had to find a new name for this approach. At that time I was attracted to behavior therapy, so I thought maybe I'd call myself a behavior therapist.

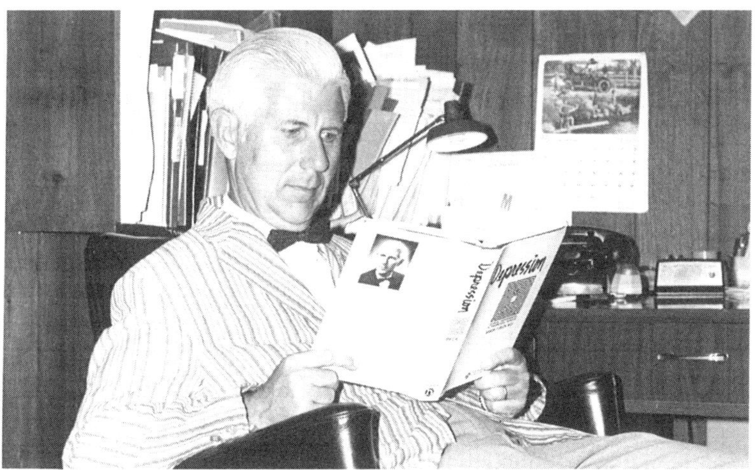

FIGURE 2.1. Aaron Beck ca. 1968 sitting in his home office looking at his new *Depression: Clinical, Experimental and Theoretical Aspects*. Used with permission of Aaron T. Beck.

[19]Aaron T. Beck, "The past and future of cognitive therapy," Unpublished manuscript, University of Pennsylvania School of Medicine, 1997, p. 7.

> I spoke to Dr. Wolpe about some of my ideas and he said, "Well, you're not a behavior therapist at all." So, I ended up with the idea of calling my approach cognitive therapy.[20]

It wasn't until Beck attracted a critical mass of residents and postdoctoral fellows in the mid-1970s—a full generation younger than he with no memory of the old psychoanalytic culture—that CT gained traction. They and successive generations catapulted Beck into a leadership role in the burgeoning cognitive-behavioral therapy movement.

These examples paint a picture, then, not of someone proactively breaking with psychoanalysis but of someone with whom the psychoanalytic establishment kept breaking. And despite his intense dislike of the culture of faith and loyalty in psychoanalysis, he continued seeking fellowship with like-minded analysts wherever he could find them. Beck emerges as a highly creative analyst intensely frustrated with a psychoanalytic establishment that kept curtailing innovation. He turned away from drive theory in an effort to break out of those restrictions. It was not in his nature, however, to rebel with a flourish but rather to plot a course that would maximize his chances of transforming psychiatry into something closer to his own image—with whomever was eager to join in (see also Bloch, 2004, p. 860, where Beck admits a "fuzzy" break with psychoanalysis and his rebellion against the autocracy of the psychoanalytic establishment).

* * * * * *

Beck and Stein did not resume contact, with the exception of a few phone calls and letters, until the Lasker Award ceremony in 2006, forty-four years after the breakup of their friendship. In his acceptance speech, Beck acknowledged Stein's crucial role in helping him become a scientist. It is tempting to speculate why Beck invited Stein to the Lasker Awards. Perhaps he still yearned for Stein's approval, keen to show him that he had made it as a scientist. He and Stein used to joke that they should create a school of psychosynthesis to put back together all of the people analyzed apart by psychoanalysis. Maybe he wanted to celebrate with Stein the realization of this vision. It's likely, too, that Beck felt the political situation in psychiatry had changed enough and they were old enough now to mend fences. I first made contact with Stein (by serendipity) in 1997, almost a decade before Beck's Lasker Award, and even then Stein was eager to share his story and help with my historical research on Beck. Clearly Stein, too, was eager to mend fences.

Whatever his motives, Stein's presence at the Lasker Award ceremony brought Beck's journey with CT full circle: to the time before the political

---

[20]Ibid.

fallout when he believed his new ideas about thinking and depression might revolutionize psychodynamics. A constant theme in Beck's work has been a quest for common ground. Neither he nor Stein had asked for the political crisis that destroyed their friendship, soured (even more) their feelings toward psychoanalysis, and launched Beck on the road to cognitive-behavioral therapy. In the case of telling his history, it may well be that a détente with psychoanalysis is in order if only because it facilitates a fuller remembering of the complicated truths of Beck's early years.

REFERENCES

Beck, A. T. (1952). Successful outpatient psychotherapy of a chronic schizophrenic with a delusion based on borrowed guilt. *Psychiatry, 15,* 305–312.

Beck, A. T. (1963, October). Thinking and depression: I. Idiosyncratic content and cognitive distortions. *Archives of General Psychiatry, 9,* 324–333.

Beck, A. T. (1964, June). Thinking and depression: II. Theory and therapy. *Archives of General Psychiatry, 10,* 561–571.

Beck, A. T. (1967). *Depression: Clinical, experimental and theoretical aspects.* New York: Harper & Row.

Beck, A. T. (1970a). Cognitive therapy: Nature and relation to behavior therapy. *Behavior Therapy, 1*(1), 184–200.

Beck, A. T. (1970b). The core problem in depression: The cognitive triad. *Science and Psychoanalysis, 17,* 47–55.

Beck, A. T. (1972). The phenomena of depression: A synthesis. In D. Offer & D. X. Freedman (Eds.), *Modern psychiatry and clinical research: Essays in honor of Roy R. Grinker Sr.* (pp. 136–158). New York: Basic Books.

Beck, A. T. (1976). *Cognitive therapy and the emotional disorders.* New York: International Universities Press.

Beck, A. T., & Hurvich, M. (1959). Psychological correlates of depression: I. Frequency of "masochistic" dream content in a private practice sample. *Psychosomatic Medicine, 21*(1), 50–55.

Beck, A. T., Sethi, B., & Tuthill, R. (1963). Childhood bereavement and adult depression. *Archives of General Psychiatry, 9,* 295–302.

Beck, A. T., & Ward, C. H. (1961). Dreams of depressed patients: Characteristic themes in manifest content. *Archives of General Psychiatry, 5,* 462–467.

Beck, A. T., Ward, C. H., Mendelson, M., Mock, J., & Erbaugh, J. (1961). An inventory for measuring depression. *Archives of General Psychiatry, 4,* 561–571.

Bloch, S. (2004). A pioneer in psychotherapy research: Aaron Beck. *Australian and New Zealand Journal of Psychiatry, 38,* 855–867.

Friedman, L. J. (1991). *Menninger: The family and the clinic.* Lawrence: University Press of Kansas.

Grinker, R. R. (1958). A philosophical appraisal of psychoanalysis. In J. H. Masserman (Ed.), *Science and psychoanalysis: Integrative studies* (Vol. 1, pp. 126–142). New York: Grune & Stratton.

Grinker, R. R., Miller, J., Sabshin, M., Nunn, R., & Nunnally, J. C. (1961). *The phenomena of depressions*. New York: Hoeber.

Hale, N. G. (1995). *The rise and crisis of psychoanalysis in the United States: Freud and the Americans, 1917–1985*. Oxford, UK: Oxford University Press.

Jacoby, R. (1975). *Historical amnesia: A critique of contemporary psychology*. Boston: Beacon Press.

Klein, G. S. (1976/1969). Freud's two theories of sexuality. Reprinted in *Psychological Issues, 36*, 14–70.

Klein, G. S. (1976). *Psychoanalytic theory*. New York: International Universities Press.

Knight, R. P., & Friedman, C. R. (Eds). (1954). *Psychoanalytic psychiatry and psychology: Clinical and theoretical papers, Austen Riggs Center, Vol. 1*. Oxford, UK: International Universities Press.

Loeb, A., Feshbach, S., Beck, A. T., & Wolf, A. (1964). Some effects of reward upon the social perception and motivation of psychiatric patients varying in depression. *Journal of Abnormal and Social Psychology, 68*, 609–616.

Rapaport, D. (1951). *Organization and pathology of thought: Selected sources*. New York: Columbia University Press.

Rosner, R. I. (1999). *Between science and psychoanalysis: Aaron T. Beck and the emergence of cognitive therapy*. Doctoral dissertation, York University, Toronto, Ontario, Canada.

Rosner, R. I. (2005). Psychotherapy research and the National Institute of Mental Health, 1948–1980. In W. E. Pickren & S. F. Schneider (Eds.), *Psychology and the National Institute of Mental Health* (pp. 113–150). Washington, DC: American Psychological Association.

Rosner, R. I. (2012). Aaron T. Beck's drawings and the psychoanalytic origin story of cognitive therapy. *History of Psychology, 15*(1), 1–18.

Rosner, R. I. (2014). The "splendid isolation" of Aaron T. Beck. *Isis, 105*, 734–758.

Rubenstein, E. A., & Parloff, M. B. (Eds.). (1959). *Research in psychotherapy*. Washington, DC: American Psychological Association.

Ward, C. H., Beck, A. T., Mendelson, M., Mock, J. E., & Erbaugh, J. K. (1962). The psychiatric nomenclature: Reasons for diagnostic disagreement. *Archives of General Psychiatry, 7*, 198–205.

Ward, C. H., Beck, A. T., & Rascoe, E. (1961). Typical dreams: Incidence among psychiatric patients. *Archives of General Psychiatry, 5*, 606–615.

Weishaar, M. (1993). *Aaron T. Beck*. Thousand Oaks, CA: SAGE.

CHAPTER 3

The Fundamental Cognitive Model

Keith S. Dobson
Julia C. Poole
Judith S. Beck

The cognitive model of psychopathology asserts that individuals who are in distress tend to experience distorted thinking and/or unrealistic cognitive appraisals of events (Beck, 1976), which in turn negatively affect their behaviors, feelings, and even physiological responses (J. S. Beck, 2011). Although the model was originally formulated for depression, its demonstrated theoretical and therapeutic value led to increased interest in its relevance to other areas, such as suicide (Beck et al., 1974), anxiety disorders and phobias (Beck, Emery, & Greenberg, 1985), personality disorders (Beck & Freeman, 1990), and substance abuse (Beck, Wright, & Newman, 1993). This chapter reviews major developments in the history of the cognitive model, outlines basic concepts and principles of the cognitive model, and describes the current status of the cognitive model.

HISTORICAL BASES OF THE COGNITIVE MODEL

Prior to the 1960s, behavior therapy was regarded as the predominant approach in scientific clinical psychology. Generally speaking, behaviorists utilized classical and operant conditioning principles to explain and modify behavior without referring to inner thoughts, beliefs, or emotions. Through the use of objective measures and carefully controlled experiments, the behavioral approach moved the field of psychology toward a more empirical science. During the 1960s and 1970s, however, the field of psychology underwent a major paradigm shift. The "cognitive revolution" marked a shift in focus from the study of observable behaviors to the study of thought content and the processes involved in thinking (Kovacs & Beck, 1978). The cognitive revolution was predicated on several shortcomings in the behaviorist approach. First, it was increasingly clear that a nonmediational approach (i.e., one that did not account for internal experiences) was insufficient to account for all human behavior (Mahoney, 1974). Critics of behaviorism, for instance, noted that children learned grammatical rules well outside the ability of most parents and educators to reinforce discriminatively, following a "language acquisition device" (Chomsky, 1975; Vygotsky, 1962). Second, the absence of observable behavior related to some psychiatric symptoms (e.g., obsessions) made noncognitive theories and interventions irrelevant. An exclusive focus on behavior was insufficient for the full range of psychiatric disorders.

Cognitive theories also provided an alternative to the psychodynamic model of personality and therapy. Although psychoanalytic models had long been highly influential, considerable dissatisfaction and skepticism had arisen by the early 1960s. It was argued that central components of the psychoanalytic model (e.g., unconscious processes) could not be empirically examined, as these components could not be operationally defined. When experimental research *was* attempted, predictions derived from the psychoanalytic model often were not validated (Clark & Beck, 1999). Indeed, early cognitive theorists explicitly rejected many of the primary psychoanalytic principles (e.g., Beck, 1967; Ellis, 1973).

Once enunciated, the cognitive model quickly garnered the interest of many theorists and therapists, some of whom had been behaviorally or psychoanalytically oriented (Clark & Beck, 1999). For example, although Aaron T. Beck was originally trained in psychoanalysis, he had become increasingly disillusioned by both psychoanalytical and strictly behaviorist formulations, particularly with respect to depression. In speaking with his patients, he noticed specific and characteristic thought patterns that could not be appropriately explained or treated through the psychoanalytical or behavioral frameworks. His depressed patients, for instance, tended to view events in terms of loss ("Nobody loves me anymore"), failure ("I didn't get promoted because I'm lazy"), and defeat ("I'm not smart enough to pass exams"), while his anxious patients tended to view events in terms of imminent threat ("My boss is acting cold, so I'm likely to get fired soon"; Beck, 1976). Beck developed a classification of cognitive distortions (Beck, 1970; Beck, Rush, Shaw, & Emery, 1979). He argued that schemas serve to filter information in a manner that continually produces cognitive distortions, which reinforce biased and inaccurate appraisal of events. Many of these cognitive distortions remain important theoretical constructs within the current cognitive model (see Table 3.1).

Beck outlined the essence of the cognitive model in *Depression: Causes and Treatment* (Beck, 1967). The model utilizes an information-processing framework, which postulates that individuals with psychiatric disorders tend to experience rigid and distorted patterns of thinking and are thus less able to process information accurately when exposed to stressful or negative experiences. These information-processing errors lead to distorted and inaccurate thoughts, which serve to maintain psychiatric problems. In a related article, Beck described how aspects of cognitive therapy and

TABLE 3.1. Common Cognitive Distortions

Title	Description
All-or-nothing thinking	Also called black-and-white, or dichotomous, thinking. Viewing a situation as having only two possible outcomes.
Catastrophization	Predicting future calamity; ignoring a possible positive future.
Fortune telling	Predicting the future with limited evidence.
Mind reading	Predicting or believing you know what other people think.
Disqualifying the positive	Not attending to, or giving due weight to, positive information. Similar to a negative "tunnel vision."
Magnification/ minimization	Magnifying negative information; minimizing positive information.
Selective abstraction	Also called *mental filter*. Focusing on one detail rather than on the large picture.
Overgeneralization	Drawing overstated conclusions based on one instance or on a limited number of instances.
Misattribution	Making errors in the attribution of causes of various events.
Personalization	Thinking that you cause negative outcomes, rather than examining other causes.
Emotional reasoning	Arguing that because something feels bad, it must be bad.
Labeling	Putting a general label on someone or something, rather than describing the behaviors or aspects of the thing.

Note. From Dobson and Dobson (2017).

behavior therapy could be integrated (Beck, 1970), while his second book, *Cognitive Therapies and the Emotional Disorders* (Beck, 1976), provided detailed descriptions of cognitive distortions common to a variety of disorders.

By the 1980s, the cognitive model of depression had become increasingly recognized as a valid and evidence-based approach to the conceptualization and treatment of depression. Beck's ongoing commitment to the advancement of the cognitive theory and its applied treatment manuals have led to fundamental changes in the formulation and treatment of a wide array of psychiatric problems and disorders. Throughout his career, Beck has assisted in the development of nineteen diagnostic scales for the symptom severity of a range of psychiatric disorders, published more than 500 research articles, and authored or co-authored seventeen books. His commitment to evidence-based research has inspired greater rigor in basic research and clinical trials across fields of mental health. Although the cognitive model itself has certainly grown over decades of empirical research, the model has maintained an emphasis on a number of common principles that describe the ways in which cognitive distortions and unrealistic appraisals of events can adversely affect feelings, behaviors, and physiological sensations.

BASIC OVERVIEW OF THE COGNITIVE MODEL OF PSYCHOPATHOLOGY

Imagine that three car passengers experience a near-fatal car accident, but all leave the accident free of any injuries. Over the next few weeks, each passenger experiences a different reaction to the near-death experience. The first feels crushed with worry because he fears he will be in another car accident; the second feels angry because she believes the accident was due to the driver's carelessness; and the third (the driver) feels grateful and relieved because everyone left the car unscathed. These vastly different emotional reactions underscore the cornerstone of the cognitive model, which is that our idiosyncratic thoughts and beliefs influence our emotional responses to events.

Hierarchical Organization of Thinking

The cognitive model of psychopathology follows the formulation outlined in Figure 3.1. The conceptualization of a clinical case and the subsequent development of appropriate therapeutic interventions require information regarding factors involved in the development and maintenance of symptoms. According to this formulation, three primary levels of thinking require examination.

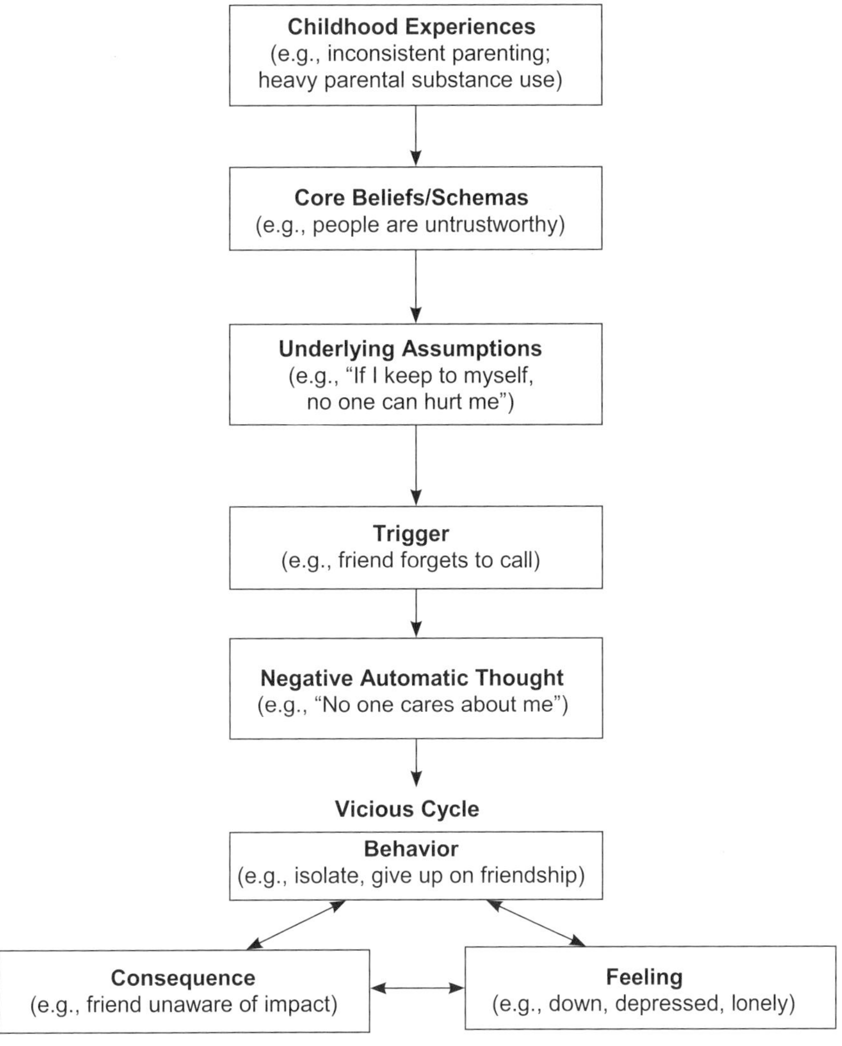

FIGURE 3.1. Example of brief cognitive model formula.

Schemas/Core Beliefs

Schemas are relatively enduring cognitive structures that become activated in response to external events (e.g., experiences of trauma) or internal events (e.g., elevated heart rate) in order to select, encode, and retrieve information. They are primarily developed early in life but can also develop and evolve in response to later life circumstances. Cognitive schemas, which contain the highest order and most general levels of cognition (or thinking) within the cognitive model, are the lenses through which we view the world; they influence both *what* we think (i.e., cognitive content) and *how* we think (i.e., information processing; Beck, 1964; Clark & Beck, 1999).

If you consider the word *examination,* the ideas, concepts, and images that you associate with an examination will arise in your mind. You have just activated a schema, which contains the concept of examination. While adaptive schemas allow for realistic appraisals of incoming information ("I can pass most examinations if I just study"), maladaptive schemas tend to foment distorted, biased, and/or dysfunctional perceptions and faulty problem solving (Beck, 1976; Dozois & Beck, 2008). The thought, "There is no way I can pass any examination!" may then lead to giving up. Thus, maladaptive schemas represent vulnerability factors for the development of psychological disorders (Clark & Beck, 2010; see Table 3.2).

Core beliefs are important components of cognitive schemas. *Core beliefs* are fixed, absolute, and generalized beliefs that people hold about themselves (e.g., "I am unlovable"), others (e.g., "No one wants to get to know me"), and the world in general ("It's dangerous"; J. S. Beck, 2011; Dobson, 2012). These negative, demeaning views of oneself, others, and the world are commonly referred to as the "negative cognitive triad." Within the cognitive model, core beliefs are largely influential in determining how individuals interact with the world, and they represent the core cognitive variables in the development and maintenance of psychopathology (J. S. Beck, 2011).

When a schema and its corresponding negative core belief(s) are

TABLE 3.2. Examples of Adaptive and Maladaptive Schemas

Adaptive	Maladaptive
No matter what happens, I can manage somehow.	I must be perfect to be accepted.
If I work at something, I can master it.	If I choose to do something, I must succeed.
I'm a survivor.	I'm a fake.
Others can trust me.	Without a woman, I'm nothing.
I'm lovable.	I'm stupid.
People respect me as I am.	People can't be trusted.
I like challenge.	The world is too frightening for me.

Note. Wright et al. (2006, p. 145). Reprinted with permission from Learning Cognitive-Behavior Therapy: An Illustrated Guide, (Copyright © 2005). American Psychiatric Association.

activated in response to a negative or stressful event, information is processed in a biased fashion that serves to reinforce the activated belief. Specifically, information that is consistent with the schema is attended to and encoded, while inconsistent information is ignored (Wenzel, 2012). Consequently, a bidirectional relationship exists between information processing and core beliefs, wherein information biases serve to reinforce core beliefs, and core beliefs reinforce information biases.

Underlying Assumptions

The next level of cognition within the hierarchy of thinking is an individual's underlying assumptions. *Underlying assumptions* are conditional propositions that direct an individual's everyday choices and reflect their standards, values, and rules for living. They are often in the form of an "if–then" statement, expressed either in a positive or negative direction (e.g., "If I am on guard around other people, I can keep myself safe" and/or "If I trust others, then I will get hurt"). Or they may be stated as a rule of living (e.g., "I must protect myself from others") or as an attitude ("Trusting others is foolish"; Beck, 1964; J. S. Beck, 2011). It has been proposed that maladaptive assumptions tend to focus on three major issues: acceptance (e.g., "I must be liked by everyone I meet"); competence (e.g., "If I get this promotion then I am capable"); and control (e.g., "I must do it all on my own"; Beck et al., 1985; Neenan & Dryden, 2011). In some instances, assumptions serve to protect people from painful core beliefs. For instance, "I should always be busy and productive" may be a protective assumption in that it would encourage the individual to keep active and thus help to ward off thoughts related to failure or inadequacy. Further, always being busy and productive could protect against the effects of a perfectionism schema that contains a core belief such as "I am not good enough" (Needleman, 1999). Given that negative core beliefs are activated when terms of assumptions are not met, underlying assumptions serve to maintain or reinforce negative core beliefs rather than to change them.

Negative Automatic Thoughts

As noted earlier, the latent patterns of cognition entailed in schemas, beliefs, and assumptions are triggered by external life events. This activation results in one or more *negative automatic thoughts* (NATs) (see Figure 3.1), which are ideas, images, and intuitions that arise spontaneously, rapidly, and involuntarily. Unlike core beliefs and assumptions, which are typically general in nature, NATs tend to be situation-specific and are therefore the least durable and least central of the cognitions. Upon stuttering during a presentation, for instance, one might have the NAT, "The audience thinks I'm an idiot!" NATs negatively affect an individual's emotions (e.g., shame), behaviors (e.g., avoidance of public speaking), and/or physiological reactions (e.g., sweating).

NATs can be triggered by both external events (e.g., upon not receiving an invitation to a social gathering: "No one thinks I am fun"; "I'm a loser") and/or internal events (e.g., upon noticing a rapid heartbeat: "I am having a heart attack!"). Three general types of questions can be used to modify NATs (Dobson & Dobson, 2017): (1) What is the evidence for and against this thought? (2) What are the alternative ways to think in this situation? and (3) What are the implications of thinking this way?

EXPANSION OF THE COGNITIVE MODEL

Modes

In the late 1990s, Aaron Beck and his colleagues proposed that schemas, which may have emotional, behavioral, physiological, and motivational components, in addition to their core belief aspects, may be correlated into more general and encompassing *modes* (Clark & Beck, 1999; Beck, 1996). A *mode* represents an interrelated network of schemas: embedded beliefs, rules, and expectancies, in addition to complex concepts such as self-esteem. Thus, a mode may consist of several cohesive systems of schemas, core beliefs, underlying assumptions, and automatic thoughts (Beck, 1996).

Three types of modes have been proposed. *Primal modes* are the most basic and immediate kinds of operation and serve to meet necessities, such as preservation and security. *Constructive modes* influence the ability to increase the life resources available to an individual, such as effective relationships, creativity, and life satisfaction. Finally, *minor modes* influence everyday activities, such as reading, writing, and recreational activities (Clark & Beck, 1999). It is not uncommon for individuals with unhelpful belief systems to demonstrate impaired functioning in all three of these modal domains. For example, while adaptive primary, constructive, and minor modes might be reflected by beliefs such as "I want adequate housing for me and my family," "I would like to be a contributing member of society, to the best of my ability and training," and "I enjoy being active most days," examples of potentially maladaptive modes in these domains include "I must have absolute security at all times," "I have to fulfil myself in everything I try," and "I cannot stand it when I am idle," respectively.

Modes are neither inherently maladaptive nor adaptive. For example, activation of the fear mode during a natural disaster may allow an individual to escape a potentially life-threatening event, whereas activation of the fear mode on a first date may result in stuttering, stammering, and loss of a romantic opportunity. Once activated, though, a mode maintains itself through feedback within the system, the selection of consistent incoming information, and the disregard or discounting of inconsistent incoming information. Therefore, the degree of adaptation of the mode is dependent on the situation in which the mode is activated and how the mode influences ongoing thoughts, feelings, and behaviors (Needleman, 1999).

The Generic Cognitive Model

An updated generic cognitive model (GCM) has recently been proposed (Beck & Haigh, 2014). Consistent with previous cognitive models, the GMC points to faulty information processing as the primary means by which disorders occur: "When information processing provides faulty information, other systems (e.g., affective, motivational, behavioral) no longer function in an adaptive way. Errors can result in other cognitive biases (e.g., interpretation, attention, memory), excessive or inappropriate affect, and maladaptive behavior" (Beck & Haigh, 2014, p. 4). The GCM expands upon many of the common principles of the original model and introduces several novel concepts described in the following.

Dual Information Processing

The concept of dual information processing proposes that effective information processing relies on the interaction of two subsystems, the automatic (or primary) processing system and the reflective (or secondary) processing system. The *automatic processing system* is responsible for the rapid intake of stimuli that may indicate personal threats, gains, or losses, while the *reflective processing system* is responsible for the intake of stimuli in a more comprehensive, nuanced, and controlled manner. The automatic processing system is efficient but is prone to judgmental heuristics and error. For example, a person hiking in the mountains might be hypersensitive to threats from wild animals, which *could* be adaptive, but that person may suffer the consequence of being startled easily and often by birds and other small and nonthreatening animals. In contrast, the reflective system processes stimuli more slowly but produces meanings that are more objective and refined. Such processes are often seen in psychotherapy, when patients reconsider their original appraisal of an event through guided questions, and say such things in therapy as, "I have never thought of it that way before," or "Hmm, that's a new point of view." The two systems work collaboratively; the rapid, often subjective, interpretations assigned by the automatic system may be made more objective by the reflective system (i.e., "reality testing").

Attentional Focus

Attentional focus refers to automatic attention to detail and context, which can facilitate reflective processing and modifies behavioral responses.

Inappropriate or inflexible focus can lead to maladaptive reactions, but attentional focus can foster adaptive responses to stimulus situations through the facilitation of accurate processing of stimuli and corrective reality testing. Beck and Haigh (2014) use panic disorder to illustrate how attentional focus can lead to maladaptive reactions in that the involuntary and often rigid focus on subjective internal experiences in panic disorder often preclude objective evaluation of such experiences.

Energizing of Schemas

As reviewed earlier in this chapter, the concept of schematic processing is a central theoretical underpinning of the cognitive model. The GCM maintains that schematic content is crucial for processing and interpreting stimuli situations. The GCM emphasizes the concept of *assimilation,* in which preexisting schemas accept new information. While a moderate degree of assimilation is necessary for adaptive functioning, schemas that are excessively permeable to new information may lead to a "loose, disorganized style of thinking" (Beck & Haigh, 2014, p. 6). In contrast, rigid thinking and delusions may emerge from impermeable schemas.

The process of *accommodation,* through which schemas are modified in order to integrate new information, is also emphasized in the GCM. A schema becomes more "dense" with repeated activation. Dense schemas are also reinforced by habitual behavior and tend to be more durable and less sensitive to change. When the process of accommodation forces schema change, the schemas become "energized" and control information processing. Energized, dysfunctional schemas are associated with psychological problems, while adaptively modified schemas can "deactivate dysfunctional schemas and lead to a reduction in symptoms" (Beck & Haigh, 2014, p. 6). As one example, patients with panic disorder typically enter treatment with an exaggerated focus on physical sensations and symptoms, as these symptoms represent a threat to the patient and are energized, and demand attention. In treatment, the patient might encounter their internal sensations repeatedly through interoceptive exposure, which can help him or her to adopt a new and more adaptive schema such as "My physical sensations do not necessarily mean I will suffer imminent death or injury; I do not need to pay as much attention to them as before," and so deactivate the dysfunctional schemas.

Cognitive Specificity

As has been previously noted, the cognitive model has been successfully applied to a variety of psychological disorders. While the general principles of the cognitive model have been largely maintained throughout its adaptions, the concept of *cognitive specificity* states that various psychological disorders can be differentiated on the basis of unique cognitive content. This concept has been fundamental in the development of distinctive conceptualizations and therapeutic intervention strategies for each disorder (J. S. Beck, 2005; Beck & Perkins, 2001; Beck & Haigh, 2014; see Table 3.3). In response to an aversive event, for instance, the depressive attribution may be, "It's my fault," while the paranoid attribution may be, "They did this to me deliberately" (Beck & Haigh, 2014). Examples of core beliefs specific to each disorder are described in Table 3.3.

TABLE 3.3. Key Themes of Core Beliefs of Varying Psychological Disorders

Psychological disorder	Core beliefs	References
Depression	Negative self-evaluation, hopelessness, loss, failure, deprivation	A. T. Beck et al., 1979; Clark, Beck, & Stewart, 1990
Generalized anxiety disorder	Worry, unrelenting standards, need to self-sacrifice, negative beliefs about uncertainty	Koerner et al., 2015
Panic disorder	Fear of a medical catastrophe (e.g., stroke, heart attack) or a mental health catastrophe (e.g., go crazy or lose control)	A. T. Beck et al., 1992; Clark, 1986; Clark et al., 1994; Sokol et al., 1989
Social phobia	Fear of failing publicly and being rejected, criticized, or humiliated	Chambless & Hope, 1996
Obsessive–compulsive disorder	Fear of losing mental or behavioral control that results in harm to oneself or others (e.g., violent thoughts will be acted upon if not suppressed)	Clark & Beck, 2010
Bipolar disorder	Beliefs that undermine medication compliance (e.g., "the medication destroys my creativity, makes me dull"), manic beliefs (e.g., "I have exceptional powers and I should use them"), and basic depressive beliefs	Ball et al., 2003
Substance abuse	A series of "need" beliefs (e.g., "I can't stand my feelings without a fix") and "permission" beliefs (e.g., "it's okay to have a smoke this one time")	A. T. Beck, 1993
Anorexia nervosa	Disconnection, impaired autonomy, impaired limits, overcontrol	Dingemans et al., 2006
Suicidal ideation and intent	Unlovability, shame, isolation, alienation, failure, defectiveness	Berk et al., 2004; Dutra et al., 2008

VALIDITY OF THE COGNITIVE MODEL

Validity of the Applied Cognitive Model

One of the most important outcomes of Beck's research has been the development of cognitive therapy (CT). Although CT was originally developed for the treatment of depression, modified forms have since allowed its application to an array of psychological problems and disorders (J. S. Beck, 2011). A central tenet of all forms of CT is the reliance on the cognitive formulation and therapeutic principles and strategies of operationalized treatment manuals that center on the identification and evaluation of distorted cognitions and dysfunctional beliefs for a particular psychiatric disorder or psychological problem. As such, CT is based on the cognitive model and fundamental assumptions about the processes responsible for therapeutic change, such as the importance of schema modification (Garratt, Ingram, Rand, & Sawalani, 2007).

Research has examined CT in the treatment of problems such as depression (e.g., Hollon, Stewart, & Strunk, 2006), anxiety disorders and phobias (e.g., Stewart & Chambless, 2009), suicidal behavior (e.g., Brown et al., 2005), personality disorders (e.g., Ng, 2005; Weinberg et al., 2006, 2010), and schizophrenia (e.g., Rector, 2004; Grant, Huh, Perivoliotis, Stolar, & Beck, 2012). Trials generally have shown CT to be as effective as other commonly used treatments (e.g., medication, alternative psychotherapies); more effective than nontreatment controls; and, in some cases, more effective than placebo control groups. In 2006, Butler and colleagues conducted a review of meta-analyses on outcome studies of CT and reported its efficacy for the treatment and relapse prevention of a wide range of problems. Large effect sizes were found for adult and adolescent unipolar depression, panic disorder, generalized anxiety disorder, social phobia, and posttraumatic stress disorder (Butler, Chapman, Forman, & Beck, 2006). Moderate effect sizes were found for a range of other disorders, including anger, childhood somatic disorders, and several chronic pain variables (Butler et al., 2006). More recent meta-analyses of the general field of CT and the broader area of cognitive-behavioral therapy (cf. Hofmann, Asnaani, Vonk, Sawyer, & Fang, 2012; Tolin, 2010) also support the overall efficacy of this model and suggest that it is at least as effective as other treatment approaches. These general meta-analyses are supported by a vast array of meta-analyses for specific models of CT and CBT, and for specific disorders (see Dobson & Dobson, 2017).

The substantial body of research that supports the efficacy of CT, in conjunction with the large number of evaluated treatment manuals, has led to the designation of CT as an empirically supported treatment for several disorders (see Chambless & Ollendick, 2001). Further research is required to evaluate the relative efficacy of CT and pharmacotherapy and other evidence-based psychotherapies. Research is also needed to examine the efficacy of CT for prevention of relapse, for use with diverse populations, and for use with comorbid disorders (Dobson, 2009).

Validity of the Theoretical Cognitive Model

Although the efficacy of CT is relatively undisputed, evidence for the theoretical assumptions and structure of the cognitive model itself is somewhat less clear. As much of the research to examine the validity of the cognitive model has focused on depression, this literature is discussed here in more detail.

In the early 1990s, Haaga, Dyck, and Ernst (1991) conducted one of the most comprehensive evaluations of the model's validity. The group derived thirteen testable hypotheses based on Beck's cognitive model of depression, including predictions based on *descriptive* elements of the model (i.e., that depressed individuals think a certain way) and on *causal* elements of the model (i.e., that cognitions lead to depression). Generally, empirical support was established for many of the theory's descriptive elements, such as the negativity hypothesis (i.e., that depressed individuals tend to experience a greater number of negative thoughts than nondepressed individuals), the cognitive triad (i.e., negative thoughts tend to extend to views of self, others, and the world), and biases in information processing (i.e., the tendency to draw negative conclusions about the self, regardless of circumstance; see also Mathews & MacLeod, 2005; Gotlib, Krasnoperova, Yue, & Joormann, 2004). In contrast, the support was less consistent for the causal elements of the cognitive model. For example, the proposition that modifications in basic cognitive processes are critical for symptom recovery was only demonstrated inconsistently (Garratt et al., 2007), as some studies yielded significant symptom reduction without documented improvement in cognitive functioning or changes in schematic processes.

The cognitive model is based on the stress-diathesis framework, which asserts that psychological dysfunction is a consequence of cognitive vulnerability (i.e., negative schemas) that becomes problematic (or activated) in the face of relevant, external stressors. Critics of the cognitive model have long argued that the stress-diathesis framework does not adequately address other possible etiological explanations, such as genetic, neurobiological, interpersonal, and emotional factors (Clark, 1995; Krantz, 1985). Nevertheless, experimental research has demonstrated considerable support for the stress-diathesis framework, specifically, that negative schemas do become activated in response to stressful or negative situations (e.g., Dozois & Back-Dermott, 2000; Abela & D'Alessandro, 2002; Scher, Ingram, & Segal, 2005; Kwon & Oei, 1992). Research has also provided evidence for causal processes in depression that are linked to the emergence of negative schemas, which may play a role in the recurrence of depressive symptoms (e.g., Segal et al., 2006).

Research related to the cognitive model has been compromised by disparate research methodologies, cognitive measures, and statistical techniques (Garratt et al., 2007). Further, most studies employ cross-sectional designs, which cannot adequately examine causational elements of the cognitive theory (Abela & D'Alessandro, 2002). Future research to examine the theoretical propositions of the cognitive model would benefit from measurement of a wide range of cognitive symptoms, use of measures sensitive to change, statistical techniques specific to causal models (e.g., standard error of measurement [SEM]), recruitment of larger sample sizes, and use of longitudinal designs (Garratt et al., 2007; Abela & D'Alessandro, 2002).

CONCLUSIONS

The cognitive model of psychopathology has instigated a major shift in the conceptualization, classification, and treatment of psychological disorders. Although the model itself has undergone substantial elaborations (e.g., Apsche & Ward Bailey, 2003; Ingram & Hollon, 1986; J. S. Beck, 1995, 2005, 2011), its theoretical underpinnings have remained predominantly unchanged. At its core, cognitive theory postulates that dysfunctional beliefs are largely responsible for psychiatric symptoms and disorders, and that the remedy lies in modification of the cognitive set (Beck, 1967; J. S. Beck, 2005).

This chapter has traced the historical development of the cognitive model from its emergence in the 1960s and 1970s to its advancement as one of the most important and well-validated contemporary theoretical and psychotherapeutic approaches. Key principles of the cognitive model assert that vulnerability toward psychological dysfunction lies in core schemas, beliefs, assumptions, and automatic thoughts. These principles have been elaborated over time, through concepts such as "modes" within the generic cognitive model. The addition of genetic, neurobiological, and emotional components to the model addresses the concern that a complete understanding of the etiology and treatment of psychopathology requires a multilevel, process-based approach to psychopathology (e.g., Forgeard et al., 2011).

The concept of cognitive specificity and the manner in which various disorders can be differentiated based on their thought content and belief structure were described and illustrated. Finally, evidence for the validity of cognitive therapy, the therapeutic paradigm based on the cognitive model, and the validity of the theoretical underpinnings of the cognitive model itself were outlined. A continued emphasis on outcome research that has used empirical guidelines and sound measures has allowed cognitive researchers to make substantial advancements in both research and practice.

As the cognitive model continues to evolve, applied areas that require further conceptualization and experimentation include the efficacy of CT as compared to that of pharmacotherapy and other evidence-based psychotherapies, and the efficacy of CT in the prevention of relapse, for use with diverse populations and with comorbid disorders. Research to examine the theoretical underpinnings of the cognitive model may focus on causal descriptions of the model and the development of more complex, transdiagnostic models. As with any theoretical approach, adaptations to the cognitive model will involve consideration of its relationship to other prevailing theoretical models of therapy (e.g., mindfulness, acceptance commitment therapy, dialectical behavioral therapy, psychodynamic psychotherapy), its relevance to diagnostic manuals of psychiatric disorders that evolve over time, and the optimal strategies for effective and wide-reaching dissemination.

REFERENCES

Abela, J., & D'Alessandro, D. U. (2002). Beck's cognitive theory of depression: A test of the diathesis-stress and causal mediation components. *British Journal of Clinical Psychology, 41*(2), 111–127.

Apsche, J. A., & Ward Bailey, S. R. (2003). Mode deactivation therapy and cognitive behavior therapy: A description of treatment results for adolescents with personality beliefs, sexual offending and aggressive behaviors. *The Behavior Analyst Today, 3*(4), 460–470.

Ball, J., Mitchell, P., Malhi, G., Skillecorn, A., & Smith, M. (2003). Schema-focused cognitive therapy for bipolar disorder: Reducing vulnerability to relapse through attitudinal change. *Australian and New Zealand Journal of Psychiatry, 37*(1), 41–48.

Beck, A. T. (1964). Thinking and depression: II. Theory and therapy. *Archives of General Psychiatry, 10*(6), 561–571.

Beck, A. T. (1967). *Depression: Causes and treatment.* Philadelphia: University of Pennsylvania Press.

Beck, A. T. (1970). Cognitive therapy: Nature and relation to behavior therapy. *Behavior Therapy, 1*(2), 184–200.

Beck, A. T. (1976). *Cognitive therapy and the emotional disorders.* New York: International Universities Press.

Beck, A. T. (Ed.). (1979). *Cognitive therapy of depression.* New York: Guilford Press.

Beck, A. T. (1996). Beyond belief: A theory of modes, personality, and psychopathology. In P. M. Salkovskis (Ed.), *Frontiers of cognitive therapy* (pp. 1–25). New York: Guilford Press.

Beck, A. T., Emery, G., & Greenberg, R. L. (1985). *Anxiety disorders and phobias: A cognitive approach.* New York: Basic Books.

Beck, A. T., & Freeman, A. (1990). *Cognitive therapy of personality disorders.* New York: Guilford Press.

Beck, A. T., & Haigh, E. A. (2014). Advances in cognitive theory and therapy: The generic cognitive model. *Annual Review of Clinical Psychology, 10,* 1–24.

Beck, A. T., Rush, A. J., Shaw, B. F., & Emery, G. (1979). *Cognitive therapy of depression.* New York: Guilford Press.

Beck, A. T., Sokol, L., Clark, D. A., Berchick, R., & Wright, F. (1992). A crossover study of focused cognitive therapy for panic disorder. *American Journal of Psychiatry, 149*(6), 778–783.

Beck, A. T., Wright, F. D., Newman, C. F., & Liese, B. S. (1993). *Cognitive therapy of substance abuse.* New York: Guilford Press.

Beck, J. S. (1979). *Cognitive therapy.* New York: Wiley.

Beck, J. S. (1995). *Cognitive therapy: Basics and beyond.* New York: Guilford Press.

Beck, J. S. (2005). *Cognitive therapy for challenging problems: What to do when the basics don't work.* New York: Guilford Press.

Beck, J. S. (2011). *Cognitive behavior therapy: Basics and beyond* (2nd ed.). New York: Guilford Press.

Beck, R., & Perkins, T. S. (2001). Cognitive content-specificity for anxiety and depression: A meta-analysis. *Cognitive Therapy and Research, 25*(6), 651–663.

Berk, M. S., Henriques, G. R., Warman, D. M., Brown, G. K., & Beck, A. T. (2004). A cognitive therapy intervention for suicide attempters: An overview of the treatment and case examples. *Cognitive and Behavioral Practice, 11*(3), 265–277.

Blatt S., Zuroff, D., Bondi C., & Sanisolow, C. (2000). Short- and long-term effects of medication and psychotherapy in the brief treatment of depression: Further analyses of data from the NIMH TDCRP. *Psychotherapy Research, 10*(2), 215–234.

Brown, G. K., Ten Have, T., Henriques, G. R., Xie, S. X., Hollander, J. E., & Beck, A. T. (2005). Cognitive therapy for the prevention of suicide attempts: A randomized controlled trial. *Journal of the American Medical Association, 294* (5), 563–570.

Butler, A. C., Chapman, J. E., Forman, E. M., & Beck, A. T. (2006). The empirical status of cognitive-behavioral therapy: A review of meta-analyses. *Clinical Psychology Review, 26*(1), 17–31.

Chambless, D. L., & Hope, D. A. (1996). Cognitive approaches to the psychopathology and treatment of social phobia. In P. M. Salkovskis (Ed.), *Frontiers of cognitive therapy* (pp. 345–382). New York: Guilford Press.

Chambless, D. L., & Ollendick, T. H. (2001). Empirically supported psychological interventions: Controversies and evidence. *Annual Review of Psychology, 52,* 685–716.

Chomsky, N. (1975). *Reflections on language.* New York: Pantheon Press.

Clark, D. A. (1995). Perceived limitations of standard cognitive therapy: A consideration of efforts to revise Beck's theory and therapy. *Journal of Cognitive Psychotherapy,* 9(3), 153–172.

Clark, D. A., & Beck, A. T. (2010). Cognitive theory and therapy of anxiety and depression: Convergence with neurobiological findings. *Trends in Cognitive Sciences, 14,* 418–424.

Clark, D. A., & Beck, A. T. (with Alford, B. A.). (1999). *Scientific foundations of cognitive theory and therapy of depression.* New York: Wiley.

Clark, D. A., Beck, A. T., & Stewart, B. L. (1990). Cognitive specificity and positive–negative affectivity: Complementary or contradictory views on anxiety and depression? *Journal of Abnormal Psychology, 99*(2), 148–155.

Clark, D. M. (1986). A cognitive approach to panic. *Behaviour Research and Therapy, 24*(4), 461–470.

Clark, D. M., Salkovskis, P. M., Hackmann, A., Middleton, H., Anastasiades, P., & Gelder, M. (1994). A comparison of cognitive therapy, applied relaxation and imipramine in the treatment of panic disorder. *British Journal of Psychiatry, 164*(6), 759–769.

Dingemans, A. E., Spinhoven, P., & Van Furth, E. F. (2006). Maladaptive core beliefs and eating disorder symptoms. *Eating Behaviors, 7*(3), 258–265.

Dobson, D. J. G., & Dobson, K. S. (2017). *Evidence-based practice of cognitive-behavioral therapy* (2nd ed.). New York: Guilford Press.

Dobson, K. S. (Ed.). (2009). *Handbook of cognitive-behavioral therapies.* New York: Guilford Press.

Dobson, K. S. (2012). *Cognitive therapy.* Washington, DC: American Psychological Association.

Dozois, D. J. A., & Back-Dermott, B. J. (2000). Sociotropic personality and information processing following imaginal priming: A test of the congruency hypothesis. *Canadian Journal of Behavioural Science, 32*(2), 117–126.

Dozois, D. J., & Beck, A. T. (2008). Cognitive schemas, beliefs and assumptions. *Risk Factors in Depression, 1,* 121–143.

Dutra, L., Callahan, K., Forman, E., Mendelsohn, M., & Herman, J. (2008). Core schemas and suicidality in a chronically traumatized population. *Journal of Nervous and Mental Disease, 196*(1), 71–74.

Ehlers, A., & Clark, D. M. (2000). A cognitive model of posttraumatic stress disorder. *Behaviour Research and Therapy, 38*(4), 319–345.

Ellis, A. (1973). *Humanistic psychotherapy.* New York: McGraw-Hill.

Forgeard, M. J., Haigh, E. A., Beck, A. T., Davidson, R. J., Henn, F. A., Maier, S. F., . . . Seligman, M. E. (2011). Beyond depression: Toward a process-based approach to research, diagnosis, and treatment. *Clinical Psychology: Science and Practice, 18*(4), 275–299.

Garratt, G., Ingram, R. E., Rand, K. L., & Sawalani, G. (2007). Cognitive processes in cognitive therapy: Evaluation of the mechanisms of change in the treatment of depression. *Clinical Psychology: Science and Practice, 14*(3), 224–239.

Gotlib, I. H., Krasnoperova, E., Yue, D. N., & Joormann, J. (2004). Attentional biases for negative interpersonal stimuli in clinical depression. *Journal of Abnormal Psychology, 113*(1), 127.

Grant, P. M., Huh, G. A., Perivoliotis, D., Stolar, N. M., & Beck, A. T. (2012). Randomized trial to evaluate the efficacy of cognitive therapy for low-functioning patients with schizophrenia. *Archives of General Psychiatry, 69*(2), 121–127.

Haaga, D. A., Dyck, M. J., & Ernst, D. (1991). Empirical status of cognitive theory of depression. *Psychological Bulletin, 110*(2), 215.

Hofmann, S. G., Asnaani, A., Vonk, I. J. J., Sawyer, A. T., & Fang, A. (2012). The efficacy of cognitive-behavioral therapy: A review of meta-analyses. *Cognitive Therapy and Research, 36,* 427–440.

Hollon, S. D., Stewart, M. O., & Strunk, D. (2006). Enduring effects for cognitive behavior therapy in the treatment of depression and anxiety. *Annual Review of Psychology, 57,* 285–315.

Ingram, R. E., & Hollon, S. D. (1986). Cognitive therapy for depression from an information processing perspective. In R. E. Ingram (Ed.), *Information processing approaches to clinical psychology* (pp. 255–281). San Diego, CA: Academic Press.

Kingdon, D. G., & Turkington, D. (2005). *Cognitive therapy of schizophrenia.* New York: Guilford Press.

Koerner, N., Tallon, K., & Kusec, A. (2015). Maladaptive core beliefs and their relation to generalized anxiety disorder. *Cognitive Behaviour Therapy,* 1–15.

Kovacs, M., & Beck, A. T. (1978). Maladaptive cognitive structures in depression. *American Journal of Psychiatry, 135*(5), 525–533.

Krantz, S. E. (1985). When depressive cognitions reflect negative realities. *Cognitive Therapy and Research, 9,* 595–610.

Kwon, S., & Oei, T. P. S. (1992). Differential causal roles of dysfunctional attitudes and automatic thoughts in depression. *Cognitive Therapy and Research, 16,* 309–328.

Mahoney, M. J. (1974). *Cognition and behavior modification.* Cambridge, MA: Ballinger.

Mathews, A., & MacLeod, C. (2005). Cognitive vulnerability to emotional disorders. *Annual Review of Clinical Psychology, 1,* 167–195.

Needleman, L. D. (1999). *Cognitive case conceptualization: A guidebook for practitioners.* London: Routledge.

Neenan, M., & Dryden, W. (2011). *Cognitive therapy in a nutshell.* London: SAGE.

Ng, R. M. K. (2005). Cognitive therapy for obsessive–compulsive personality disorder—A pilot study in Hong Kong Chinese patients. *Hong Kong Journal of Psychiatry, 15*(2), 50–53.

Rector, N. A. (2004). Cognitive theory and therapy of schizophrenia. In R. L. Leahy (Ed.), *Contemporary cognitive therapy: Theory, research, and practice* (pp. 244–265). New York: Guilford Press.

Scher, C. D., Ingram, R. E., & Segal, Z. V. (2005). Cognitive reactivity and vulnerability: Empirical evaluation of construct activation and cognitive diatheses in unipolar depression. *Clinical Psychology Review, 25,* 487–510.

Segal, Z. V., Kennedy, M. D., Gemar, M., Hood, K., Pedersen, R., & Buis, T. (2006). Cognitive reactivity to sad mood provocation and the prediction of depressive relapse. *Archives of General Psychiatry, 63,* 749–755.

Sokol, L., Beck, A. T., Greenberg, R. L., Wright, F. D., & Berchick, R. J. (1989). Cognitive therapy of panic disorder: A nonpharmacological alternative. *Journal of Nervous and Mental Disease, 177*(12), 711–716.

Stewart, R. E., & Chambless, D. L. (2009). Cognitive-behavioral therapy for adult anxiety disorders in clinical practice: A meta-analysis of effectiveness studies. *Journal of Consulting and Clinical Psychology, 77*(4), 595.

Stone, E. R., Dodrill, C. L., & Johnson, N. (2001). Depressive cognition: A test of depressive realism versus negativity using general knowledge questions. *Journal of Psychology, 135*(6), 583–602.

Strack, S. (Ed.). (2005). *Handbook of personology and psychopathology.* New York: Wiley.

Tolin, D. F. (2010). Is cognitive-behavioral therapy more effective than other therapies?: A meta-analytic review. *Clinical Psychology Review, 30,* 710–720.

Vygotsky, L. S. (1962). *Thought and language.* Cambridge, MA: MIT Press.

Weinberg, I., Gunderson, J. G., Hennen, J., & Cutter, C. J., Jr. (2006). Manual assisted cognitive treatment for deliberate self-harm in borderline personality disorder patients. *Journal of Personality Disorders, 20*(5), 482–492.

Weishaar, M. E. (1996). Developments in cognitive therapy. In *Developments in psychotherapy: Historical perspectives.* London: SAGE.

Wenzel, A. (2012). Modification of core beliefs in cognitive therapy. In I. R. De Oliveira (Ed.), *Standard and innovative strategies in cognitive behavior therapy* (pp. 17–33). Rijeka, Croatia: InTech. Available from *www.intechopen.com/books/standard-and-innovative-strategies-in-cognitive-behavior-therapy/modification-of-core-beliefs-in-cognitive-therapy.*

Wills, F. (2013). *Beck's cognitive therapy: Distinctive features.* London: Routledge.

Wright, J. H., Basco, M. R., & Thase, M. E. (2006). *Learning cognitive-behavior therapy: An illustrated guide.* Washington, DC: American Psychiatric Publishing.

CHAPTER 4

Outcome Studies in Cognitive Therapy

Steven D. Hollon
Robert J. DeRubeis

OUTCOME STUDIES IN COGNITIVE THERAPY

In the fifty years since cognitive therapy (CT) first burst upon the scene, it has become the most extensively investigated psychosocial intervention (Hollon & Beck, 2013). It is most clearly efficacious for the nonpsychotic disorders (mood, anxiety, stress, and eating disorders) but it also has been applied with positive results to the personality disorders and the psychoses (the latter usually as an adjunct to medications) (Butler, Chapman, Forman, & Beck, 2006). Cognitive therapy even has been used to prevent the first onset of mood and anxiety disorders in at-risk children and adolescents (Garber et al., 2009). This is an unprecedented array of clinical successes.

In this chapter, we provide an illustrative overview of some of the best of this literature. Our goal is not to be exhaustive but rather to highlight the best of the outcome studies with CT across a number of different disorders and life problems. We start with a brief overview of the basic cognitive model and then describe the therapeutic strategies that form the core of the intervention. We then proceed to a description of some of the most informative of the outcome studies that have been done across a variety of different diagnostic categories, describing in the process the way the basic model needed to be elaborated and the therapeutic strategies modified to fit the specifics of the particular disorder. This is not a systematic review of the evidence in a given area but rather an explication of what can be accomplished in a well-executed trial in which CT is conducted well and appropriately.

COGNITIVE THEORY OF DISORDER

Cognitive theory posits that it is not just what happens to people that determines how they feel and what they do but rather the way that they interpret those events (Beck, 2005). People prone to psychopathology are seen as falling prey to a number of inaccurate beliefs and maladaptive information-processing strategies that influence affect and behavior in a deleterious fashion. Automatic negative thoughts in specific situations are seen as being driven by latent schemas laid down in youth in a manner that interacts with individual differences in genes and temperament (Beck, 2008).

Schemas are organized knowledge structures that consist of core beliefs ("I am incompetent" or "I am unlovable" for depression and "the world is a dangerous place" for anxiety) that influence the way the individual processes new information in novel situations. Core beliefs give rise to conditional assumptions ("if I let others get close to me, they will not like me, so better to be standoffish and keep my distance") that are designed to cut one's losses in a world that is unlikely to give us all the things that we want. Compensatory strategies are the ways that people go about trying to get what they want out of life while simultaneously protecting themselves against the consequences of their own perceived deficiencies or the predations of the outside world (Beck, Freeman, Davis, & Associates, 2004). Compensatory strategies range from the safety behaviors intended to protect one's self from harm, common in those with anxiety or stress disorders, to the problematic acting-out behaviors engaged in by those with personality disorders. The key point is that they are all designed to protect the individual from harm or to facilitate the pursuit of appetitive goals even in the context of erroneous beliefs about the nature of the self, the world, and the future (the negative cognitive triad).

COGNITIVE THEORY OF THERAPY

CT focuses on teaching patients how to examine the accuracy of their own beliefs. This is often best accomplished by encouraging the patients to run experiments in which they act in ways that are inconsistent with their initial inclinations so as to test whether what they believe is really true. For example, people who are certain that no one will hire them might be encouraged to apply for jobs (with a little guidance) to see if their expectations really are true. Some disorders like depression put a premium on behavioral activation for its own sake (it is good to get active if only to overcome the inertia found in the disorder), but such activation is set up as a test of the notion that the patient could not do, or would not enjoy, engaging in the activity. Other beliefs, such as that the symptoms of a panic attack indicate that one is about to die from a heart attack or that looking flushed and anxious means that others will think less of you, lend themselves to more immediate tests. In the former case, the patient can engage in behaviors that he or she expects will lead to cardiac failure; in the latter, the patient can act in such a way that he or she expects will provoke others' disapproval. Cognitive restructuring is a common tool that is used in many of the disorders, especially depression, but may be less necessary when clear-cut behavioral tests of those beliefs present themselves as they do in panic disorder or in the eating disorders. The basic approach always involves encouraging patients to test the accuracy of their beliefs, but exactly how that is done depends on the nature of the disorder. It is this emphasis on accuracy that allows the therapy to take advantage of behavioral tests; there is an external reality against which idiosyncratic beliefs can be tested. It is the emphasis on the acquisition of basic skills that enables CT to have an enduring effect; the patient develops the tools to become his or her own cognitive therapist (Hollon, Stewart, & Strunk, 2006).

COGNITIVE THERAPY FOR DEPRESSION

CT was first tested in the treatment of depression. Two decades of research starting in the late 1950s involving several hundred placebo-controlled trials had established that the antidepressant medications, at that time largely the monoamine oxidase inhibitors (MAOIs) and the tricyclic antidepressants (TCAs), were efficacious in the treatment of unipolar major depression. However, psychosocial interventions had not been found to be as efficacious as medications or even superior to pill-placebo. That changed with the publication of a study conducted at the University of Pennsylvania, which found CT superior to the widely used TCA imipramine in the treatment of acute depression (Rush, Beck, Kovacs, & Hollon, 1977). When a subsequent study conducted in Edinburgh Scotland, found CT superior to two other TCA antidepressant medications among depressed patients in a general medical setting, CT was taken to be efficacious and generated considerable excitement in the field (Blackburn et al., 1981).

The problem with both of these early studies was that pharmacotherapy was not implemented in a manner that represented good pharmacotherapy management. Subsequent trials in which both CT and medications were implemented to a good standard typically found no differences between them, but none were placebo-controlled. The first with a placebo condition was the National Institute of Mental Health Treatment of

Depression Collaborative Research Program (NIMH TDCRP). CT was not found to be more efficacious than pill-placebo, and it was less efficacious than antidepressant medications (again the TCA imipramine) among patients with more severe depressions (Elkin et al., 1995). However, the quality of CT in that trial has been questioned (see Jacobson & Hollon, 1996). A subsequent placebo-controlled trial in which both monotherapies were adequately implemented found that CT was as efficacious as paroxetine, a selective serotonin reuptake inhibitor (SSRI), in the treatment of patients with severe depression, and that both were superior to pill-placebo (DeRubeis et al., 2005).

In that trial, as in others before it, CT was shown to have an enduring effect not found for medications. Patients treated to remission with CT were only about half as likely to relapse following treatment termination relative to patients treated to remission on medications, and they were no more likely to relapse than patients kept on continuation medications (Hollon et al., 2005). This robust effect was obtained in seven of the eight trials in which CT was tested (Cuijpers et al., 2013).

The bottom line from research thus far is that CT can be as efficacious as antidepressant medications when it is adequately implemented and that, unlike medication, its benefits persist after treatment ceases. Whether this is true of other comparably efficacious psychosocial interventions, such as behavioral activation or interpersonal psychotherapy, remains to be seen.

One caveat is in order. CT has demonstrated an enduring effect when provided in the absence of medications but thus far has not proven to have this effect when provided along with medications. In a recent trial, we found that adding CT to medications enhanced rates of recovery for nonchronic patients who were more severe (about one-third of those in our sample) but had little effect on patients who were chronic (another third of the sample) and was not necessary for nonchronic patients who were not severe (the remaining third of the sample; Hollon et al., 2014). These findings speak to the power of moderation: different response for patients with different characteristics (DeRubeis et al., 2014). What was striking was the absence of any indication that exposure to CT, which in this trial was always provided in the context of medication treatment, served to forestall recurrences (onsets of new episodes; DeRubeis, 2014). It is well documented that combining cognitive–behavioral therapy with medications inhibits any enduring effect for the psychosocial intervention in the treatment of panic (Barlow, Gorman, Shear, & Woods, 2000). In the Barlow study, combined treatment with a pill-placebo did not interfere with the subsequent enduring effect of cognitive-behavioral therapy but combined treatment with an active medication did. This finding suggests that the underlying mechanism was pharmacological and not purely psychological.

Maier, Amat, Baratta, Paul, and Watkins (2006) found that exposure to controllable stress fomented cortical inhibition of the lower brainstem and limbic systems that mediated the stress response. Maier and Seligman (2016) recently reinterpreted the learned helpless phenomenon to suggest that it was exposure to controllable stress that led to learning something new (resilience), whereas exposure to uncontrollable stress triggers only the default species-specific stress response. It is quite possible that cortical activation needs to be paired with the limbic/brainstem activation for resilience to be learned. If that is the case, then providing CT in combination with active medications may inhibit the acquisition of learned resilience in much the same fashion as appeared to be the case with panic patients in the Barlow study.

COGNITIVE THERAPY FOR PANIC AND THE ANXIETY DISORDERS

A good case can be made that CT should be the treatment of choice for panic disorder. As described in a now classic article by David Clark, panic disorder involves the catastrophic misinterpretation of otherwise benign physical symptoms or mental experiences (Clark, 1986). For example, an individual who misconstrues physical sensations associated with stress or arousal as an indication of an impending heart attack is likely to go on to experience panic at the prospect of imminent death. The same can occur in an individual who misconstrues random ideation as a harbinger of impending psychotic decompensation. Such a person will typically engage in safety behaviors (aka compensatory strategies), such as ceasing all physical activity or going to the emergency room, in order to forestall the impending catastrophe. The consequence is that he or she never learns that there is no true danger. To counter this process, Clark has the patient do everything possible to bring on the anticipated catastrophe. When the patient is still alive thirty minutes later, he or she has experienced a powerful disconfirmation of the catastrophic beliefs.

Clark and colleagues found CT superior to either imipramine or applied relaxation, with each treatment superior in turn to a wait list control (Clark et al., 1994). Nearly 90% of the patients treated with CT were panic-free nine months later compared to only 50% of the patients treated with the other active modalities. These are very powerful effects that appear to endure over time. In the United States, therapists tend to teach their patients to control their panic symptoms rather than to cure them (because therapists are reluctant to push the limits) and Clark's approach has not gotten the widespread adoption that it deserves.

Clark also is in the process of revolutionizing how we treat social anxiety. Starting with the observation that people prone to social anxiety focus too much on their own internal images of themselves performing poorly in interpersonal interactions, he encourages patients to drop their safety behaviors and focus on the other person with whom they are interacting. He makes videotapes of patients interacting with others both engaging in and not engaging in their typical safety behaviors and invites them to watch the contrast (most prefer the no-safety-behavior version). He then has patients interact with others in such a way that their worst fears are likely to be realized (putting rouge on their faces, or spraying water under their armpits, to simulate anxiety) and helps them recognize that they can readily handle these situations. To paraphrase Samuel Johnson, "we would not worry so much what other people thought of us if we knew how little they thought of us."

This approach was superior to either fluoxetine or pill-placebo in one trial (Clark et al., 2003) and better than exposure plus response prevention—with both superior to wait list—in another (Clark et al., 2006). A subsequent trial conducted in Germany found CT superior to interpersonal psychotherapy at each of two different sites, including one that preferred the interpersonal approach (Stangier, Schramm, Heidenreich, Berger, & Clark, 2011). A recent network analysis conducted as part of a systematic review by the National Institute for Health and Clinical Excellence (NICE) found that individual cognitive-behavioral therapy (CBT), particularly the variant implemented by Clark, was the treatment of choice (in terms of maximizing effect sizes while minimizing side effects) of the available treatments for social anxiety (Mayo-Wilson et al., 2014). In the United States, we tend to focus more on behavioral skills training and less on the specific cognitive propensities that Clark has uncovered. Perhaps for this reason, findings from studies conducted in the United States have been somewhat less impressive, but they are largely consistent with what has been found in Europe.

One comment is in order about how Clark gets these effects. As in the case of both panic disorder and social anxiety, he starts with clinical observation to identify the distinctive features of the relevant syndrome: catastrophic cognitions in the case of panic and internal imagery regarding the self in social anxiety. He then conducts a series of descriptive psychopathology studies to confirm their presence in clinical cases and to refine his conceptualization. He next proceeds to trials in which he attempts to alter the proclivity experimentally. Once he has a set of strategies in place, he builds them into a clinical intervention that can readily be tested in controlled trials. He has outlined this approach in a conceptual methodological piece in the journal *Behavioural Research and Therapy* (Clark, 2004). Judging from the results, it is a most compelling and successful approach.

As a treatment of generalized anxiety disorder (GAD), CT is at least as efficacious, and quite possibly longer lasting, than alternative approaches, including more purely behavioral interventions. It is recommended as a first-line treatment in the clinical guidelines in use in the United Kingdom (NICE, 2011). GAD appears to be less a problem of generalized arousal than one of chronic worry. This recognition led Ladouceur and colleagues to drop relaxation training entirely and focus on more purely cognitive targets, such as intolerance of uncertainty and cognitive avoidance (Ladouceur et al., 1999). Recent trials suggest that this approach may be superior to and longer lasting than more purely behavioral relaxation (Dugas et al., 2010; Wells et al., 2010).

PTSD AND THE STRESS DISORDERS

There is an emerging consensus that trauma-focused approaches that involve exposure to the traumatic memory are the treatment of choice for PTSD (Bisson et al., 2007; see also Resick, Chapter 20 of this volume). In a major theoretical paper, Ehlers and Clark (2000) proposed that PTSD becomes persistent when individuals process trauma in a way suggesting that a prior experience represents a current threat. They encourage patients to relive the traumatic memory (as is done in other trauma-focused therapies) but largely in the service of accessing the underlying meaning that has been ascribed to the prior trauma so that it can be evaluated for accuracy through cognitive restructuring. This more cognitive approach typically requires fewer repeated instances of reliving than the more purely behavioral prolonged exposure. They also assist patients in identifying the classically conditioned cues that trigger activation of the latent memories and encourage them to refrain from engaging in the safety behaviors such as avoiding reminders or suppressing recollections that they have used to suppress distress. Cognitive therapy for PTSD has been found to be superior to a wait list control, and its gains have been maintained across a six-month follow-up (Ehlers, Clark, Hackmann, McManus, & Fennell, 2005). It has also been tested successfully in a general clinical setting with patients suffering from a range of different types of trauma (Ehlers et al., 2013).

In a recent trial, an intensive seven-day course of CT was as efficacious as the standard three months of weekly CT, with each superior to emotion-focused supportive therapy, which was in turn superior to a wait list control (Ehlers et al., 2014). There were no indications of any increment in problematic adverse events in the intensive treatment condition. In essence, cognitive therapy for PTSD is at least as efficacious as other trauma-focused approaches. Some patients may find it less aversive, as it quickly addresses the problematic beliefs that serve to maintain the distress.

COGNITIVE THERAPY FOR OBSESSIVE–COMPULSIVE DISORDER

Exposure plus response prevention is the best established treatment for obsessive–compulsive disorder (OCD), but there is an increasing sense that cognitive processes play an important role in the disorder and in its treatment. In a major theoretical statement, Salkovskis (1999) stressed the role of perceived personal responsibility in the etiology and maintenance of the disorder. In essence, it is not simply the content of the obsessions that drives the disorder, but what it means to the patient to have the obsession in the first place. The newer cognitive approaches retain the emphasis on exposure and response prevention but emphasize the process of uncovering the meaning of the obsessions to the patient and the undue responsibility taken for personal welfare (in the case of contamination fears) or others (in the case of concerns about causing harm to others). An example of a belief that instantiates a contamination fear is: "it would be irresponsible of me not to protect myself from contamination." A "checking" behavior is likely to be related to a belief such as "I may have caused harm to others." This opens the way for cognitive restructuring amidst exposure (see Sookman, Chapter 19 of this volume). CT (termed "integrative cognitive-behavior therapy" when it incorporates a greater emphasis on meaning of the obsessions) appears to be about as efficacious as more purely behavioral approaches among patients with overt compulsions, but the evidence suggests that it provides a distinct advantage for those without overt compulsions (Whittal, Woody, McLean, Rachman, & Robichaud, 2010). Whether there are any advantages in terms of the long-term stability of change remains to be determined.

COGNITIVE THERAPY FOR THE EATING DISORDERS

Cognitive-behavioral therapy (CBT) is the clear treatment of choice for bulimia and possibly other eating disorders. As practiced by Fairburn and colleagues, CBT is more behavioral than cognitive in the procedures that it uses (for example, there is no explicit effort to engage in cognitive restructuring), but aberrant beliefs about shape and weight form the theoretical core of the intervention (Fairburn, 1981). In brief, Fairburn posits that patients (typically young women) become focused on shape and weight in the pursuit of interpersonal relationships and as a consequence engage in restrictive dieting in an effort to control their weight. This leaves them vulnerable to "loss-of-control" eating under stress (binges), which in turn leads them to engage in self-induced vomiting (purges) or excessive exercising in an effort to rid themselves of the excess calories. Therapy involves laying out this basic rationale, identifying the aberrant beliefs, and normalizing eating behaviors while dropping the compensatory strategies (dieting and purging).

Recent trends view aberrations in food intake as a transdiagnostic disorder uniting bulimia with anorexia and perhaps binge eating as well. A recent trial found that conventional CBT was sufficient for less complicated eating disorders but that an enhanced version that addressed issues like mood intolerance and perfectionism was more efficacious with patients with more complex disorders (Fairburn et al., 2009). In a subsequent trial, enhanced CBT was superior to interpersonal psychotherapy in the treatment of a transdiagnostic sample of patients with any of a variety of different eating disorders (Fairburn et al., 2015).

In a recent trial, twelve weeks of CBT proved more than twice as efficacious as two years of psychodynamic treatment (Poulsen et al., 2014). This is one of the biggest differences between active interventions in the treatment literature. These findings were even more remarkable given that all the allegiance effects favored dynamic therapy. The therapists who implemented the psychodynamic approach were experienced with it prior to the trial, whereas the therapists who conducted CBT were trained for the purpose of the study and received only remote supervision (from Fairburn) during the trial. Nonetheless, CBT was markedly superior at the end of only twelve weeks of active treatment (half the patients in that modality no longer binged), and dynamic therapy never approached the rates of response shown by CBT even when continued for two full years.

Anorexia remains the most difficult of the eating disorders to treat, but it, too, may yield to CBT. A recent inpatient trial comparing conventional to enhanced CBT found significant improvements in weight and eating disorders, with only modest evidence of deterioration following discharge from the hospital (the usual bane of inpatient programs) (Dalle Grave et al., 2013). How CBT compares to more behavioral inpatient programs remains to be determined. Similar encouraging findings were produced by an open trial with outpatient treatment of anorexia nervosa (Fairburn et al., 2013). Fairburn and colleagues have a trial currently underway comparing enhanced CBT with the Maudsley anorexia treatment program and each with specialist-supportive clinical management (Andony et al., 2015).

SCHEMA-FOCUSED COGNITIVE THERAPY FOR PERSONALITY DISORDERS

CT has been adapted for use with patients with long-standing personality disorders. In this adaptation, greater attention is given to the underlying schema, childhood reconstruction techniques are employed, and the therapeutic relationship is used as a basis for working through problematic interpersonal behaviors (Beck et al., 2004). In the one trial in which it has been tested, schema-focused CT was superior to dynamic transference-focused psychotherapy in the treatment of patients with borderline personality disorders (BPDs; Giesen-Bloo et al., 2006). Treatment was intensive and prolonged, consisting of twice-weekly sessions over a three-year span. Treatment gains were maintained beyond the end of treatment, such that schema-focused CT was found to be significantly more cost effective than dynamic therapy (van Asselt et al., 2008). It remains to be seen how schema therapy compares to more widely utilized approaches such as dialectic behavior therapy, with which it shares many features, or how it fares in the treatment of patients with personality disorders other than BPD (see Arntz, Chapter 5 of this volume and Davis, Chapter 21).

COGNITIVE THERAPY FOR THE SCHIZOPHRENIAS

Aaron Beck's first publication was a case study of a patient with paranoid schizophrenia (Beck, 1952). However, Beck soon shifted his attention to depression, and the development of CT was largely focused on other non-psychotic disorders. The bulk of the work with the schizophrenias was conducted in the United Kingdom and did not really take off until the 1990s. Nonetheless, that work prospered, and a little more than a decade generated over thirty trials of CT, usually as an adjunct to medications (Wykes, Steel, Everitt, & Tarrier, 2008). The upshot was that adding CT enhanced response to medication (with modest-sized effects), leading to its being recommended as an adjunct to medications in both the United States (APA, 2004) and the United Kingdom (NICE, 2009).

Beck, aware and supportive of this work, returned to his first interest in the last decade (see Beck, Chapter 1 of this volume), with a focus on low-functioning patients with chronic schizophrenia. In order to adapt the approach to such patients, Beck and colleagues shifted from the symptom-focused approach prominent in the United Kingdom to a more person-oriented approach that emphasizes the individual patient's interests and strengths (Beck, Rector, Stolar, & Grant, 2009). Treatment is focused on identifying and promoting concrete goals that improve the quality of life and facilitate reintegration into society. The focus is on overcoming "defeatist" thinking and encouraging patients to pursue the things they value (Grant & Beck, 2009).

In a randomized controlled trial, this recovery-oriented approach to CT led to meaningful change in functional outcomes when added to medications, relative to standard medication treatment with supportive counseling, across an eighteen-month interval (Grant, Huh, Perivoliotis, Stolar, & Beck, 2012). There was little change over time in standard treatment, but changes were observed in both positive and negative symptoms in CT. These findings suggest a role for CT in even the most refractory patients.

CONCLUSIONS

In the nearly fifty years since it was first formulated, cognitive therapy has emerged as one of the most efficacious of the treatment interventions. It is at least as efficacious as medications in the treatment of depression, and it has an enduring effect that pharmacology simply cannot match. It is the treatment of choice for panic disorder and social anxiety and quite possibly GAD as well. It is as efficacious as some of the purely behavioral exposure approaches in PTSD, and it is typically experienced as less aversive. It is the clear treatment of choice for bulimia and perhaps the other eating disorders as well. Schema-focused CT is efficacious in the treatment of borderline personality disorder, and recovery-oriented CT can be a useful adjunct in the treatment of schizophrenia. All of these conclusions are based on high-quality outcome studies. This is a record that no other psychosocial intervention can match.

REFERENCES

American Psychiatric Association. (2004). Practice guideline for the treatment of patients with schizophrenia (2nd ed.). *American Journal of Psychiatry, 161*(Suppl. 2), 1–56.

Andony, L. J., Tay, E., Allen, K. L., Wade, T. D., Hay, P., Touyz, S., . . . Byrne, S. M. (2015). Therapist adherence in the strong without anorexia nervosa (SWAN) study: A randomized controlled trial of three treatments for adults with anorexia nervosa. *International Journal of Eating Disorders, 48,* 1170–1175.

Barlow, D. H., Gorman, J. M., Shear, M. K., & Woods, S. W. (2000). Cognitive-behavioral therapy, imipramine, or their combination for panic disorder: A randomized controlled trial. *Journal of the American Medical Association, 283,* 2529–2536.

Beck, A. T. (1952). Successful out-patient psychotherapy of a chronic schizophrenic with a delusion based on borrowed guilt. *Psychiatry, 15,* 205–212.

Beck, A. T. (2005). The current state of cognitive therapy: A 40-year retrospective. *Archives of General Psychiatry, 62,* 953–959.

Beck, A. T. (2008). The evolution of the cognitive model of depression and its neural correlates. *American Journal of Psychiatry, 165,* 969–977.

Beck, A. T., Freeman, A., Davis, D. D., & Associates. (2004). *Cognitive therapy of personality disorders* (2nd ed.). New York: Guilford Press.

Beck, A. T., Rector, N. A., Stolar, N. M., & Grant, P. M. (2009). *Schizophrenia: Cognitive theory, research and therapy.* New York: Guilford Press.

Bisson, J. I., Ehlers, A., Matthews, R., Pilling, S., Richards, D., & Turner, S. (2007). Psychological treatments for chronic post-traumatic stress disorder: Systematic review and meta-analysis. *British Journal of Psychiatry, 190,* 97–104.

Blackburn, I. M., Bishop, S., Glen, A. I. M., Whalley, L. J., & Christie, J. E. (1981). The efficacy of cognitive therapy in depression: A treatment trial using cognitive therapy and pharmacotherapy, each alone and in combination. *British Journal of Psychiatry, 139,* 181–189.

Butler, A. C., Chapman, J. E., Forman, E. M., & Beck, A. T. (2006). The empirical status of cognitive-behavioral therapy: A review and meta-analysis. *Clinical Psychology Review, 26,* 17–31.

Clark, D. M. (1986). A cognitive approach to panic. *Behaviour Research and Therapy, 24,* 461–470.

Clark, D. M. (2004). Developing new treatments: On the interplay between theories, experimental science and clinical innovation. *Behaviour Research and Therapy, 42,* 1089–1104.

Clark, D. M., Ehlers, A., Hackmann, A., McManus, F., Fennell, M., Grey, N., . . . Wild, J. (2006). Cognitive therapy versus exposure and applied relaxation in social phobia: A randomized controlled trial. *Journal of Consulting and Clinical Psychology, 74,* 568–578.

Clark, D. M., Ehlers, A., McManus, F., Hackmann, A., Fennell, M. J. V., Campbell, H., . . . Louis, B. (2003). Cognitive therapy versus fluoxetine in generalized social phobia: A randomized placebo-controlled trial. *Journal of Consulting and Clinical Psychology, 71,* 1058–1067.

Clark, D. M., Salkovskis, P. M., Hackmann, A., Middleton, H., Anastasiades, P., & Gelder, M. (1994). A comparison of cognitive therapy, applied relaxation and imipramine in the treatment of panic disorder. *British Journal of Psychiatry, 164,* 759–769.

Cuijpers, P., Hollon, S. D., van Straten, A., Bockting, C., Berking, M., & Andersson, G. (2013). Does cognitive behavior therapy have an enduring effect that is superior to keeping patients on continuation pharmacotherapy? *BMJ Open, 3*(4), E002542.

Dalle Grave, R., Calugi, S., Conti, M., Doll, H., & Fairburn, C. G. (2013). Inpatient cognitive behavior therapy for anorexia nervosa: A randomized controlled trial. *Psychotherapy and Psychosomatics, 82,* 390–398.

DeRubeis, R. J. (2014, March). *Cognitive therapy and medication in the prevention of recurrence in depression.* Symposium at the Anxiety Depression Association of America conference, Chicago, IL.

DeRubeis, R. J., Gelfand, L. A., German, R. E., Fournier, J. C., & Forand, N. R. (2014). Understanding processes of change: How some patients reveal more than others—and some groups of therapists less—about what matters in psychotherapy. *Psychotherapy Research, 24,* 419–428.

DeRubeis, R. J., Hollon, S. D., Amsterdam, J. D., Shelton, R. C., Young, P. R., Salomon, R. M., . . . Gallop, R. (2005). Cognitive therapy vs. medications in the treatment of moderate to severe depression. *Archives of General Psychiatry, 62,* 409–416.

Dugas, M. J., Brillon, P., Savard, P., Turcotte, J., Gaudet, A., Ladouceur, R., . . . Gervais, N. J. (2010) A randomized clinical trial of cognitive-behavioral therapy and applied relaxation for adults with generalized anxiety disorder. *Behavior Therapy, 41,* 46–58.

Ehlers, A., & Clark, D. M. (2000). A cognitive model of posttraumatic stress disorder. *Behaviour Research and Therapy, 38,* 319–345.

Ehlers, A., Clark, D. M., Hackmann, A., McManus, F., & Fennell, M. (2005). Cognitive therapy for post-traumatic stress disorder: Development and evaluation. *Behaviour Research and Therapy, 43,* 413–431.

Ehlers, A., Grey, N., Wild, J., Stott, R., Liness, S., Deale, A., . . . Clark, D. M. (2013). Implementation of cognitive therapy for PTSD in routine clinical care: Effectiveness and moderators of outcome in a consecutive sample. *Behaviour Research and Therapy, 51,* 742–752.

Ehlers, A., Hackmann, A., Grey, N., Wild, J., Liness, S., Albert, I., . . . Clark, D. M. (2014). A randomized controlled trial of 7-day intensive and standard weekly cognitive therapy for PTSD and emotion-focused supportive therapy. *American Journal of Psychiatry, 171,* 294–304.

Elkin, I., Gibbons, R. D., Shea, T., Sotsky, S. M., Watkins, J. T., Pilkonis, P. A., . . . Hedeker, D. (1995). Initial severity and differential treatment outcome in the national institute of mental health treatment of depression collaborative research program. *Journal of Consulting and Clinical Psychology, 63,* 841–847.

Fairburn, C. G. (1981). A cognitive behavioral approach to the treatment of bulimia. *Psychological Medicine, 11,* 707–711.

Fairburn, C. G., Bailey-Straebler, S., Basden, S., Doll, H. A., Jones, R., Murphy, R., . . . Cooper, Z. (2015). A transdiagnostic comparison of enhanced cognitive behaviour therapy (CBT-E) and interpersonal psychotherapy in the treatment of eating disorders. *Behaviour Research and Therapy, 70,* 64–71.

Fairburn, C. G., Cooper, Z., Doll, H. A., O'Connor, M. E., Bohn, K., Hawker, D. M., . . . Palmer, R. L. (2009). Transdiagnostic cognitive behavioral therapy for patients with eating disorders: A two-site trial with 60-week follow-up. *American Journal of Psychiatry, 166,* 311–319.

Fairburn, C. G., Cooper, Z., Doll, H. A., O'Connor, M. E., Palmer, R. L., & Dalle Grave, R. (2013). Enhanced cognitive behaviour therapy for adults with anorexia nervosa: A UK-Italy study. *Behaviour Research and Therapy, 51,* R2–R8.

Garber, J., Clarke, G. N., Weersing, V. R., Beardslee, W. R., Brent, D. A., Gladstone, T. R., . . . Iyengar, S. (2009). Prevention of depression in at-risk adolescents: A randomized controlled trial. *Journal of the American Medical Association, 301,* 2215–2224.

Giesen-Bloo, J., van Dyck, R., Spinhoven, P., van Tilburg, W., Dirksen, C., van Asselt, T., . . . Arntz, A. (2006). Outpatient psychotherapy for borderline personality disorder: Randomized trial of schema-focused therapy vs. transference-focused psychotherapy. *Archives of General Psychiatry, 63,* 649–658.

Grant, P. M., & Beck, A. T. (2009). Defeatist beliefs as a mediator of cognitive impairment, negative symptoms, and functioning in schizophrenia. *Schizophrenia Bulletin, 35,* 798–806.

Grant, P. M., Huh, G. A., Perivoliotis, D., Stolar, N. M., & Beck, A. T. (2012). Randomized trial to evaluate the efficacy of cognitive therapy for low-functioning patients with schizophrenia. *Archives of General Psychiatry, 69,* 121–127.

Hollon, S. D., & Beck, A. T. (2013). Cognitive and cognitive-behavioral therapies. In M. J. Lambert (Ed.), *Garfield and Bergin's handbook of psychotherapy and behavior change* (6th ed., pp. 393–442). New York: Wiley.

Hollon, S. D., DeRubeis, R. J., Fawcett, J., Amsterdam, J. D., Shelton, R. C., Zajecka, J., . . . Gallop, R. (2014). Effect of cognitive therapy with antidepressant medications vs. antidepressants alone on the rate of recovery in major depressive disorder: A randomized clinical trial. *Journal of the American Medical Association Psychiatry, 71*(10), 1157–1164.

Hollon, S. D., DeRubeis, R. J., Shelton, R. C., Amsterdam, J. D., Salomon, R. M., O'Reardon, J. P., . . . Gallop, R. (2005). Prevention of relapse following cognitive therapy versus medications in moderate to severe depression. *Archives of General Psychiatry, 62,* 417–422.

Hollon, S. D., Stewart, M. O., & Strunk, D. (2006). Cognitive behavior therapy has enduring effects in the treatment of depression and anxiety. *Annual Review of Psychology, 57,* 285–315.

Jacobson, N. S., & Hollon, S. D. (1996). Prospects for future comparisons between drugs and psychotherapy: Lessons from the CBT-versus-pharmacotherapy exchange. *Journal of Consulting and Clinical Psychology, 64,* 104–108.

Ladouceur, R., Dugas, M. J., Freeston, M. H., Rheaume, J., Blais, F., Gagnon, F., . . . Boisvert, J. M. (1999). Specificity of generalized anxiety disorder symptoms and processes. *Behavior Therapy, 30,* 191–207.

Maier, S. F., Amat, J., Baratta, M. V., Paul, E., & Watkins, L. R. (2006). Behavioral control, the medial prefrontal cortex, and resilience. *Dialogues in Clinical Neuroscience, 8,* 353–373.

Maier, S. F., & Seligman, M. E. P. (2016). Learned helplessness at fifty: Insights from neuroscience. *Psychological Review, 123,* 349–367.

Mayo-Wilson, E., Dias, S., Mavranezouli, I., Kew, K., Clark, D. M., Ades, A. F., . . . Pilling, S. (2014). Psychological and pharmacological interventions for social anxiety disorder in adults: A systematic review and network meta-analysis. *Lancet Psychiatry, 1,* 368–376.

National Institute for Health and Clinical Excellence (NICE). (2009). *Schizophrenia: Core interventions in the treatment and management of schizophrenia in adults in primary and secondary care.* NICE Clinical Guideline 82.

National Institute for Health and Clinical Excellence (NICE). (2011). *Generalised anxiety disorder in adults: Management in primary, secondary and community care.* NICE Clinical Guideline 113.

Poulsen, S., Lunn, S., Daniel, S. I., Folke, S., Mathiesen, B. B., Katznelson, H., . . . Fairburn, C. G. (2014). A randomized controlled trial of psychoanalytic psychotherapy or cognitive-behavioral therapy for bulimia nervosa. *American Journal of Psychiatry, 171,* 109–116.

Rush, A. J., Beck, A. T., Kovacs, M., & Hollon, S. D. (1977). Comparative efficacy of cognitive therapy and pharmacotherapy in the treatment of depressed outpatients. *Cognitive Therapy and Research, 1,* 17–37.

Salkovskis, P. M. (1999). Understanding and treating obsessive–compulsive disorder. *Behaviour Research and Therapy, 37*(Suppl. 1), S29–S52.

Stangier, U., Schramm, E., Heidenreich, T., Berger, M., & Clark, D. M. (2011). Cognitive therapy vs. interpersonal psychotherapy in social anxiety disorder: A randomized controlled trial. *Archives of General Psychiatry, 68,* 692–700.

Van Asselt, A. D., Dirksen, C. D., Arntz, A., Giesen-Bloo, J. H., van Dyck, R., Spinhoven, P., . . . Severens, J. L. (2008). Out-patient psychotherapy for borderline personality disorder: Cost-effectiveness of schema-focused therapy v. transference-focused psychotherapy. *British Journal of Psychiatry, 192,* 450–457.

Wells, A., Welford, M., King, P., Papageorgiou, C., Wisely, J., & Mendel, E. (2010). A pilot randomized trial of metacognitive therapy vs. applied relaxation in the treatment of adults with generalized anxiety disorder. *Behaviour Research and Therapy, 48,* 429–434.

Whittal, M. L., Woody, S. R., McLean, P. D., Rachman, S. J., & Robichaud, M. (2010). Treatment of obsessions: A randomized controlled trial. *Behaviour Research and Therapy, 48,* 295–303.

Wykes, T., Steel, C., Everitt, B., & Tarrier, N. (2008). Cognitive behavior therapy for schizophrenia: Effect sizes, clinical models, and methodological rigor. *Schizophrenia Bulletin, 34*(3), 523–537.

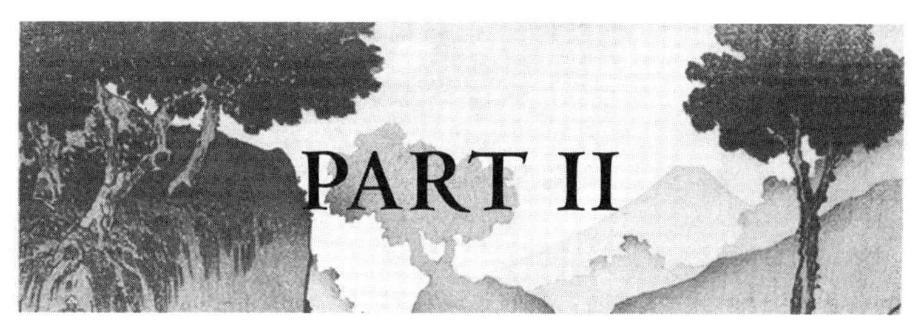

ETIOLOGY AND MECHANISMS OF CHANGE

CHAPTER 5

Schema Therapy

Arnoud Arntz

In the 1990s, schema therapy (ST) developed from cognitive therapy in an attempt to provide a treatment that was better suited to long-standing problems that have their roots in the patient's personality. For patients with chronic depression, chronic anxiety disorders, and personality disorders, the clinical observation was that the usual "rational" cognitive therapy (CT) techniques, like Socratic questioning and behavioral experiments, did not have enough impact. A typical response is "I see what you mean, but I don't feel it." A second problem that was encountered was that some of the patients had difficulties maintaining a focus on one target. Their instability was also reflected in changes in what their request for help was. In some of them, the instability during the session interfered so strongly with systematically addressing a specific topic during a session that regular cognitive-behavioral therapy (CBT) seemed impossible. Their problems seemed too complex for an approach that was initially developed to treat depression or anxiety disorders in patients who functioned quite well until the disorder developed, and who despite the disorder still have functional capacities like systematically collaborating with the therapist on a specific topic.

Already in the 1980s, some of Beck's pupils became interested in the power of experiential techniques, like those used in Gestalt therapy (Edwards, 1989, 1990; Edwards & Arntz, 2012; Young, 1990), and Beck himself started to integrate the use of imagery work in CT for anxiety disorders (Beck & Emery, 1985). It took about another two decades before imagery work and other experiential techniques were less a taboo for mainstream CT researchers and practitioners. Experiential techniques draw attention because they are so powerful in eliciting emotions and therefore have the potential to bring about cognitive changes on a "felt level" and not only on a reasoning level.

Another important development was that the taboo on focusing therapy on childhood experiences (one of the central characteristics of psychodynamic therapy that was heavily criticized by CBT theorists) started to fall apart. The empirical evidence that many chronic problems have their roots in abusive and neglectful experiences in childhood could not be denied. Moreover, the understanding that cognitive schemas and biases have their roots in such early experiences and that it might be helpful to address the memories of such experiences, like one does in the treatment of posttraumatic stress disorder (PTSD), gained ground.

Still another development was the recognition that highly unstable patients can be better understood in terms of "modes," temporary expressions of activated schemas and coping, than by stable trait-like schemas. It was Beck who introduced this schema–mode concept during a workshop in Oxford, United Kingdom, in the 1980s when he interviewed a patient with borderline personality disorder (David M. Clark, personal communication, cited in Arntz, 2015). The mode concept was further developed by Young and became very central in the modern applications of ST.

A last development was the realization that the therapeutic relationship can serve more goals than collaboration, as in the traditional "collaborative empiricism" concept in CT. For instance, personality problems will become manifest in the therapeutic relationship, and raise feelings and opinions in the therapist. Instead of trying to work around them and only focus on the collaboration in addressing issues outside therapy, the therapeutic relationship can also be used to help patients change their maladaptive interpersonal patterns. Moreover, as patients with chronic personality-related problems generally had a problematic childhood, the therapeutic relationship can also be used as a direct means to "repair" what went wrong in early development.

Although these considerations had their impact on various CT models that were developed to treat chronic characterological problems, it was Jeffrey Young who developed the most articulated and integrated model (Young, 1990; Young, Klosko, & Weishaar, 2003). In a cognitive model, he integrated techniques and views of different schools, including CT, behavior therapy, Gestalt therapy, and other experiential approaches, attachment theory and other developmental views, and psychodynamic views.

COGNITIVE MODEL

In ST, the basic idea is that maladaptive schemas can develop when basic emotional childhood needs are not adequately met. In the absence of a comprehensive model of the essential emotional needs of children, Young proposed a list that makes sense for many cases clinicians see. According to Young (Young et al., 2003, p. 10), the major emotional needs of children can be grouped as follows:

1. safety and nurturance (including secure attachment)
2. autonomy, competence and sense of identity
3. freedom to express needs, emotions, and opinions
4. spontaneity and play
5. realistic limits and self-control

If such needs are not adequately met, chances are great that the child develops fundamental representations of the self, of other people or the world in general, and of the meaning of emotions and needs, that are understandable in the given circumstances but are not necessarily adaptive in other circumstances—for instance, when the child is grown up and no longer dependent on the family of origin. For example, if the child is systematically punished by verbal (shouting, denigrating) or physical (hitting, of being locked up) means when showing negative emotions, the child learns that it is dangerous and wrong to show emotions. In other words, the child will develop a schema containing a negative meaning of emotions and an expectation that others will punish you when you show negative emotions. Moreover, as it is an inborn need of children to turn toward caregivers to reduce their arousal and find safety when experiencing negative emotions, the child might also develop a distrust schema and a loneliness schema.

As schemas can develop on the basis of very early experiences, before the age when verbal abilities are developed, the content of schemas need not be verbal (e.g., insecure attachment representations). Rather, the schema might have more of a felt-sense quality: the activation of the schema might become apparent primarily through bodily feelings and action tendencies, and not so much through verbal cognitions.

The original ST formulation contained an important additional construct: coping style. The idea is that people can differ in the way they deal with schema activation. Three groups of coping styles are distinguished, akin to the primitive stress responses of fight, flight, or freeze: overcompensation, avoidance, and surrender. Overcompensating is characterized by attempts to fight the underlying schema by pretending and behaving in the opposite manner. For example, one can compensate for an inferiority schema by pretending to be superior to other people and trying to believe that this is actually the case. Avoidance-coping is characterized by various kinds of situational, cognitive, and emotional avoidance maneuvers so that full activation of the schema is avoided. As an example, somebody with an inferiority schema can avoid contact with other people as a way of preventing people from discovering the inferiority. Lastly, surrender is characterized by giving in to the activation of the schema. A typical surrender coping with the inferiority schema would be fully believing that one is inferior.

As has been noted, the schema–mode concept was introduced to better understand and deal with difficult patients. It helps patients and therapists alike understand the current emotional-cognitive-behavioral state of the patient and to choose the appropriate treatment technique. It also helps to understand that incompatible states can occur in one and the same patient—for instance, in a patient who is at one time feeling and acting superior, at another time inferior. Lastly, specific models of schema modes for personality disorder have been developed and empirically tested (Arntz, 2012; Lobbestael, Arntz, & Sieswerda, 2005; Lobbestael, van Vreeswijk, & Arntz, 2008; Bamelis, Evers, Spinhoven, & Arntz, 2011). Such models help therapists in formulating idiosyncratic mode models for specific patients. ST theory states that a schema mode results from an activated schema through the person's coping style at the moment. Studies indeed support the model that coping style mediates the relationship between schemas and schema modes (Rijkeboer & Lobbestael, 2012).

CLINICAL APPLICATION

ST may be used between about 20 and 200 sessions, depending on the severity of the disorder and the aims of treatment (Arntz, 2015). For instance, for patients with very severe borderline or forensic personality pathology, studies have investigated up to three years of treatment with two sessions per week (usually with gradual reduction in treatment frequency at the end). However, attempts to speed up treatment have been made, and the current model for severe borderline personality disorder is a two-year trajectory, with two sessions a week in year one, one session a week in the first six months of the second year, with gradual further reduction in the last six months of the second year. (This format is being tested in a group and combined group–individual format in an international trial; Wetzelaer et al., 2014).

In the therapeutic relationship, the concept of *limited reparenting* is central. The idea is that the therapist offers the patient a relationship during therapy that offers at least a partial antidote to what went wrong in important childhood relationships. In other words, the therapist tries to offer direct corrective experiences for emotional needs that were not adequately met during childhood–notably, safe attachment, guidance, stimulation of autonomy, and realistic limits. This therapy should be offered within professional boundaries and should never lead to therapists transgressing personal limitations. For example, although emergency telephone calls between sessions can be offered, they should not lead to endless telephone calls that cause the therapist to resent the patient or create the risk of therapist burnout. Thus, the therapist should be able to set limits for patients who ask for more than they are able or willing to give. *Limited reparenting* also involves creating frustration by confronting patients with, for instance, lack of discipline or impulsive risky actions, just as real parenting does. During therapy, the therapist gradually changes the therapeutic stance, increasingly stimulating the patient's autonomy and responsibility in the later phases of treatment, as one would do with real parenting when the child develops too much dependence on an adult. Also, ST therapists tend to be more open about their feelings about the patient and use personal disclosure more often than therapists with other orientations, if the disclosure is deemed to be helpful for the patient (Boterhoven De Haan & Lee, 2014).

The first four to six sessions usually focus on getting acquainted, introducing the ST model and aims, and especially formulating a case conceptualization in schema mode terms. The idiosyncratic schema mode model should summarize the most important modes of the patient, relating these modes to developmental factors that played a role in their origin and to current problems. Figure 5.1 presents an example of a schema mode model of a patient with both an avoidant and an obsessive–compulsive personality disorder.

In the period after these 4–6 introductory sessions, patients are further stimulated to recognize and understand their modes. The historical origins of the modes are further explored, and attention is given to the emotional processing of childhood experiences related to them. However, often at least two barriers must first be addressed.

First, *coping modes* might block the access to vulnerable child modes that are associated with the childhood memories. For instance, patients might show a massive detached protector mode in the session, blocking access to any vulnerable feeling. Other examples are overcompensating modes, for instance, a paranoid or perfectionistic overcontroller, or a self-aggrandizer mode used to control the therapy, including the working alliance and the therapist. These barriers can be addressed in various ways:

- The therapist explores with the patient what event during the last days or weeks triggered the coping mode, understanding and empathizing with its function (i.e., to deal with the emotional impact of the event), and invites the patient to address the vulnerable feelings that were initially triggered. For instance, the therapist might ask the patient to imagine the triggering event, to experience the vulnerable feelings, and to use an affect-bridge to detect a childhood memory with a similar emotional tone, all of which may start imagery rescripting with the memory (see below).

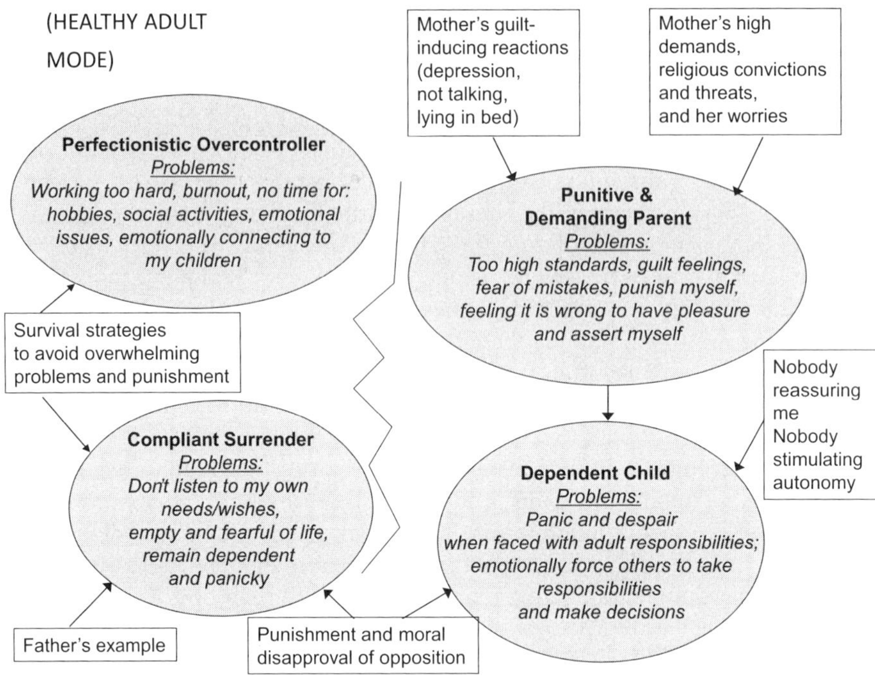

FIGURE 5.1. Idiosyncratic schema mode model of a patient with avoidant and obsessive–compulsive personality disorder.

• The therapist uses a cognitive technique, *reviewing the pros and cons* of maintaining the coping mode in therapy and, if necessary, reminding patients of their initial reasons for requesting therapy. If this motivational interviewing-like technique leads to an opening in the barriers, therapists can negotiate with the patient about (initial) measures to guarantee safety in the session. Note that with this technique understanding is expressed for the reasons of using the coping mode, and patients are reassured that it is not the aim of treatment to suddenly deprive the patients of their coping modes, which for good reason became their most important survival strategy.

• A more experiential technique is the *multiple-chair technique,* during which patients are invited to express views, emotions, and needs from different modes on different chairs. For this particular use of the multiple-chair technique, it is important that patients express these views, emotions, and needs for the coping mode, for the vulnerable child mode, and for the healthy adult mode. Expressing these different modes helps to break through the barrier of rigid coping modes.

• Using the therapeutic relationship, especially the idea of *limited reparenting,* the therapist might explore the reasons for maintaining the coping mode (usually these are fears about what could happen if the coping mode is lowered) and reassure the patient that the therapists will guarantee that that what is feared won't happen. Through the limited reparenting approach, this reassurance will be given in a personal way, showing genuine care for the patient's need for safety.

• Another interpersonal technique is *empathic confrontation.* When this technique is used in this context, the therapist expresses genuine empathy for the rigid use of the coping mode, usually also pointing out previous (e.g., childhood) experiences as justification. In addition to this empathy, the therapist confronts the patient with the need for change, if the patient wants to profit from therapy. If the patient starts to open up, the therapist can start negotiating about what safety measures will help the patient bypass the coping mode.

The second major barrier to accessing vulnerable feelings and their childhood origins might be the punitive and demanding (parent) modes. These modes might criticize and punish patients for accessing, showing, and sharing vulnerable feelings (e.g., "You don't deserve any attention for this, you just make them up to manipulate others. You should be punished for them."). To prevent full activation of these modes, the patient might resist opening up. Or, when trying to open up, patients might slip into a fully activated punitive mode, experiencing shame, guilt, and worthlessness. It is important that therapists develop a sense of activation of these modes, inquire with the patient whether the mode is indeed activated, and address the mode actively. The most important technique therapists can use to accomplish these goals is the *empty chair technique,* during which the punitive or demanding mode is symbolically placed on an empty chair to help patients take a distance from these modes, which, after all, are based on internalization of *external* responses to their expressions of needs and opinions. After what the mode on the empty chair is stating is expressed, the therapist starts to combat the mode by talking in a firm voice to the empty chair, disagreeing with the position of the mode and standing up for the needs of the patient. After a first round, the mode is usually not silent, so the therapist asks what the mode is responding, and then further combats it. This is repeated until the mode is silent, or if it doesn't remain silent after repeated and more forceful attempts, the empty chair is put in the corridor, telling it that it is no longer needed and that it can come back when it becomes of real help to the patient. While the therapist should not expect that punitive and demanding modes are open to rational arguments, rational arguments and psychoeducation should be weaved into what is said to these modes, as patients will take these in from the points of view of the vulnerable child and healthy adult modes. Combating the punitive and demanding modes themselves is a power struggle that the therapist can win only by taking a consistent and determined stance. Through this technique, the patient will feel protected against these modes and supported in the right to make mistakes, to have needs and emotions, and to express opinions. When patients feel that the parent who is being echoed in the combated mode is overly criticized, it is important that the therapist not address the parent as a whole but just its excessive punitive or demanding behavior.

When it is possible to access the vulnerable child mode, experiential techniques are recommended to emotionally process and correct dysfunctional meanings of childhood memories related to that mode. One of the most powerful techniques to do this is imagery rescripting. With this technique, the patient imagines a negative situation from childhood that contributed to development of the current problems, as if it is happening in the here-and-now. When the unmet needs of the child are identified, the therapist steps into the image and intervenes, to help the child meet its needs. While all this "rescripting" is imagined in fantasy, it has powerful emotional and cognitive effects. Usually, the primary need is one of safety; thus, the therapist protects the child and stops the threat, for instance, by stopping emotional, physical, or emotional abuse. The next usual needs relate to safety in the longer term, justice, and comfort. Thus, the therapist helps the child to find safety (e.g., when living in a dangerous environment, by moving in fantasy to a family of a friend where there is safety). When safety is experienced and needs for justice are met, there might be room for sadness accompanied by the need of being soothed. The patient can imagine a trustworthy person soothing him or her as a child, or the therapist can do this in the image, if the patient wishes so. During the rescripting, the therapist weaves in corrective messages and psychoeducation. For instance, when addressing a perpetrator, the therapist will state that the perpetrator is not allowed to abuse the child, and the therapist will explain why and will tell the perpetrator that he or she should feel ashamed. As occurs when addressing the punitive and demanding modes, this will usually not convince the perpetrator, but the patient, from the child's perspective, will listen and remember what is said. When turning to the child, again the therapist actively explains to the child that he or she is not to blame, thereby reducing guilt and shame. Later in therapy, the patient will be invited to lead the rescripting by entering the image from childhood as an adult and rescript like the therapist did before.

As we found out that corrective measures taken by the adult self are not always fully integrated by the child and that the adult does not always sense all of the child's needs, we added an extra step to the procedure by starting the imagery rescripting again, with patients now experiencing the actions by their adult self from their child perspective. After the rescripting of the adult is complete, the child is stimulated to express any further needs and ask the adult self to meet them. Therapists might need to coach patients when they rescript themselves as adults, sometimes in the image by also entering the scene and collaborating with the adult patient in rescripting. For more details about the procedures, see Arntz (2011), Arntz and Weertman (1999), and Arntz and van Genderen (2012).

Instead of using imagery, drama therapy can be used to rescript childhood memories. This technique can be helpful for patients who report having difficulties with imagery—for instance, they cannot imagine the rescripting or they cannot maintain focus on one scene (e.g., Arntz & Weertman, 1999).

The core techniques of imagery rescripting and drama rescripting can be supplemented with other experiential techniques, such as the multiple-chair technique; writing letters to caregivers (without posting them); expressing needs to an empty chair where a caregiver is symbolically seated; and so on. As to the most important *cognitive* techniques, psychoeducation is the most often used. Thus, instead of challenging possible misinterpretations, therapists more often rely on educating the patient about normal emotional needs and the function of emotions, as most patients with severe personality pathology lack healthy knowledge in these areas.

Regarding the angry, impulsive, and undisciplined child modes, a slightly different approach is chosen. One of the common problems with the angry child mode is that the patient fears its activation, often because it has been associated with interpersonal difficulties that resulted from angry outbursts, and hence the patient tries to suppress it. This suppression in turn leads to a buildup of inhibited anger that might suddenly come into the open in a way that is even more difficult to control—because all the past irritations contribute to it. Thus, the patient should feel safe to express anger in the session, after which the issue of how the patient can express irritation earlier can be addressed, as a way of preventing too much anger buildup and, in more functional ways, preventing interpersonal difficulties. Anger often relates to a moment of experienced vulnerability (Beck, 1999), so it is always good when anger has been vented, to focus on the underlying vulnerable feelings and explore and process painful childhood experiences related to them (e.g., using imagery techniques). Just as the angry child mode is a poorly controlled way for patients to stand up for their rights and protest against maltreatment, the impulsive child mode is often a poorly controlled way to meet emotional needs. Thus, patients might rebel against the punitive or demanding parent mode, and just take the right to have a good feeling, to feel loved, to get a treat, and the like. And so they might impulsively buy things they cannot afford, have impulsive sex to feel special and loved, or eat or drink too much to get a good feeling. Here the main technique is that of empathic confrontation: empathy is expressed about the underlying intention to stand up for the right to have nice experiences and the like. At the same time, patients are confronted with the impulsive way they organize this, which will create further problems and fuel the punitive mode. As an alternative, patients are invited to discuss how they can organize their lives in such a way that their needs are better met without creating new problems.

Lastly, the undisciplined child mode needs a quite different approach, at least when it is not driven by anger because of perceived maltreatment. This mode usually has its roots in severe neglect and/or materialistic spoiling, and can be very difficult to address because patients usually don't see any short-term profit from learning discipline. Repeated psychoeducation, empathic confrontation, and limit setting might be needed to create an understanding in patients that they should learn more discipline.

So far, the healthy adult mode has not been extensively discussed. However, this mode is very important, for it is the basis for the therapeutic relationship and the mode that helps the patient continue therapy even in difficult times. The therapist should create a firm bond with this aspect of the patient, and here it is that the cognitive therapy concept of collaborative empiricism (Beck et al., 1979) comes in. However, in most patients with severe personality disorders, this mode is weak and needs further development. The most important ways to achieve development of the healthy adult mode are the following. First, the therapist should be a model for the healthy adult. Everything that the therapist does and says, within or outside techniques, can contribute to its development. That is one reason why rational things are said even to irrational others (like abusers in imagery rescripting): the patient listens and will incorporate what is said in the healthy adult mode. Psychoeducation is also provided to strengthen this mode. In the later phases of treatment, to further strengthen the healthy adult mode, the therapist will give more responsibility to patients and will stimulate their autonomous development.

This brings us to the later parts of treatment. Whereas in the previous part a lot of attention was given to childhood experiences that contributed to the development of the problems, later in treatment the focus will be more on the patient's present and future life. While some patients will make major changes as a result of the more experiential work focusing on childhood experiences in the previous phase, many are quite stuck in their behavioral patterns. Thus, for an ultimate change, it is necessary to start with "behavioral pattern breaking," that is, changing habitual ways of behaving and trying out new, more functional behaviors (Young et al., 2003). Therapist and patient discuss problems in present life, how modes, schemas, and childhood experiences are related, and what new behaviors are indicated, so that the patient's present needs are better met. For instance, when patients suffer from a pattern of dysfunctional partner choice, discussion can be started on what signals possible repetition of the old pattern (e.g., a date being interested only in sex) and what signals possible healthy relationships (e.g., a date being interested in the patient's views and feelings). New behaviors can be discussed and tried out using role plays and imagery techniques (trying out new behaviors in imagery), such as showing assertiveness, expressing emotional needs, and sharing emotions. Also, more traditional cognitive challenging techniques can be used in this phase.

In the concluding phase of treatment, it is recommended that the therapy not be ended suddenly, but rather that a number of booster sessions, spread over several months, be planned, so that patients can practice with relying on their own and using newly acquired insights and strategies from treatment. Any problem encountered can be discussed during the booster sessions and related to the mode model, but patients are given more and more responsibility to choose how they want to address the problem (Arntz, 2012). Thus, instead of viewing a return to an old pattern as a fully automatic mechanism, the patient is asked to make an active choice for either a new or an old pattern.

RESEARCH

Research has generally supported the factorial validity of early maladaptive schemas, assessed with the Young Schema Questionnaire, across cultures, although there is less consistency as to the higher order factor structure (Calvete et al., 2013). Similarly, the most important schema modes assessed with self-report have also received empirical support (Lobbestael et al., 2008; Bamelis et al., 2011; Reiss et al., 2012, 2016). Two studies have now found support for the assumption that coping style mediates the relationship between schemas and schema modes (Rijkeboer & Lobbestael, 2012; van Wijk-Herbrink et al., 2017). Moreover, one study also found evidence for the theory that similar schemas might underlie externalizing and internalizing psychopathology, and that it depends on the coping styles and hence the schema mode whether a specific schema results in externalizing or internalizing psychopathology (van Wijk-Herbrink et al., 2017). In other words, depending on the person's preferred way(s) of dealing with schema activation, the person will show, for instance, aggressive and impulsive problems, and/or fear and depression, in response to activation of an abandonment schema.

Furthermore, research has supported the hypothesis that schemas mediate the relationship between childhood adverse events and (personality) psychopathology, both internalizing and externalizing (Arntz et al., 1999; Atmaca et al., 2016; Calvete, 2014; Crawford et al., 2007; Cukor & McGinn, 2006; Gay et al., 2013; Estévez et al., 2016; Jenkins et al., 2013; O'Dougherty-Wright et al., 2009; Varnaseri et al., 2016). This indicates that problematic experiences in childhood affect later personality problems only when they have given rise to maladaptive schemas.

Although the evidence base for the effectiveness of ST as a treatment for chronic characterological problems is still limited, the initial findings are positive. The most studied is ST for borderline personality disorder (BPD). So far, five studies have been conducted on outpatient ST for BPD, two small-scale uncontrolled trials and three randomized controlled trials (RCTs).As to the RCTs, one study compared ST to transference focused psychotherapy (TFP), a psychodynamic treatment, and found ST to be superior on primary and secondary outcomes, as well as resulting in less attrition (Giesen-Bloo et al., 2006). Another RCT found the superiority of group ST over treatment as usual, again on both outcomes and attrition (Farrell, Shaw, & Webber, 2009). The third RCT compared individual ST for BPD with and without telephone availability outside office hours, without finding evidence for improved effects with telephone availability (Nadort et al., 2017). Figure 5.2 shows a meta-analysis of the pre–post effect sizes of change in indicators of BPD severity and reveals remarkably consistent high-effect sizes. The difference between studies depends largely

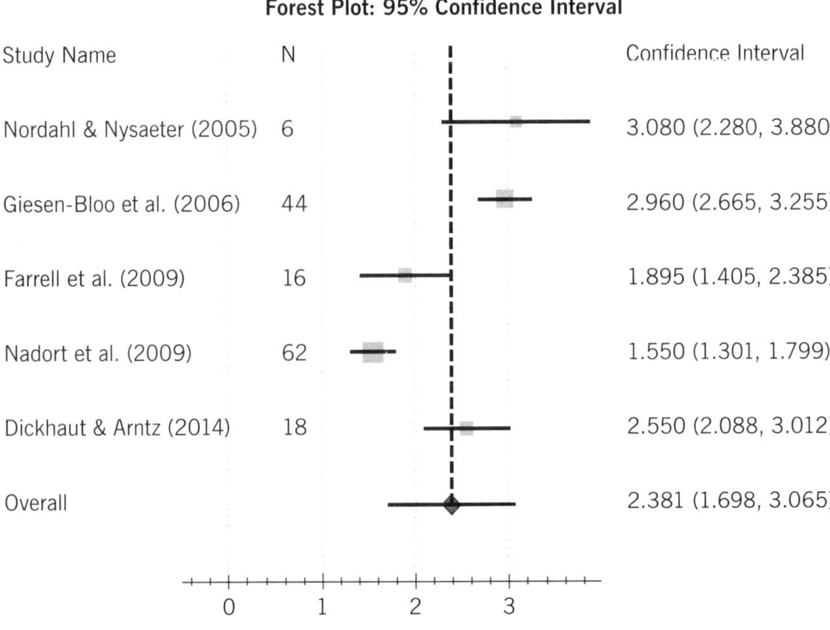

FIGURE 5.2. Meta-analysis of outpatient studies of schema therapy for borderline personality disorder: Pre–post changes. Reprinted with permission from Jacob, G. A., & Arntz, A. (2013). Schema therapy for personality disorders—A review. *International Journal of Cognitive Therapy*, 6, 171–185. Copyright © 2013 by The Guilford Press.

on the number of sessions provided to the patients: the more sessions, the higher the effect (Jacob & Arntz, 2013).

Following the successful studies on application of ST to BPD, ST variants were developed based on schema mode models for other personality disorders. For instance, ST protocols for cluster-C, paranoid, narcissistic, and histrionic personality disorders were developed, as was a specialized form of ST for high-risk forensic personality disorders patients. A large RCT of ST for six non-BPDs demonstrated the superiority of ST over the usual psychological treatment (which was in majority psychodynamic) in recovery from diagnosis, comorbid depression, and increase in Global Assessment of Functioning (GAF) and Social and Occupational Functioning Assessment Scale (SOFAS) scores. Again, treatment dropout was smaller in ST, and at three-year follow-up, fewer ST patients were still in treatment than patients in the comparison group (Bamelis et al., 2014). However, the superiority of ST was not reflected in self-report measures, possibly because more objectifiable indices of personality disorder pathology are more sensitive in picking up improvement than self-reports, which might still be influenced by the old ideas participants have about the self and the world. The same study also had a second experimental treatment, clarification-oriented psychotherapy (COP), a variant of client-centered therapy for personality disorders developed by Rainer Sachse (2001). Indicating that it was not the heightened expectations of an innovative therapy that lead to the superior effects, ST as compared to COP was also significantly better in terms of recovery from personality disorder diagnosis, GAF and SOFAS scores, and being treatment-free at three years.

A special form of ST has also been developed for forensic high-risk patients (Bernstein et al., 2007, 2012). This treatment was tested by comparing it to Treatment as Usual (TAU) in high-security forensic hospitals in the Netherlands. In these clinics, treatment is already quite highly developed, including a therapeutic milieu, verbal and nonverbal psychological treatments, and systematic preparation for return to society.

Nevertheless, ST was shown to be superior to TAU in the primary outcomes: (1) reduction of personality disorder features as assessed by three raters (employees of the clinic who knew the patients), and by the patients themselves; and (2) time until permission for a short-term leave from the clinic was attained—which is based on a decision by an independent review committee that reviews leave requests using outcomes from systematic risk assessment and other sources of information. ST again turned out to be superior to TAU in treatment retention, as well as in a couple of secondary outcomes, such as assessments of risks, strengths, and vulnerabilities, and maladaptive schemas.

In addition to individual ST, group forms have been developed. Farrell and Shaw developed a form of group ST for BPD that uses group dynamics in a very special way, emphasizing the safety in the group and keeping all members involved in the process as much as possible (2012). The developers tested this format in a small RCT and found it to be superior to TAU (Farrell et al., 2009). A somewhat different format is the combination of weekly group and individual ST, in decreasing frequency over time, which was found to be effective in open trials by Dickhaut and Arntz (2014) and Fassbinder et al. (2016). The strong effects in a relatively short time has inspired others to test group ST as a more generic treatment for all kinds of personality disorders; an open trial suggests that it has good effects (Skewes, Samson, Simpson, & van Vreeswijk, 2014; Simpson, Skewes, van Vreeswijk, & Reid, 2015). More training-like short forms of group ST have also been developed, but they miss the typical use of experiential techniques and the specific use of the group dynamics. They are therefore generally not considered as real ST. For that reason, the protocol developed by Broersen and van Vreeswijk (2012) is labeled differently ("schema-based cognitive-behavioral group therapy"). Research has been uncontrolled so far and suggests effectiveness, though not as strong as that of "real ST" (van Vreeswijk, Spinhoven, Eurelings-Bontekoe, & Broersen, 2012; Renner et al., 2013). It is not known whether this lesser effectiveness is caused by the relatively shorter duration or by the difference in techniques used.

Inpatient ST for BPD has been tested in three open trials and has also been found to be effective (Reiss et al., 2014), although its long-term results are not completely clear (future research should add follow-ups after inpatient treatment termination). Special variants of ST for personality disorders have now been developed and tested for the elderly with personality disorders (Videler et al., 2016, 2017) and youngsters.

The success of ST with personality disorders has inspired others to try ST for other chronic complex disorders that often have a lot in common with personality disorders: chronic depression; treatment-resistant obsessive–compulsive disorder (OCD), complex PTSD, and eating disorders. Two case-series studies, with a control by repeated assessments during baseline, delivered first evidence that ST might be effective for chronic depression (Malogiannis et al., 2014; Renner, Arntz, Peeters, Lobbestaal, & Huibers, 2016). However, in one RCT that compared ST to CBT as a treatment for depression, ST did not outperform CBT, as also it did not in the chronically depressed subgroup—although statistical power was too low for that subanalysis and ST was rather short, questioning whether the study represented the true effects of ST (Carter et al., 2013). Heileman, Pieters, Kehoe, and Yang (2011) piloted ST in Latina women suffering from severe depression, with good effects. Simpson, Skewes, van Vreeswijk, and Reid (2010) have piloted group ST for patients with eating disorder and reported good effects. An RCT found no difference between individual ST, CBT, and appetite-focused CBT for binge-eating problems, with all treatments achieving good results (McIntosh et al., 2016). However, because of recruitment problems, only 56% of the planned sample size was obtained.

As to complex PTSD, ST was found to be more effective than usual CBT for veterans with PTSD in an Australian study (Cockram et al., 2010). Interestingly, participants reported that the connection that was made during ST between the recent war-related trauma, childhood experiences, and schemas was experienced as helpful. Treatment-resistant OCD has been treated with a combination of ST and the standard exposure with response prevention approach to OCD in a German inpatient study. This uncontrolled study reported promising effects, as patients previously not responsive to CBT and pharmacotherapy showed a good response with high effect sizes (Thiel et al., 2016). Often, personality disorder is comorbid to other highly complex disorders and then remains untreated, despite the clinically obvious problems the personality disorder creates, or the disorder has qualities that resemble personality disorder. Examples are psychosis, autism, dissociative identity disorder, eating disorders, and substance dependence. Adjusted forms of ST for such populations have been developed and tested by specialists (Vuijk & Arntz, 2017; Boog, 2015; Huntjens, 2014). It must be admitted that early attempts to apply ST for the "double diagnosis" of substance dependence and personality disorder have not been very successful (Ball, Maccarelli, La Paglia, & Ostrowski, 2011), but it has been argued that this failure might relate to methodological problems (e.g., a too high dropout from the study driven by legal consequences of return to drug use) and the content of the ST given (e.g., not enough experiential elements) (Lee & Arntz, 2013).

Both quantitative and qualitative research has shed some light on the elements of ST that contribute to its effectiveness. First, it has been repeatedly found that patients appreciate the therapeutic relationship in ST more than in comparison conditions (Spinhoven, Giesen-Bloo, van Dyck, Kooiman, & Arntz, 2007; Bamelis et al., 2014). This already becomes apparent starting in the third session (Bamelis et al., 2014) and contributes to less chance of dropout from treatment (Spinhoven et al., 2007). Qualitative studies on patients' and therapists' perspectives have indicated that the schema mode model is viewed as especially helpful as it gives a metacognitive understanding of the present problems and helps patients to understand when a problem pops up, what is underlying it, and how they can deal with it. Moreover, for many patients, linking childhood experiences to present problems is positively valued and the therapeutic techniques to process these childhood experiences are reported to be very powerful (de Klerk, Bamelis, & Arntz, 2016).

Last, but not least, the cost effectiveness of ST is the subject of two studies. In cost-effectiveness research, all costs that are made related to the disorder and its treatment are compared between treatments and are related to the difference in effects between the treatments. It is important to take a societal perspective on costs, that is, to take all costs into account, independent of who pays the costs, to prevent a seeming cost reduction by moving costs from one sector to the other. In the first study, Van Asselt et al. (2008) compared the cost effectiveness of ST and TFP for BPD from the Giesen-Bloo et al. (2006) study and found that both in costs and in clinical effectiveness ST was superior to TFP. As to quality of life, the effects were less clear but still favored ST. Similarly, in the second study, Bamelis et al. (2015) found schema therapy to be superior to TAU and COP in the randomized controlled trial of treatment of six personality disorders other than borderline BPD, in terms of both costs and effects. One factor driving the lower societal costs of ST was the earlier return to work of those who were on sick leave. This finding is in line with the higher social and societal functioning scores the ST patients attained during the three-year investigation (Bamelis et al., 2014). In many countries, cost effectiveness underlies decisions about which treatments should be delivered. In other words, in attempts to make rational decisions about health care that should or should not be provided, cost effectiveness is an important issue. It is therefore important knowledge that, although ST is apparently quite costly to deliver, its effects on costs (on a societal level), clinical outcome, and quality of life are so good that it has been found to be cost effective.

CONCLUSIONS

Schema therapy developed from Beck's cognitive therapy as specialized treatment for chronic severe psychopathology with roots in personality problems. Still based on a cognitive model of psychopathology, it has enriched the model by integrating developmental viewpoints, and insights and techniques from other schools. It is increasingly popular among therapists and patients, and various clinical trials support its effectiveness and cost effectiveness, especially for the more severe forms of psychopathology. Given the comprehensive focus of what is addressed in ST and the wide range of techniques used, explanation for the low dropout rates and the strong effects of ST remains unclear. Qualitative research has given rise to some hypotheses, including the following: the integrative character of ST that leads to the use of multiple channels of change (experiential, cognitive, and behavioral); the therapeutic relationship, which is more personal and caring than usual and in which the concept of limited reparenting plays an important role; the triple focus on childhood experiences, the therapeutic relationship, and the present and future; and lastly, the schema mode model, which offers a strong organizing metacognitive framework for patients that helps them to understand their problems and choose functional alternative responses. Future research will clarify the essential ingredients of ST.

REFERENCES

Arntz, A. (2011). Imagery rescripting for personality disorders. *Cognitive and Behavioral Practice, 18,* 466–481.

Arntz, A. (2012). Schema therapy for cluster C personality disorders. In M. Van Vreeswijk, J. Broersen, & M. Nadort (Eds.), *The Wiley–Blackwell handbook of schema therapy: Theory, research and practice* (pp. 397–414). Chichester, UK: Wiley–Blackwell.

Arntz, A. (2015). Borderline personality disorder. In A. T. Beck, D. D. Davis, & A. Freeman (Eds.), *Cognitive therapy of personality disorders* (3d ed., pp. 366–390). New York: Guilford Press.

Arntz, A., Dietzel, R., & Dreessen, L. (1999). Assumptions in borderline personality disorder: Specificity, stability and relationship with etiological factors. *Behaviour Research and Therapy, 37,* 545–557.

Arntz, A., Klokman, J., & Sieswerda, S. (2005). An experimental test of the schema mode model of borderline personality disorder. *Journal of Behavior Therapy and Experimental Psychiatry, 36,* 226–239.

Arntz, A., & van Genderen, H. (2012). *Schema therapy for borderline personality disorder.* Oxford, UK: Wiley–Blackwell.

Arntz, A., & Weertman, A. (1999). Treatment of childhood memories; theory and practice. *Behaviour Research and Therapy, 37,* 715–740.

Atmaca, S., & Gençöz, T. (2016). Exploring revictimization process among Turkish women: The role of early maladaptive schemas on the link between child abuse and partner violence. *Child Abuse and Neglect, 52,* 85–93.

Ball, S. A., Maccarelli, L. M., LaPaglia, D. M., & Ostrowski, M. J. (2011). Randomized trial of dual-focused vs. single focused individual therapy for personality disorders and substance dependence. *Journal of Nervous and Mental Disease, 199,* 319–328.

Bamelis, L. M., Evers, S. M. A. A., Spinhoven, P., & Arntz, A. (2014). Results of a multicenter randomized controlled trial of the clinical effectiveness of schema therapy for personality disorders. *American Journal of Psychiatry, 171,* 305–322.

Bamelis, L. M., Renner, F., Heidkamp, D., & Arntz, A. (2011). Extended schema mode conceptualizations for specific personality disorders: An empirical study. *Journal of Personality Disorders, 25,* 41–58.

Beck, A. T. (1999). *Prisoners of hate: The cognitive basis of anger, hostility, and violence.* New York: HarperCollins.

Beck, A. T., & Emery, G. (with Greenberg, R. L.). (1985). *Anxiety disorders and phobias: A cognitive perspective.* New York: Basic Books.

Beck, A. T., Rush, A. J., Shaw, B. F., & Emery, G. (1979). *Cognitive therapy of depression.* New York: Guilford Press.

Bernstein, D. P., Arntz, A., & de Vos, M. (2007). Schema focused therapy in forensic settings: theoretical model and recommendations for best clinical practice. *International Journal of Forensic Mental Health, 6*(2), 169–183.

Bernstein, D., Keulen-de Vos, M., Jonkers, P., de Jonge, E., & Arntz, A. (2012). Schema therapy in forensic settings. In M. van Vreeswijk, J. Broersen, & M. Nadort (Eds.), *The Wiley–Blackwell handbook of schema therapy, Theory, research, and practice* (pp. 425–438). Chichester, UK: Wiley.

Boog, M. (2015). Are there indications for the effectiveness of schema therapy for patients suffering from borderline personality disorder and alcohol dependency? (Netherlands Trial Register NTR5218). Available at *www.trialregister.nl/trialreg/admin/rctview.asp?TC=5218*.

Boterhoven De Haan, K. L., & Lee, C. W. (2014). Therapists' thoughts on therapy: Clinicians' perceptions of the therapy processes that distinguish schema, cognitive behavioural and psychodynamic approaches. *Psychotherapy Research, 24*(5), 538–549.

Broersen, J., & Van Vreeswijk, M. F. (2012). Schema therapy in groups: A short-term schema CBT protocol. In M. F. Van Vreeswijk, J. Broersen, & M. Nadort (Eds.), *The Wiley–Blackwell handbook of schema therapy theory, research, and practice* (pp. 373–381). Chichester, UK: Wiley.

Calvete, E. (2014). Emotional abuse as a predictor of early maladaptive schemas in adolescents: Contributions to the development of depressive and social anxiety symptoms. *Child Abuse and Neglect, 38*(4), 735–746.

Calvete, E., Orue, I., & González-Diez, Z. (2013). An examination of the structure and stability of early maladaptive schemas by means of the Young Schema Questionnaire-3. *European Journal of Psychological Assessment, 29*(4), 283–290.

Carter, J. D., McIntosh, V. V., Jordan, J., Porter, R. J., Frampton, C. M., & Joyce, P. R. (2013). Psychotherapy for depression: A randomized clinical trial comparing schema therapy and cognitive behavior therapy. *Journal of Affective Disorders, 151*(2), 500–505.

Cockram, D. M., Drummond, P. D., & Lee, C. W. (2010). Role and treatment of early maladaptive schemas in Vietnam veterans with PTSD. *Clinical Psychology and Psychotherapy, 17*(3), 165–182.

Crawford, E., & O'Dougherty-Wright, M. (2007). The impact of childhood psychological maltreatment on interpersonal schemas and subsequent experiences of relationship aggression. *Journal of Emotional Abuse, 7*, 93–116.

Cukor, D., & McGinn, L. K. (2006). History of child abuse and severity of adult depression: The mediating role of cognitive schema. *Journal of Child Sexual Abuse: Research, Treatment, and Program Innovations for Victims, Survivors, and Offenders, 15*, 19–34.

de Klerk, N., Abma, T. A., Bamelis, L. L. M., & Arntz, A. (2016). Schema therapy for personality disorders: A qualitative study of patients' and therapists' perspectives. *Behavioural and Cognitive Psychotherapy*. Under review.

Dickhaut, V., & Arntz, A. (2014). Combined group and individual schema therapy for borderline personality disorder: A pilot study. *Journal of Behavior Therapy and Experimental Psychiatry, 45*(2), 242–251.

Edwards, D. (1989). Cognitive restructuring through guided imagery: Lessons from Gestalt therapy. In A. Freeman, K. M. Simon, L. E. Beutler, & H. Arkowitz (Eds.), *Comprehensive handbook of cognitive therapy* (pp. 283–297). Boston: Springer.

Edwards, D. J. (1990). Cognitive therapy and the restructuring of early memories through guided imagery. *Journal of Cognitive Psychotherapy, 4*, 33–50.

Edwards, D., & Arntz, A. (2012). Schema therapy in historical perspective. In M. van Vreeswijk, J. Broersen, & M. Nadort (Eds.), *The Wiley–Blackwell handbook of schema therapy* (pp. 3–26). Chichester, UK: Wiley.

Estévez, A., Ozerinjauregi, N., Herrero-Fernández, D., & Jauregui, P. (2016). The mediator role of early maladaptive schemas between childhood sexual abuse and impulsive symptoms in female survivors of CSA. *Journal of Interpersonal Violence*, 1–22.

Farrell, J. M., & Shaw, I. A. (2012). *Group schema therapy for borderline personality disorder: A step-by-step treatment manual with patient workbook*. Hoboken, NJ: Wiley.

Farrell, J. M., Shaw, I. A., & Webber, M. A. (2009). A schema-focused approach to group psychotherapy for outpatients with borderline personality disorder: A randomized controlled trial. *Journal of Behavior Therapy and Experimental Psychiatry, 40*, 317–328.

Fassbinder, E., Schuetze, M., Wedemeyer, N., Marten, E., Kranich, A., Sipos, V., . . . Schweiger, U. (2016). Feasibility of group schema therapy for outpatients with severe borderline personality disorder in Germany: A pilot study with three year follow-up. *Frontiers in Psychology, 7*, 1851.

Gay, L. E., Harding, H. G., Jackson, J. L., Burns, E. E., & Baker, B. D. (2013). Attachment style and early maladaptive schemas as mediators of the relationship between childhood emotional abuse and intimate partner violence. *Journal of Aggression, Maltreatment and Trauma, 22*(4), 408–424.

Giesen-Bloo, J., van Dyck, R., Spinhoven, P., van Tilburg, W., Dirksen, C., van Asselt, T., . . . Arntz, A. (2006). Outpatient psychotherapy for borderline personality disorder: Randomized trial of schema-focused therapy vs. transference-focused psychotherapy. *Archives of General Psychiatry, 63*, 649–658.

Farrell, J. M., Shaw, I. A., & Webber, M. A. (2009). A schema-focused approach to group psychotherapy for outpatients with borderline personality disorder: A randomized controlled trial. *Journal of Behavior Therapy and Experimental Psychiatry, 40*(2), 317–328.

Heilemann, M. V., Pieters, H. C., Kehoe, P., & Yang, Q. (2011). Schema therapy, motivational interviewing, and collaborative-mapping as treatment for depression among low income, second generation Latinas. *Journal of Behavior Therapy and Experimental Psychiatry, 42*(4), 473–480.

Holt, S. L. (2013). *Childhood maltreatment as a predictor of subsequent social avoidance, revictimization, and perpetration of aggression in young adulthood: The mediating role of maladaptive schemas*. Unpublished thesis, Bowling Green State University, Bowling Green, OH.

Huntjens, R. J. C. (2014). Innovation in the treatment of dissociative identity disorder: The application of schema therapy (Netherlands Trial Register NTR5218). Available at *www.trialregister.nl/trialreg/admin/rctview.asp?TC=4496*.

Jacob, G. A., & Arntz, A. (2013). Schema therapy for personality disorders—A review. *International Journal of Cognitive Therapy, 6*, 171–185.

Jenkins, P. E., Meyer, C., & Blissett, J. M. (2013). Childhood abuse and eating psychopathology: The mediating role of core beliefs. *Journal of Aggression, Maltreatment and Trauma, 22*(3), 248–261.

Lee, C. W., & Arntz, A. (2013). A commentary on Ball et al.'s (2011) study on dual focused versus single focused therapy for personality disorders and substance dependence: What can we really conclude? (Letter to the editor). *Journal of Nervous and Mental Disease, 201*(8), 712–713.

Lobbestael, J., Arntz, A., & Bernstein, D. P. (2010). Disentangling the relationship between different types of childhood maltreatment and personality disorders. *Journal of Personality Disorders, 24*(3), 285–295.

Lobbestael, J., Arntz, A., & Sieswerda, S. (2005). Schema modes and childhood abuse in borderline and antisocial personality disorders. *Journal of Behavior Therapy and Experimental Psychiatry, 36,* 240–253.

Lobbestael, J., Vreeswijk van, M., & Arntz, A. (2008). An empirical test of schema mode conceptualizations in personality disorders. *Behaviour Research and Therapy, 46,* 854–860.

Lobbestael, J., Vreeswijk van, M., Spinhoven, P., Schouten, E., & Arntz, A. (2010). Reliability and validity of the Short Schema Mode Inventory (SMI). *Behavioural and Cognitive Psychotherapy, 38,* 437–458.

Malogiannis, I. A., Arntz, A., Spyropoulou, A., Tsartsara, E., Aggel, A., Karveli, S., . . . Zervas, I. (2014). Schema therapy for patients with chronic depression: A single case series study. *Journal of Behavior Therapy and Experimental Psychiatry, 45,* 319–329.

McIntosh, V. V., Jordan, J., Carter, J. D., Frampton, C. M., McKenzie, J. M., Latner, J. D., . . . Joyce, P. R. (2016). Psychotherapy for transdiagnostic binge eating: A randomized controlled trial of cognitive-behavioural therapy, appetite-focused cognitive-behavioural therapy, and schema therapy. *Psychiatry Research, 240,* 412–420.

Nadort, M., Arntz, A., Smit, J. H., Giesen-Bloo, J., Eikelenboom, M., Spinhoven, P., . . . van Dyck, R. (2009). Implementation of outpatient schema therapy for borderline personality disorder with versus without crisis support by the therapist outside office hours: A randomized trial. *Behaviour Research and Therapy, 47*(11), 961–973.

Nordahl, H. M., & Nysæter, T. E. (2005). Schema therapy for patients with borderline personality disorder: A single case series. *Journal of Behavior Therapy and Experimental Psychiatry, 36*(3), 254–264.

O'Dougherty-Wright, M., Crawford, E., & Del Castillo, D. (2009). Childhood emotional maltreatment and later psychological distress among college students: The mediating role of maladaptive schemas. *Child Abuse and Neglect, 33,* 59–68.

Reiss, N., Dominiak, P., Harris, D., Knörnschild, C., Schouten, E., & Jacob, G. A. (2012). Reliability and validity of the German version of the revised Schema Mode Inventory (SMI). *European Journal of Psychological Assessment, 28,* 297–304.

Reiss, N., Krampen, D., Christoffersen, P., & Bach, B. (2016). Reliability and validity of the Danish version of the Schema Mode Inventory (SMI). *Psychological Assessment, 28,* 19–26.

Reiss, N., Lieb, K., Arntz, A., Shaw, I. A., & Farrell, J. (2014). Responding to the treatment challenge of patients with severe BPD: Results of three pilot studies of inpatient schema therapy. *Behavioural and Cognitive Psychotherapy, 42,* 355–367.

Renner, F., Arntz, A., Peeters, F. P. M. L., Lobbestael, J., & Huibers, M. J. H. (2016). Schema therapy for chronic depression: Results of a multiple single case series. *Journal of Behavior Therapy and Experimental Psychiatry, 51,* 66–73.

Renner, F., van Goor, M., Huibers, M., Arntz, A., Butz, B., & Bernstein, D. (2013).

Short-term group schema cognitive-behavioral therapy for young adults with personality disorders and personality disorder features: Associations with changes in symptomatic distress, schemas, schema modes and coping styles. *Behaviour Research and Therapy, 51*, 487–492.

Rijkeboer, M. M., & Lobbestael, J. (2012, May 17–19). *The relationships between early maladaptive schemas, schema modes and coping styles: An empirical study*. Paper presented at the Fifth World Conference of Schema Therapy, New York.

Rijkeboer, M. M., & van den Berg, H. (2006). Multiple group confirmatory factor analysis of the Young Schema-Questionnaire in a Dutch clinical versus non-clinical population. *Cognitive Therapy and Research, 30*, 263–278.

Sachse, R. (Ed.). (2001). *Psychologische Psychotherapie der Persönlichkeitsstöringen*. Göttingen, Germany: Hogrefe-Verlag.

Simpson, S. G., Morrow, E., van Vreeswijk, M., & Reid, C. (2010). Group schema therapy for eating disorders: a pilot study. *Frontiers in Psychology, 1*, 182.

Simpson, S. G., Skewes, S. A., van Vreeswijk, M., & Samson, R. (2015). Commentary: Short-term group schema therapy for mixed personality disorders: An introduction to the treatment protocol. *Frontiers in Psychology, 6*.

Skewes, S. A., Samson, R. A., Simpson, S. G., & van Vreeswijk, M. (2014). Short-term group schema therapy for mixed personality disorders: A pilot study. *Frontiers in Psychology, 5*.

Spinhoven, P., Giesen-Bloo, J., van Dyck, R., Kooiman, K., & Arntz, A. (2007). The therapeutic alliance in schema-focused therapy and transference-focused psychotherapy for borderline personality disorder. *Journal of Consulting and Clinical Psychology, 75*(1), 104–115.

Thiel, N., Jacob, G. A., Tuschen-Caffier, B., Herbst, N., Külz, A. K., Hertenstein, E., . . . Voderholzer, U. (2016). Schema therapy augmented exposure and response prevention in patients with obsessive–compulsive disorder: Feasibility and efficacy of a pilot study. *Journal of Behavior Therapy and Experimental Psychiatry, 52*, 59–67.

van Asselt, A. D. I., Dirksen, C. D., Arntz, A., Giesen-Bloo, J. H., van Dyck, R., Spinhoven, P., . . . Severens, J. L. (2008). Out-patient psychotherapy for borderline personality disorder: Cost-effectiveness of schema-focused therapy v. transference-focused psychotherapy. *British Journal of Psychiatry, 192*, 450–457.

van Vreeswijk, M. F., Spinhoven, P., Eurelings-Bontekoe, E. H. M., & Broersen, J. (2014). Changes in symptom severity, schemas and modes in heterogeneous psychiatric patient groups following short-term schema cognitive-behavioural group therapy: A naturalistic pre-treatment and post-treatment design in an outpatient clinic. *Clinical Psychology and Psychotherapy, 21*(1), 29–38.

van Wijk-Herbrink, M. F., Bernstein, D. P., Broers, N. J., Roelofs, J., Rijkeboer, M. M., & Arntz, A. (2017). *Internalizing and externalizing behaviors share a common predictor: The effects of early maladaptive schemas are mediated by coping responses and schema modes*. Manuscript under review.

Varnaseri, H., Lavender, T., & Lockerbie, L. (2016). An investigation of the mediating factors in the relationship between early childhood adversity and borderline personality characteristics in forensic inpatients. *Journal of Forensic Practice, 18*(1), 17–30.

Videler, A. C., van Alphen, S. P., van Royen, R. J., van der Feltz-Cornelis, C. M., Rossi, G., & Arntz, A. (2017). Schema therapy for personality disorders in older adults: A multiple baseline study. *Aging and Mental Health*, 1–10.

Videler, A. C., van Royen, R. J., Heijnen-Kohl, S. M., Rossi, G., van Alphen, S. P., & van der Feltz-Cornelis, C. M. (2017). Adapting schema therapy for personality disorders in older adults. *International Journal of Cognitive Therapy, 10*(1), 62–78.

Vuijk, R., & Arntz, A. (2017). Schema therapy as treatment for adults with autism spectrum disorder and comorbid personality disorder. Protocol of a multiple-baseline case series study testing cognitive-behavioral and experiential interventions. *Contemporary Clinical Trials Communications, 5*, 80–85.

Wetzelaer, P., Farrell, J., Evers, S., Jacob, G. A., Lee, C. W., Brand, O., . . . Arntz, A. (2014). Design of an international multicentre RCT on group schema therapy for borderline personality disorder. *BMC Psychiatry, 14*, 319.

Young, J. E. (1990). *Cognitive therapy for personality disorders*. Sarasota, FL: Professional Resources Press.

Young, J. E., Klosko, J. S., & Weishaar, M. E. (2003). *Schema therapy: A practitioner's guide*. New York: Guilford Press.

CHAPTER 6

Emotional Schema Therapy

A Social-Cognitive Model

Robert L. Leahy

The initial cognitive model advanced by Aaron Beck emphasized the role of cognition in the activation, escalation, and maintenance of troubling emotional states such as sadness, anxiety, and anger (Beck, 1967). In contrast to the psychodynamic model that was dominant during the 1960s that emphasized overcoming repression of emotion, catharsis, working through, and uncovering unconscious conflicts, the cognitive model stressed accessible conscious cognitions or images that either resulted in emotional experiences or were the consequences of emotions that had already been activated. For example, the cognitive model of depression was based on the "negative triad" of a negative view of self, experience, and the future and proposed a cognitive "architecture" with automatic thoughts, maladaptive assumptions, and schemas about self and others that contributed to the activation and maintenance of sadness, anxiety and anger (Beck, 1967, Beck, Rush, Shaw, & Emery, 1979). Although the concept of "schema" in the cognitive model has been largely focused on beliefs about self (e.g., unworthy, helpless, unlovable) or about others (e.g., controlling, judgmental, untrustworthy), Beck and Freeman (1990) in the first edition of *Cognitive Therapy of Personality Disorders* also recognized that one can have "schemas" or concepts about a wide variety of phenomena.

In contrast to the original cognitive model that emphasizes the *content* of these personal schemas, the innovative metacognitive model advanced by

Wells places less emphasis on the content of these personal schemas and more on the individual's interpretations and responses about unwanted thoughts (Wells, 2004, 2009). According to the metacognitive model, worry, anxiety, and depression are a consequence of problematic cognitive strategies—namely, the cognitive attentional syndrome (CAS)—characterized by threat monitoring, repetitive thinking, limitation in cognitive resources, unhelpful control strategies, and continued focus on the content of thinking (Wells, 2000, 2006; Wells & Mathews, 1994). Thus, it is the *process* of responding to unwanted thoughts rather than the specific content of depressive thinking that drives worry and rumination. Wells has proposed a range of techniques that help reverse this process, and his approach has been shown to be effective in treating depression, generalized anxiety disorder (GAD), posttraumatic stress disorder (PTSD) and other disorders (Wells, 2009).

The emotional schema model draws on both the schema model and the metacognitive model, advancing a social-cognitive model of how individuals interpret, evaluate, and strategize in response to the emotions of self and others. The emotional schema model follows in a long tradition in social psychology that addresses what has been called "naïve psychology" (everyday concepts and theories about psychological processes), "social cognition," and "theory of mind." Beginning with the seminal work by Fritz Heider in *The Psychology of Interpersonal Relations,* which outlined a model of how individuals infer psychological states in self and others (Heider, 1958), emotional schema therapy (EST) model recognizes and incorporates earlier social-cognitive models of causal inference—Jones and Davis (1965) on correspondent inferences, H. H. Kelley (1973) on the covariation model of attribution, Bem's (1972) self-perception theory, and Weiner's (1986) model of causal inference. In addition, the emotional schema model draws on social-cognitive theory that focuses on "implicit psychology," causal theories of emotion, models of affect forecasting, and beliefs about the legitimacy, shame and universality of different emotions. As such, the EST therapist endeavors to understand the patient's theory of emotion and emotion regulation and to utilize this conceptualization in addressing problematic strategies (such as suppression, avoidance, rumination, blaming, and self-criticism) that arise from these unhelpful beliefs. If one can view the metacognitive model as a theory of mind, the EST model extends this to the theory of emotion.

In the theory of emotion model, emotions (for self and other) are the *object* of cognition. The EST model proposes that individuals differ in their "theory of emotion" (as a branch of theory of mind) and that these differences in the theory of emotion can account for problematic "solutions" that are recruited to "handle" unwanted emotions. These problematic solutions include a full range of psychopathology: worry, rumination, blaming others, avoidance, suppression, binge eating, binge drinking, drug abuse, and other strategies. Thus, it is not simply the intensity of an emotion that matters but rather the interpretation and evaluation of that emotion and the unhelpful coping strategies that are employed. In this sense, the patient's solutions are often the problem, but underlying those solutions are the problematic emotional schemas.

Similar to Beck's schema model, the EST model suggests that individuals differ in the content of their interpretations about emotions. In this model, emotion is the "object" of cognition—that is, people are *thinking about emotion* (Leahy, 2015). Enhancing metacognitive awareness of recognizing, labeling, and interpreting emotions is an essential component of EST. These interpretations of emotion include beliefs about legitimacy, distinctiveness, danger, and comprehensibility of an emotion—as well as other beliefs. For example, the individual might believe that his anger is shameful (illegitimate), unique to him (highly distinctive), dangerous (can harm others) and incomprehensible (makes no sense). The EST model has parallels with the metacognitive model in that the EST model stresses the importance of beliefs about the duration and uncontrollability of emotion, tolerance for ambivalence, and the difficulty in accepting an emotion. In addition, the EST model draws on models of intolerance of uncertainty in the maintenance of psychopathology (Dugas, Buhr, & Ladouceur, 2004). For example, individuals have difficulty tolerating the uncertainty about the causes of their emotion, the danger of their emotion, the comprehensibility of their emotion, and the existence of mixed feelings.

Individuals differ in how they explain their emotions and those of others. The EST model assesses the patient's beliefs by addressing a number of questions, such as whether emotions are due to a specific situation and are distinctive to the individual (Kelley, 1973), and whether they are modifiable (Dweck, 2006). The EST model draws on work on affect forecasting, which refers to the individual's predictions about emotions in the future, often reflecting biases in these predictions based on anchoring to current emotions ("emotion heuristic"), failing to recognize mitigating factors ("immune neglect"), and underestimating the ability to cope with changes (Gilbert, Pinel, Wilson, Blumberg, & Wheatley, 1998; Wilson & Gilbert, 2003). Similarly, the fundamental attribution error (attributing one's behavior and emotions to the situations, while attributing the behavior and emotions of the other person to dispositional traits) is also relevant to the interpersonal aspects of emotional schemas (Jones & Nisbett, 1972). For example, a man may attribute his wife's emotions to an "unstable personality" while attributing his own emotions to what his wife just said (the situation). The consequences of these biases in thinking can be explored where interpersonal conflict is the focus of treatment. For example, does the husband in this example blame his wife for her feelings, tell her that others would not feel this way, tell her that her emotions do not make sense, claim that she goes on forever with these feelings, and focus only on her "negative emotions" to the exclusion of a full range of emotions?

Emotional schemas are tied to implicit theories of how emotions can (or cannot be changed). For example, some individuals believe that "unpleasant emotions" cannot be accepted and must be eliminated. They may believe that the only way to change this emotion is to get other people to change—thereby blaming others or avoiding them. Others may believe that emotions can be changed by "trying to think positively," thereby activating self-talk, mantras, and reassurance seeking—often with unsatisfactory results. Still others believe that emotions can be changed by suppressing them through the use of alcohol or drugs, further complicating the emotional experience and perpetuating both anxiety and reliance on substances. Concomitant with these theories of self-change are beliefs about changing the emotions of others. These "theories" include beliefs that one has a responsibility to change the emotions of one's partner by giving unsolicited advice. Another problematic theory of change is that one should insist that another person see things rationally—or stop complaining. As a result of these underlying theories of change, interpersonal conflicts may arise leading to further escalation of emotions for both parties in the dyad.

GENERAL COGNITIVE MODEL

The EST model proposes that individuals hold specific theories—*emotional schemas*—about their emotions and the emotions of others. Emotions are viewed in terms of twelve dimensions or strategies: duration, controllability, tolerance of ambivalence, comprehensibility, similarity to the emotions of others, shame or guilt, acceptance, expression, validation, blaming, rumination, and relation to higher values. For example, let's imagine that Kevin is going through a breakup in his relationship with Rene and he notices that he feels angry, anxious, sad, and confused—but also a bit relieved. In the instance where he has negative emotional schemas about this experience, he might believe that his painful emotions will last indefinitely (duration), that they will escalate or go out of control, that he cannot tolerate having so many "conflicting" emotions since he believes he should feel only one way, that his intense emotions don't make sense to him since he was only involved for three months, that others would not have such a range of emotions, he feels ashamed about his emotions since he thinks he should be "stronger" and "more manly," he cannot accept these emotions, he believes it is not appropriate to express them, that no one would understand or validate him, he blames Rene for all of these feelings, and he ruminates about his emotional experience. In contrast, consider Michael who is going through a similar breakup. Michael has a less negative theory about his emotions. He believes that however intense his feelings are at the present moment they will pass with time. He believes that his emotions will not go out of control or drive him insane—and, therefore, he feels less of a sense of urgency to suppress these feelings. He recognizes that ambivalence about the breakup is acceptable, since there were both positive and negative qualities to the relationship and there are trade-offs for him in being on his own. His emotions make sense to him, and he believes others might also feel the same way. He doesn't think that men should not have these feelings, he can accept them, he expresses them with his friend Mark, and he finds that Mark can validate him. As a result of his interpretation of his emotion, he feels less of a need to blame Rene or to ruminate about the way he feels. The Emotional Schema Model is shown in Figure 6.1, illustrating how interpretations of emotions can result in helpful or unhelpful strategies of emotion regulation and coping.

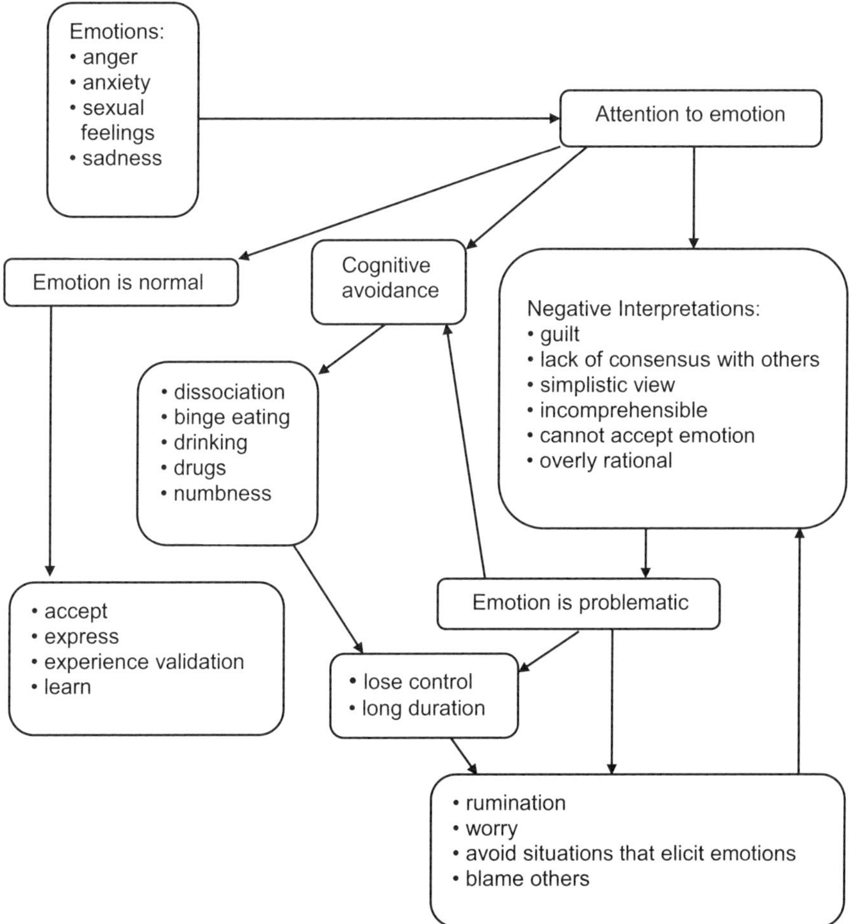

FIGURE 6.1. Metacognitive schematic of emotions.

The EST model proposes that some individuals have a belief that their emotions should be "pure" and "clear" and "univalent"—what I have called *pure mind*. This model of emotion (or intrusive thoughts in OCD or PTSD) leads the individual to attempt to "get emotions clear"—"How do I really feel?"—and therefore have difficulty tolerating mixed feelings. Moreover, part of pure mind is the belief that one should be rational, in control of one's emotions, not surprised or confused about emotion, and able to produce the "right emotions." This leads to further difficulty in accepting an emotional experience and often results in rumination about "why am I feeling this way?" which contributes to greater risk for depression. The EST model proposes that emotions are not univalent and that human existence is a kaleidoscope of emotions, much like the range of notes and harmonies and contrasts in a complex symphony. Rather than view emotional life as having purity, rationality, and simplicity, the EST model assists the patient in exploring the advantage of accepting a range of "conflicting," often transitory, emotions as part of the range of awareness of needs, perceptions, situations, and moods of everyday life. This can help individuals explore a full range of often "contradictory" emotions, normalizing their experience and obviating rumination about "how do I really feel?" or "why do I have such mixed feelings?" For example, in our example of the young man going through a breakup, his inability to accept mixed feelings (anger, anxiety, sadness, relief, and indifference) had led him to ruminate, criticize himself, and avoid friends.

Related to pure mind is the phenomenon of *emotional perfectionism* that is less about the clarity of emotional experience and more about the "legitimacy" of certain emotions. For example, individuals endorsing beliefs about emotional perfectionism often believe that they should not feel angry, sad, anxious, weak, helpless, or hopeless and, alternatively, that they should feel happy, hopeful, and fulfilled. This intolerance of unpleasant emotions can often lead to rumination about the emotions, self-criticism ("What's wrong with me that I feel this way?"), avoidance of situations that elicit these unwanted emotions, and frantic attempts to rid oneself of certain emotions. The belief that one should have "good emotions" and get rid of "bad emotions" is likely to lead to a range of difficulties, such as rumination, shame, difficulty sharing emotional experience, and unhelpful strategies to suppress or eliminate these emotions. The EST therapist helps the patient explore the costs and benefits of this belief, helps normalize a range of emotions, and links "unpleasant" emotions to values (e.g., loneliness is linked to the desire for closeness, stress due to overwork is linked to conscientiousness). The patient's belief in emotional perfectionism can be explored by asking what range of emotions admired people have, what emotions are depicted in literature and music, and how sharing, normalizing, and validating these painful experiences enhances the richness of a full emotional life. Reversing emotional perfectionism by validating a full range of emotions, while recognizing that one has the option not to act on an emotion, can be helpful.

Related to pure mind and emotional perfectionism is *existential perfectionism,* which entails beliefs about how one's life in general must proceed. For example, the individual who endorses this existential perfectionism becomes frustrated and disillusioned that work is not "fulfilling," that dreams are not always realized, that people let them down, or that their significant relationships are less than ideal. An example of existential perfectionism is a young man who felt depressed that his job was not completely fulfilling, that there were tedious tasks to do, and—in addition—that his relationship with his partner was less than ideal. While he considered options to his job and his partner, he realized that the options also had some downside. This led to his sense of futility—that no matter what he chose he would "suffer" negatives. The EST model recognizes that life is seldom—if ever—ideal for very long and that coping with the range of experiences in life leads to a recognition that there are trade-offs for almost any chosen alternative. For example, the EST therapist can normalize disillusionment and disappointment and unfairness by helping the patient realize that these may be inevitable experiences. However, they do not have to lead to cynicism, pessimism, or hopelessness. Rather, disillusionment can lead to a more balanced and realistic appraisal of the pros and cons of work and relationships or value systems and to the realization that disappointment can lead to a recognition that expectations may sometimes be inaccurate predictions but that it is not essential that expectations are always fulfilled—especially if they can be readjusted to match reality. The emotions linked to the perception of unfairness can be validated ("Yes, people should be fair"), but the therapist can assist the patient in seeing that, just as in sports, one can succeed in an unfair process.

Finally, the EST model also identifies beliefs about emotional permanence, such as the belief that an emotion will last indefinitely and that one's identity is reducible to an emotion: "I am an angry person" or "My friend is a jealous person." This tendency to equate emotions with persons (or dispositions) can lead to beliefs that emotions do not change, a negative filter on the unwanted emotion, hopelessness, and self-criticism. In contrast, the EST model encourages the patient to expand the range of emotions that one experiences and to recognize that the emotions of others are often situational and transitory. For example, the so-called angry person can recognize that her anger varies with the individual with whom she is speaking, the thoughts that she has at the moment (e.g., personalizing, mind reading, should statements), prior frustrating events that led to frustration (e.g., being stuck in traffic), and other factors. Rather than equating people with an emotion, the EST therapist assists the patient in recognizing the variability, situational dependence, and cognitive processes underlying temporary emotional experiences, thereby suggesting possibilities of change. This is especially relevant for interpersonal perception and evaluation of emotion. For example, our research indicates greater couple dissatisfaction for individuals who believe that their partner has a negative view of their emotion. Thus, if you believe that your partner thinks that your emotions go on indefinitely, are out of control, blames you for your feelings, does not validate you, and has other problematic beliefs about your emotion, then it is highly likely that you will be dissatisfied in your relationship.

Once an emotion arises (for whatever reason), the individual's interpretations, evaluations, and strategies are activated. For example, the individual who believes that her intense loneliness will last indefinitely and go out of control may turn to any number of unhelpful strategies such as binge drinking, binge eating, suicidal threats, blaming others, or self-cutting. In the event that the unwanted emotion initially decreases (e.g., drinking alcohol), the "emotion theory" that is supported is that (1) "I can't handle intense emotions" and (2) "I can get rid of these emotions by drinking." The beliefs about duration, loss of control, danger, uniqueness of emotion, and invalidation are not adequately tested. Alternatively, the EST therapist can encourage the patient to notice the emotion, take a mindful distant observer stance toward the emotion, accept the emotion for a moment, plan some distracting activities, challenge the idea that emotions are always escalating and dangerous, examine the cognitive biases that initially elicited the emotion, develop alternative interpretations of events, utilize problem solving, and develop short-term and long-term goals with action plans to be carried out. These CBT strategies are then carried out in "experiments" to test the belief that one's emotions are long-lasting, out of control, and dangerous. Similarly, the belief that my partner's emotions are of long duration, out of control, and do not make sense, and the concurrent belief that validating those emotions will only "reinforce" complaining can be tested out. These tests of interpersonal emotional schemas can include using active listening skills, providing compassionate validation of the partner, exploring the partner's interpretation of events, linking those interpretations to legitimate needs, and accepting that one does not have to "get my partner to feel better right now."

The EST model proposes that problematic coping strategies (such as worrying, rumination, blaming, avoiding, or suppressing) are a consequence of both intense emotion and unhelpful interpretations. For example, the acceptance of emotion that is predicated on beliefs about duration (emotions are temporary), escalation (emotions rise and fall), uniqueness (others have similar feelings), and other beliefs would be expected to result in less reliance on substance abuse, binge eating, avoidance, rumination, or isolation.

CLINICAL APPLICATION

The EST clinical model begins with an evaluation of the patient's emotional schemas using both the Leahy Emotional Schema Scale–II and the clinical interview. The clinician then inquires about which emotions (e.g., anger, sadness, loneliness, anxiety) are the most problematic for the patient—and why they are problematic. The inquiry may reveal that the patient believes that his anger is unacceptable because he should always be kind and thoughtful, but that he does not feel ashamed about his sadness. Or the opposite can be true. A taxonomy of "acceptable" and "unacceptable" emotions emerges, which can be extended to how the patient views the emotions of others. In addition, the clinician can inquire about why certain emotions are acceptable while others are not—and if these rules apply to both self and other.

The initial evaluation includes inquiry about the patient's beliefs about the danger and loss of control of an emotion, the guilt or shame over an emotion, the sense that one's emotions do not make sense, beliefs about whether others would have similar emotions, tolerance for mixed feelings, beliefs about the ability to express an emotion, and other beliefs. Further inquiry focuses on how the patient learned about emotions in the family of origin—for example, "Were parents (and which parent) dismissive of emotion, humiliating the patient, or overwhelmed with their own emotions?" How have significant partners and friends responded to the patient's emotions (e.g., is the spouse dismissive of emotion, blaming the patient for his or her feelings). What problematic strategies or responses does the patient employ—for example, rumination, worry, avoidance, complaining, blaming—and what is the rationale that the patient has for each strategy? What does the patient believe will happen if he or she simply accepted these emotions for the moment without recruiting these unhelpful strategies? The clinician and patient collaborate in developing a case conceptualization, linking beliefs about specific emotions, how these emotional schemas lead to problematic coping, how these beliefs were learned in the family of origin, and how these beliefs perpetuate a cycle of problematic emotion/problematic coping/problematic emotion. Cost–benefit analysis is continually applied to each set of beliefs (e.g., what is the cost and benefit of thinking you should only feel one way?).

The clinical application of EST involves identifying the universality of emotions, how emotions are linked to evolutionary adaptation, and how emotions can tell us about our needs and our values. For example, the EST model of jealousy links jealousy (and the other emotions that arise from jealousy, such as anxiety, anger, and sadness) to the evolutionary model of parental investment and competition for limited resources (Leahy & Tirch, 2008). Specifically, for romantic or sexual jealousy, the *parental investment model* advanced by Robert Trivers (1972) argues that one will be more invested in others who share more genes with the self. In the absence of certainty of paternity, the individual would be less invested. Jealousy is a strategy to protect that investment. Similarly, although females are always certain about the maternity of the offspring, they would be more likely than males to be jealous of the male who directs emotional attachment, resources, and "protection" to other females, since this would deprive her and the offspring of these potential advantages. The therapist assists the patient in realizing that all emotions have evolved to have some helpful function and that the hope to eliminate them would be senseless. The clinical question then becomes, "Is this emotion-and its intensity and the behavior linked to it—helpful today?"

Problematic emotions can also be linked to values that drive the emotion. For example, loneliness can be linked to the desire for closeness, attachment, commitment, and meaning; feeling burned out from work can be linked to conscientiousness, feelings of responsibility to others, and beliefs that one cannot let up because they will let themselves down; anger can be linked to beliefs about fairness and deservingness, which may often be frustrated in the realities of everyday life. The EST model helps the patient recognize that often our values will lead to unpleasant emotions—that we will have disappointments, disappoint others, and experience the occasional disillusionment. Yet, the model proposes that unpleasant emotions may be a necessary ingredient of a meaningful life—that it is not simply a matter of "feeling good" but more a matter of the capability of "feeling everything" in the context of a full, complicated, and often challenging existence.

The specific emotional schemas (e.g., duration, control, shame/guilt) are then examined and tested using a wide variety of CBT techniques. For example, the belief that a strong "negative" emotion will last indefinitely is examined in terms of costs and benefits of the belief. If the individual believes that a strong negative emotion will last a very long time, this belief might add to the sense of helplessness and hopelessness and may lead to the use of problematic coping strategies such as misuse of alcohol or drugs, avoidance, withdrawal, rumination, or other safety behaviors. In contrast, if one believes that a strong negative emotion only lasts a short time, then reliance on problematic coping will be less likely. Problematic coping can then be examined in terms of how it impedes disconfirmation of the belief that a strong negative emotion lasts indefinitely unless these unhelpful strategies are utilized. For example, if the patient experiments with abstaining from drinking as a coping mechanism, does the "negative emotion" last indefinitely? Further review of past emotions that have dissipated can illustrate that certain activities, ways of relating to others, new experiences, or new facts often lead emotions to dissipate. The patient can also collect information about emotion and behavior using activity scheduling, assigning activities and determining which emotions change. Safety behaviors— such as reassurance seeking about emotion, avoidance, self-talk, use of substances to suppress emotions—can be explored, with the patient experimenting with relinquishing these behaviors and observing the emotional outcome. In the use of exposure (e.g., with OCD), the EST therapist inquires about predictions regarding emotion. For example, a patient who feared contamination predicted that if he exposed himself to a feared stimulus he would decompensate, his entire week would be ruined, his anxiety would escalate to unmanageable levels, and he might have to be hospitalized. The actual exposure led to none of these feared outcomes. His belief prior to exposure was: "I am too fragile" and "I am not ready." These emotional avoidance beliefs were examined in terms of their functionality—they permitted avoidance—which did not allow him to disconfirm his beliefs. Beliefs about fragility or weakness or readiness are examined in terms of how they maintain themselves by preventing emotional exposure.

Affect forecasting, which involves predictions about emotions, can be evaluated by examining how past predictions about emotions may have been inaccurate, by eliciting predictions about emotions in the short term and long term, and by exploring which life events or new interpretations can give rise to changes in emotion. Patients often forget their past predictions of their emotions—unless they are reminded—and the therapist can encourage an ongoing "prediction log" of the duration, intensity, and tolerability of feared emotions.

Guilt and shame over an emotion can also be examined by inquiring about what the patients think the reason is for not having an emotion and about what they do once they begin feeling guilty about an emotion. Do they criticize themselves, and does that lead to further sadness and anxiety, thereby exacerbating the emotions that gave rise to the guilt? Do they refrain from sharing these emotions, and thus fail to learn that others also have these emotions, that they can be validated, and that they can learn that a wide range of unpleasant emotions is part human nature? The theory behind the guilt can be examined. This includes examining why an emotion cannot be tolerated or accepted, beliefs about thought–action fusion regarding an emotion ("If I feel angry I might harm someone"), who is actually harmed by the internal experience that one has, and if they would apply this intolerance to all other people? For example, the EST model of envy links envy to evolutionary models of competition for resources, the universal nature of dominance hierarchies, the positive aspects of envy in often motivating behavior or establishing fair distribution, and the fact that envy is a universal emotion (Leahy, 2015). "Normalizing the abnormal" is part of the EST model in acceptance, validation, universalization, and augmentation of self-compassion rather than self-criticism for emotional experiences.

As mentioned earlier, theories of change may include problematic strategies and beliefs about the intolerability of unpleasant experience.

The EST model contrasts the patient's avoidant or low-frustration tolerance approach with a model of "empowerment" that stresses "constructive discomfort" (doing uncomfortable things so that one's life can improve) and "successful imperfection" (doing imperfect behaviors that help make progress) (Leahy, 2005).

Similar to acceptance and commitment therapy (Hayes, Luoma, Bond, Masuda, & Lillis, 2006), the EST model stresses the acceptance of what is given, the emotional experience at the moment, and commitment to change, even in the face of difficulty. For example, the therapist may ask the patient to state a goal (e.g., lose 10 pounds), ask "What do you have to do to attain that goal?" (e.g., increase exercise and decrease calories, and then ask, "What are you willing to do?" The therapist may then suggest that "waiting to be ready," or "wanting to do it," or "being motivated" are not relevant to the "willingness to do what needs to be done." The therapist may ask the patient to consider a new theory of change: "You may need to do what you don't want to do to get what you want to get." By taking a history of behavior that the patient is proud of—past accomplishments, meaningful things that were done—the therapist can help the patient recognize that tolerating unpleasantness as a means to an end is the road to self-efficacy and "legitimate" self-esteem. The goal of therapy is not to eliminate unpleasant emotions but rather to accomplish important goals, realize one's values, deepen one's emotional experience, and act even in the face of discomfort.

RELEVANT RESEARCH

A number of studies provide support for the general EST model of the relationship between problematic beliefs about emotion and psychopathology. The first study on emotional schemas was conducted by Leahy (2002). Fifty-three adult psychotherapy patients were assessed, and their responses on the Leahy Emotional Schema Scale were correlated with the Beck Depression Inventory and the Beck Anxiety Inventory. Depression was related to greater guilt over emotion, expectation of longer duration, greater rumination, and view of one's emotions as less comprehensible, less controllable, and different from the emotions others have. Anxiety was related to greater guilt over emotion, a more simplistic view of emotion, greater rumination, viewing of one's emotions as less comprehensible, less acceptance of feelings, and viewing one's emotions as less controllable and as different from the emotions of others (Leahy, 2002).

In a study of 425 adult psychotherapy patients, Risk Aversion, Negative Beliefs about Emotion (a composite score on the LESS), and Psychological Flexibility were significantly related to depression and to each other (Leahy et al., 2012). Arguably, individuals might avoid taking risks—and making changes—because they have a negative view of the emotions that might arise, believing that if things do not work out, then their negative feelings will last indefinitely and might escalate even further. Thus, isolation, passivity, and procrastination may be strategies to avoid risky behavior. Silberstein, Tirch, Leahy, and McGinn (2012) tested 107 adult cognitive-behavioral outpatient participants on Dispositional Mindfulness, Psychological Flexibility, and Emotional Schemas. Individuals with higher levels of dispositional mindfulness also had higher levels of psychological flexibility and were more likely to endorse more adaptive dimensions of emotional schemas (Silberstein et al., 2012). In a study of 295 adult patients, Tirch and colleagues (Tirch, Leahy, Silberstein, & Melwani, 2012) examined the relationship between psychological flexibility (Acceptance and Action Questionnaire II [Bond et al., 2011]), Mindfulness (Mindful Attention and Awareness Scale [Brown & Ryan, 2003]) and Emotional Schemas (Leahy, 2002). All measures were significantly related to each other. Regression analysis indicated that emotional schemas regarding control of affect were the primary predictors of elevated Beck Anxiety Inventory (BAI) scores while psychological flexibility was the primary predictor of elevated anxiety scores on the MCMI-III (Tirch et al., 2012).

In a study of 425 psychotherapy patients, Leahy, Wupperman, and Shivaji (2016) explored the relationship between emotional schemas, metacognitive factors in worry (Metacognitions Questionnaire–II [MCQ-II] [Wells & Cartwright-Hatton, 2004]), depression (Beck Depression Inventory-II), and anxiety (Beck Anxiety Inventory). Negative Beliefs about Emotions was significantly correlated with each of the five Metacognitive Factors and with both depression (BDI-II) and anxiety (BAI). When controlling for anxiety, each of the MCQ factors was significantly related to Negative Beliefs about Emotion, except for Cognitive Competence, which was marginally significant ($p <. 02$). Stepwise multiple regression indicated that Uncontrollability/Danger of worry and Negative Beliefs about emotion were the best predictors of anxiety and Uncontrollability/Danger of Worry, Negative Beliefs about Emotion and Cognitive Competence were the best predictors of depression.

Several studies have explored the mediational role of emotional schemas for different forms of psychopathology. In a study by Edwards, Micek, Mottarella, and Wupperman (2016), 668 college students completed the Toronto Alexithymia Scale–20, the LESS-II, the Socialization of Emotion Scale, the Child Abuse and Trauma Scale (Sanders & Becker-Lausen, 1995), and the Trauma History Questionnaire (Green, 1996). Mediation analysis of the predictor variables on alexithymia indicated that emotion ideology (emotional schemas) completely mediated the effects of emotion socialization and child abuse. In a study of 325 adult psychotherapy outpatients by Westphal, Leahy, Pala, and Wupperman (2016), participants completed several self-report forms: the Millon Clinical Multiaxial Inventory-III (Millon, Millon, & Davis, 1994), Leahy Emotional Schema Scale (Leahy,

2002), the Self-Compassion Scale—Short Form (Raes, Pommier, Neff, & Van Gucht, 2011), and the Measure of Parenting Style (Parker et al., 1997). The subscale for Invalidation on the Leahy Emotional Schema Scale (LESS) and the subscales on the MCMI for MDD, PTSD, and BPD were of specific interest in this study. Invalidation on the LESS was strongly related to PTSD, MDD, and BPD, and self-compassion was strongly inversely associated with emotional invalidation. Both self-compassion and emotional invalidation mediated the relationship between parental indifference and mental health outcomes. Specifically, patients exposed to indifferent parenting displayed lower self-compassion and higher emotional invalidation, which mediated the risk for BPD, MDD, and PTSD.

In a study of 200 participants using a Russian version of the LESS-II, Sirota, Moskovchenko, Yaltonsky, Kochetkov, and Yaltonskaya (2013) found that emotional schemas are linked with the severity of psychopathological symptoms, early maladaptive schemes, and maladaptive cognitive emotional regulation strategies. In a study of 300 medical and dental students in Russia, Moskovchenko and colleagues found that students endorsing negative emotional schemas are characterized by higher scores on anxiety, depression, obsessive–compulsive symptoms, and somatization. Batmaz, Kaymak, Kocbiyik, and Turkcapar (2014) tested three groups of participants (166 unipolar depressed, 140 bipolar depressed, and 151 healthy controls) on the Metacognition Questionnaire–30 (MCQ-30), and the LESS. The clinicians diagnosed participants using a structured clinical interview (MINI) and rated the moods of the subjects with the Montgomery Asberg Depression Rating Scale (MADRS) and the Young Mania Rating Scale (YMRS). Of specific interest to the EST model, all three groups differed from each other on the LESS dimensions of guilt, duration, blame, validation, and acceptance of feelings. The mood-disordered groups were significantly different from the healthy controls on the LESS dimensions of simplistic view of emotions, numbness, rationality, rumination, higher values, and control.

In a study in Iran, Rezaee, Ghazanfari, and Rezaee (2016a, 2016b) tested 439 female college students on the Childhood Trauma Questionnaire (CTQ), the Early Maladaptive Schemas Questionnaire (SQ-SF), the LESS, the Acceptance and Action Questionnaire (AAQ-II), and the Beck Depression Inventory–II (BDI-II). The findings indicated that disconnection and rejection (DR) schemas mediated the relationship between CT and depression but CT did not predict depression symptoms, through the negative emotional schemas (NESs) and EA. NESs mediated the relationship between DR schemas and depression, and EA mediated the relationship between NESs and depression.

In a single subject design with two adult psychiatric patients who described years of persistent GAD, Kahleghi (unpublished manuscript) used a form of emotional schema therapy over a course of ten sessions evaluating changes on the Beck Anxiety Inventory, Hamilton Rating Scale of Anxiety, the Metacognition Questionnaire–30, and the Penn State Worry Questionnaire. There were substantial changes in overall anxiety on the Beck Anxiety Inventory (e.g., 79% and 72% for the two participants), and substantial changes on the the MCQ-30, the HARS, and the PSWQ, and these changes were maintained at two-months follow-up. In a preliminary study on the effectiveness of EST, Kahleghi (unpublished manuscript) compared a form of metacognitive therapy (MCT) with a form of EST in the treatment of generalized anxiety disorder. Both therapies were effective in reducing signs and symptoms of anxiety. Both therapies were significantly effective on negative and positive metacognitive beliefs about worry, and MCT was more effective than EST on both measures. Finally, both therapies were effective in reducing patients' worry, while MCT was relatively more effective than EST.

CURRENT ISSUES

The emotional schema model is an integrative CBT model that draws on social cognitive processes, models of affect forecasting, implicit theories of emotion, theory of mind, metacognitive processes, and other theories. Recent research suggests that emotional schemas are related to a wide range of psychopathology, to processes such as psychological flexibility, risk aversion, and early maladaptive personality schemas, and to early childhood experiences of problematic parenting and child trauma. Of particular interest is the role of negative beliefs about emotion as mediating the role of other experiences and processes in the emergence of psychopathology. The only preliminary study of the effectiveness of EST suggests that it shows efficacy in reducing anxiety, worry, and changing metacognitive factors underlying worry. However, future research will need to address the question of efficacy of treatments based on this model.

Future research can also address the issue of whether individuals have different schemas about different emotions—for example, sadness, anger, sexual desire, and anxiety—and whether different emotion-regulation strategies are activated for these different emotions. In addition, current work is being done evaluating cross-cultural differences in emotional schemas. Finally, given the assumption that individuals differ in their theories of emotion, research on the developmental course of these schemas would be of interest.

CONCLUSIONS

The emotional schema model extends the cognitive model by addressing how individuals "construct" the emotions of self and others. Once an emotion arises, the questions become, "How do you interpret that emotion?" and "What strategies of change (or acceptance) are activated?" Similarly, the EST model suggests that one's theory of the emotions of others will affect how one responds to those emotions and that these responses can either escalate, soothe, or accept the emotions of others. Although CBT has often been criticized for ignoring the importance of emotions, the EST model suggests that there may be a significant advantage to an integrative CBT model such as EST, which allows us to develop cognitive conceptualizations of how individual differences in the social construction of emotion can be implicated in psychopathology.

REFERENCES

Batmaz, S., Kaymak, S. U., Kocbiyik, S., & Turkcapar, M. H. (2014). Metacognitions and emotional schemas: A new cognitive perspective for the distinction between unipolar and bipolar depression. *Comprehensive Psychiatry, 55*(7), 1546–1555.

Beck, A. T. (1967). *Depression: Clinical, experimental and theoretical aspects.* New York: Harper & Row.

Beck, A. T., Davis, D. D., & Freeman, A. (1990). *Cognitive therapy of personality disorders.* New York: Guilford Press.

Beck, A. T., & Freeman, A. (1990). *Cognitive therapy of personality disorders.* New York: Guilford Press.

Beck, A. T., Rush, A. J., Shaw, B. F., & Emery, C. (1979). *Cognitive therapy of depression.* New York: Guilford Press.

Bem, D. J. (1972). Self-perception theory. *Advances in Experimental Social Psychology, 6,* 1–62.

Bond, F. W., Hayes, S. C., Baer, R. A., Carpenter, K. C., Guenole, N., Orcutt, H. K., . . . Zettle, R. D. (2011). Preliminary psychometric properties of the Acceptance and Action Questionnaire—II: A revised measure of psychological flexibility and acceptance. *Behavior Therapy, 42,* 676–688.

Brown, K. W., & Ryan, R. M. (2003). The benefits of being present: Mindfulness and its role in psychological well-being. *Journal of Personality and Social Psychology, 84,* 822–848.

Dugas, M. J., Buhr, K., & Ladouceur, R. (2004). The role of intolerance of uncertainty in the etiology and maintenance of generalized anxiety disorder. In R. G. Heimberg, C. L. Turk, & D. S. Mennin (Eds.), *Generalized anxiety disorder: Advances in research and practice* (pp. 143–163). New York: Guilford Press.

Dweck, C. S. (2006). *Mindset: The new psychology of success.* New York: Random House.

Edwards, E. R., Micek, A., Mottarella, K., & Wupperman, P. (2016). Emotion ideology mediates effects of risk factors on alexithymia development. *Journal of Rational-Emotive and Cognitive-Behavior Therapy,* 1–24.

Gilbert, D. T., Pinel, E. C., Wilson, T. D., Blumberg, S. J., & Wheatley, T. P. (1998). Immune neglect: A source of durability bias in affective forecasting. *Journal of Personality and Social Psychology, 75*(3), 617–638.

Green, B. L. (1996). Trauma history questionnaire. *Measurement of Stress, Trauma, and Adaptation, 1*, 366–369.

Hayes, S. C., Luoma, J. B., Bond, F. W., Masuda, A., & Lillis, J. (2006). Acceptance and commitment therapy: Model, processes and outcomes. *Behaviour Research and Therapy, 44*(1), 1–25.

Heider, F. (1958). *The psychology of interpersonal relations.* Hoboken, NJ: Wiley.

Jones, E., & Davis, K. E. (1965). From acts to dispositions: The attribution process in person perception. In L. Berkowitz (Ed.), *Advances in experimental social psychology* (Vol. 2, pp. 219–266). New York, Academic Press.

Jones, E. E., & Nisbett, R. E. (1972). The actor and the observer: Divergent perceptions of the causes of the behavior. In E. E. Jones, D. E. Kanouse, H. H. Kelley, et al. (Eds.), *Attribution: Perceiving the causes of behavior* (pp. 79–94). Morristown, NJ: General Learning Press.

Kelley, H. H. (1973). The processes of causal attribution. *American Psychologist, 28*(2), 107–128.

Leahy, R. L. (2002). A model of emotional schemas. *Cognitive and Behavioral Practice, 9*(3), 177–190.

Leahy, R. L. (2005). *The worry cure: Seven steps to stop worry from stopping you.* New York: Crown Publishing.

Leahy, R. L. (2012). *Leahy Emotional Schema Scale II (LESS II).* Unpublished manuscript, American Institute for Cognitive Therapy.

Leahy, R. L. (2015). *Emotional schema therapy.* New York: Guilford Press.

Leahy, R. L., & Tirch, D. (2008). Cognitive behavioral therapy for jealousy. *International Journal of Cognitive Therapy, 1*, 18–32.

Leahy, R. L., Tirch, D. D., & Melwani, P. S. (2012). Processes underlying depression: Risk aversion, emotional schemas, and psychological flexibility. *International Journal of Cognitive Therapy, 5*(4), 362–379.

Leahy, R. L., Wupperman, P., & Shivaji, S. (2016). *Metacognition and emotional schemas.* Poster session presented at the Anxiety and Depression Association of America Conference, Philadelphia, PA.

Millon, T., Millon, C., & Davis, R. D. (1994). *MCMI-III manual.* Piscataway Township, NJ: National Computer Systems.

Parker, G., Roussos, J., Hadzi-Pavlovic, D., Mitchell, P., Wilhelm, K., & Austin, M. P. (1997). The development of a refined measure of dysfunctional parenting and assessment of its relevance in patients with affective disorders. *Psychological Medicine, 27*(5), 1193–1203.

Raes, F., Pommier, E. M., Neff, K. D., & Van Gucht, D. (2011). Construction and factorial validation of a short form of the self-compassion scale. *Clinical Psychology and Psychotherapy, 18*(3), 250–255.

Rezaee, M., Ghazanfari, F., & Rezaee, F. (2016a). The role of childhood trauma, early maladaptive schemas, emotional schemas and experimental avoidance on depression: A structural equation modeling. *Psychiatry Research, 246*, 407–414.

Rezaee, M., Ghazanfari, F., & Reazee, F. (2016b). Effectiveness of emotional schema therapy on severity of depression and rumination in people with major depressive disorder. *Journal of Shahid Sadoughi University of Medical Sciences, 24*(1), 41–54.

Sanders, B., & Becker-Lausen, E. (1995). The measurement of psychological maltreatment: Early data on the child abuse and trauma scale. *Child Abuse and Neglect, 19*(3), 315–323.

Silberstein, L. R., Tirch, D., Leahy, R. L., & McGinn, L. (2012). Mindfulness, psychological flexibility and emotional schemas. *International Journal of Cognitive Therapy, 5*(4), 406–419.

Sirota, N., Moskovchenko, D. V., Yaltonsky, V. M., Kochetkov, Y. A., & Yaltonskaya, A. V. (2013). *Psychodiagnostics of emotional schemas: The results of transcultural adaptation and assessment of psychometric properties of Russian version of Leahy Emotional Schema Scale II.* Unpublished manuscript.

Tirch, D. D., Leahy, R. L., Silberstein, L. R., & Melwani, P. S. (2012). Emotional schemas, psychological flexibility, and anxiety: The role of flexible response patterns to anxious arousal. *International Journal of Cognitive Therapy, 5*(4), 380–391.

Trivers, R. L. (1972). Parental investment and sexual selection. In B. Campbell (Ed.), *Sexual selection and the descent of man, 1871–1971* (pp. 136–179). Chicago: Aldine.

Weiner, B. (1986). *An attributional theory of motivation and emotion.* New York: Springer-Verlag.

Wells, A. (2000). *Emotional disorders and metacognition: Innovative cognitive therapy.* New York: Wiley.

Wells, A. (2004). A cognitive model of GAD: Metacognitions and pathological worry. In R. G. Heimberg, C. Turk, & D. Mennin (Eds.), *Generalized anxiety disorder: Advances in research and practice* (pp. 3–28). New York: Guilford Press.

Wells, A. (2006). The metacognitive model of worry and generalized anxiety disorder. In G. C. L. Davey & A. Wells (Eds.), *Worry and psychological disorders: Assessment and treatment* (pp. 179–216). Chichester, UK: Wiley.

Wells, A. (2009). *Metacognitive therapy for anxiety and depression.* New York: Guilford Press.

Wells, A., & Cartwright-Hatton, S. (2004). A short form of the metacognitions questionnaire: Properties of the MCQ-30. *Behaviour Research and Therapy, 42*(4), 385–396.

Wells, A., & Matthews, G. (1994). *Attention and emotion: A clinical perspective.* Hove, UK: Jason Erlbaum.

Westphal, M., Leahy, R. L., Pala, A. N., & Wupperman, P. (2016). Self-compassion and emotional invalidation mediate the effects of parental indifference on psychopathology. *Psychiatry Research, 242,* 186–191.

Wilson, T. D., & Gilbert, D. T. (2003). Affective forecasting. *Advances in Experimental Social Psychology, 35,* 345–411.

CHAPTER 7

Cognitive Vulnerability to Depression and Bipolar Disorder

Lauren B. Alloy
Taylor A. Burke
Jared O'Garro-Moore
Lyn Y. Abramson

Cognitive models have aided our understanding of the etiology, course, and treatment of mood disorders and have been the subject of intensive investigation for four decades. In this chapter, we discuss the role of cognitive vulnerabilities in unipolar and bipolar mood disorders. We begin by presenting the Beck (1967) and hopelessness (Abramson, Metalsky, & Alloy, 1989) theories of depression and their extension to bipolar disorder. Next, we review empirical studies testing whether cognitive vulnerabilities featured in these two theories predict the onset and course of depression and bipolar disorders, alone or in interaction with stressful life events. Our review is not meant to be comprehensive. Information-processing biases and rumination, also found to be cognitive vulnerabilities (e.g., Gotlib & Joormann, 2010; Wisco & Nolen-Hoeksema, 2008), are not covered in this review. Finally, we discuss the clinical implications of cognitive vulnerabilities to mood disorders and directions for future research.

BECK AND HOPELESSNESS THEORIES OF MOOD DISORDERS

Unipolar Depression

Cognitive theories of unipolar depression suggest that the way in which an individual interprets his or her world, or one's cognitive style, influences his or her vulnerability to depression. These theories generally suggest that cognitive styles interact with environmental stimuli to predict depression, a vulnerability-stress perspective. This perspective holds that a cognitive vulnerability may be activated and thus, result in depression when an individual confronts a negative event. According to Beck's (1967) model, activation of negative cognitive self-schemas, such as those characterized by themes of worthlessness, failure, and inadequacy, serve as a *mechanism* through which depression may develop. Such negative self-schemas are often represented by dysfunctional attitudes in which the person believes that his or her worth and happiness depend on others' approval or being perfect. Beck (1967) hypothesized that when activated by negative events, these negative self-schemas can lead to negatively biased cognitions about one's self, world, and future (i.e., the negative cognitive triad) and, in turn, the onset of depression. Beck believed that these negative schemas are formed early in individuals' lives and become more rigid over time. Moreover, even when depressive episodes remit, negative self-schemas can remain stable, thus continuing to serve as risk factors for the recurrence of depression (Beck, 1967). More recently, Beck (1987) expanded this cognitive model of depression, suggesting that there are specific personality types that serve as additional cognitive risk factors for the onset and/or recurrence of depression. Individuals who exhibit elevated levels of sociotropy and autonomy are at risk for depression when they experience stressors that are personality-congruent. Thus, individuals high on sociotropy are vulnerable to depression when they experience life events involving interpersonal loss or rejection ("sociotropic traumas"), whereas individuals high on autonomy are at risk for depression when they experience stressors characterized by threats to their independence, control, or achievement ("autonomous stressors").

A second prominent cognitive vulnerability-stress model with some similarity to Beck's theory, hopelessness theory (Abramson et al., 1989), proposes that a negative inferential or cognitive style involving three components increases individuals' vulnerability to depression when they experience negative life events. The three components are the tendency to (1) attribute negative life events to internal as opposed to external causes, global as opposed to specific causes, and stable as opposed to unstable causes, (2) infer negative self-characteristics due to the occurrence of the event, and (3) infer that the negative event will lead to negative consequences. Individuals with this negative inferential style who encounter negative life events are most likely to develop hopelessness, the proximal cause of depressive symptoms (Abramson et al., 1989). In addition, like Beck's model, hopelessness theory has a specific vulnerability hypothesis in which life events that match the domain in which an individual possesses a negative inferential style are most likely to trigger hopelessness and depression (e.g., interpersonal rejection or loss for a person with a negative inferential style in the interpersonal domain).

Whereas the original learned helplessness theory of depression (Seligman, 1975) viewed the expectation that one could not control events as the cause of depression, the hopelessness theory (Abramson et al., 1989) proposes that it is the expectation of uncontrollability, combined with the expectation that negative outcomes are highly likely to occur and/or desired outcomes are very unlikely to occur (i.e., hopelessness), that is the proximal cause of depression. Thus, uncontrollable positive events would be expected to lead to depression in the helplessness theory, but only uncontrollable negative events would predict depression in the hopelessness theory, a prediction that better fits with the empirical evidence (Monroe & Harkness, 2005). Moreover, an important advantage of the hopelessness theory compared to the original helplessness theory is that it also specifies a sequence of processes in a causal chain hypothesized to culminate in hopelessness and depression, and thus, identifies distal vulnerabilities for depression (i.e., negative inferential style).

Bipolar Disorder

Cognitive vulnerability-stress models of unipolar depression have been extended to bipolar spectrum disorders (BSDs) as well (Alloy et al., 2005; Alloy, Abramson, Walshaw, Keyser, & Gerstein, 2006a; Alloy, Abramson, Walshaw, & Nereen, 2006b; Alloy, Abramson, Urosevic, Bender, & Wagner, 2009a). The same negative cognitive styles hypothesized to confer risk for unipolar depressive episodes also may increase vulnerability to the depressive episodes of BSDs. With respect to hypomanic and manic (hereafter referred to as "hypomanic") episodes of BSD, Beck (1976) suggested that mania-prone individuals have latent positive self-schemas involving unrealistically positive attitudes about the self, world, and future. The occurrence of positive life events can activate these optimistic self-schemas, leading to hypomanic symptoms. Similarly, in hopelessness theory, positive inferential styles for positive life events should promote vulnerability to hopefulness and, in turn, hypomanic symptoms when individuals experience positive events. In addition, given that negative life events have been found to predict hypomanic episodes as well as depressive episodes in people with BSDs (e.g., Alloy et al., 2005; 2006a, 2006b; Johnson & Roberts, 1995), bipolar individuals' self-schemas and cognitive styles for interpreting negative events also may be relevant to affecting their risk for hypomania.

In applying the cognitive models of depression to BSDs, theorists (e.g., Alloy et al., 2005, 2006a, 2006b, 2009b) have suggested that these cognitive models need to be integrated with theory and evidence that individuals with BSD possess a hypersensitive behavioral approach system (BAS) or reward system, a motivational system involved in goal-striving and attainment of rewards (Alloy & Abramson, 2010; Alloy, Nusslock, & Boland, 2015; Depue & Iacono, 1989; Johnson, Edge, Holmes, & Carver, 2012; Urosevic, Abramson, Harmon-Jones, & Alloy, 2008). The BAS has been linked to a dopaminergic fronto-striatal neural circuit sensitive to reward-relevant stimuli (e.g., Haber & Knutson, 2010) and is activated by goal- or reward-relevant cues that may be internal (e.g., expectation of winning an award) or external (e.g., job promotion). BAS activation is associated with increased motor activity, incentive motivation, and positive goal-striving emotions such as hope and happiness (e.g., Gray, 1994). Thus, cognitive styles relevant to predicting bipolar symptoms and episodes should be characterized by distinctive BAS features related to high drive and incentive motivation such as perfectionism, autonomy, and overly ambitious goal-striving, as well as self-criticism when the ambitious goals are not met (Alloy et al., 2006a, 2006b, 2009b).

Research on Cognitive Vulnerabilities to Unipolar Depression and Bipolar Disorder

Much research has tested the cognitive vulnerability hypotheses of Beck's theory and hopelessness theory for both unipolar and bipolar mood disorders. As reviewed here, whereas cross-sectional studies have established associations between the cognitive styles featured in Beck's and hopelessness theories and depression and BSDs, studies of individuals remitted from depression or BSDs indicate whether maladaptive cognitive patterns exhibit some stability independent of current mood symptoms. More powerful tests of the cognitive vulnerability hypotheses are provided by prospective longitudinal studies. As described here, several prospective studies have indicated that certain dysfunctional attitudes, self-schemas, and inferential styles do, in fact, predict depressive and hypomanic symptoms and episodes (and even first lifetime onset of depression and BSD) alone or in combination with relevant life events.

Unipolar Depression

Cross-sectional studies have demonstrated associations between the dysfunctional attitudes and self-schemas featured in Beck's theory and the negative inferential styles from hopelessness theory and depressive symptoms and disorders in children, adolescents, and adults (see Alloy, Abramson,

Keyser, Gerstein, & Sylvia, 2008, 2012b, for reviews). Some studies also show that individuals in remission from a previous depressive episode continue to exhibit dysfunctional attitudes and negative inferential styles; however, other studies find that remitted depressives only exhibit these negative cognitive patterns when the styles are activated or "primed" by a depressive mood induction or exposure to stressors (see Ingram, Miranda, & Segal, 1998; Just, Abramson, & Alloy, 2001; Persons & Miranda, 1992, for reviews). Explicit priming appears to be less important for observing negative inferential styles than dysfunctional attitudes in remitted depressives, perhaps because the typical measure of negative inferential styles (i.e., Cognitive Style Questionnaire [CSQ] and its variants; Alloy et al., 2000) may contain built-in hypothetical life event primes (Haeffel et al., 2005). Moreover, when studies select samples of remitted depressives who have not received treatments that may ameliorate their negative cognitive styles, dysfunctional attitudes and negative inferential styles are observed in remission (e.g., Abela, Stolow, Zhang, & McWhinnie, 2012; Haeffel et al., 2005). Indeed, Romens, Abramson, and Alloy (2009) found that dysfunctional attitudes and negative inferential styles were relatively stable over seven years.

More powerful evidence supporting Beck's and hopelessness theory's cognitive vulnerability hypotheses comes from prospective longitudinal studies. For example, dysfunctional attitudes have been found to predict depressive symptoms in adults prospectively (e.g., Zuroff, Igreja, & Mongrain, 1990) and mediate the prospective relationship between anxious attachment and depressive symptoms in youth (e.g., Lee & Hankin, 2009). Negative self-schemas also predict depressive symptoms prospectively in adolescents (Connolly, Abramson, & Alloy, 2016). Additional research supports the vulnerability-stress conceptualization of Beck's model, suggesting that dysfunctional attitudes predict depression in interaction with experiences of life stressors in adults (e.g., Joiner, Metalsky, Lew, & Klocek, 1999; Olinger, Kuiper, & Shaw, 1987) and youth (e.g., Abela & Skitch, 2007; Hankin, Wetter, Cheely, & Oppenheimer, 2008).

Although there is considerable support for Beck's original cognitive model, evidence for the sociotropy and autonomy aspects of Beck's model (Beck, 1987) has been mixed. For example, levels of sociotropy and autonomy were found to be higher in currently depressed than remitted depressed individuals, who, in turn, exhibited higher levels than healthy control individuals (Fairbrother & Moretti, 1998). In addition, Clark, Beck, and Brown (1992) found a significant interaction between sociotropy and negative interpersonal events (but not autonomous events) in predicting levels of dysphoria. Of note, however, this study also found that autonomy did not predict dysphoria. More recent studies suggest that the evidence is inconsistent for sociotropy and autonomy in interaction with personality style—congruent events as predictors of depression (e.g., Fresco, Sampson, Craighead, & Koons, 2001; Husky, Mazure, Maciejewski, & Swendsen, 2007; Iacoviello, Alloy, Abramson, & Grant, 2009).

With respect to the hopelessness theory, negative inferential style has been found to predict onset of depressive episodes (e.g., Nusslock et al., 2011). In youth, some evidence suggests that individuals' "weakest link" (their most negative inferential style dimension) predicts depressive symptoms better than a composite measure of negative inferential style (e.g., Abela & Sarin, 2002; Abela & Schleffler, 2008); however, the evidence regarding the superiority of the weakest link over a composite negative inferential style measure is mixed in adults (e.g., Haeffel, 2010; Reilly, Ciesla, Felton, Weitlauf, & Anderson, 2012; Xiao et al., 2016). There also is considerable support for hopelessness theory's vulnerability-stress component. Specifically, longitudinal studies conducted among adolescents and adults provide evidence that negative inferential styles interact with stressful life events to predict depressive symptoms and episodes as predicted by the theory (for a recent review, see Liu, Kleiman, Nestor, & Cheek, 2015). Developmental research aimed at understanding when these negative inferential styles form has provided support for the notion that they stabilize in adolescence and in turn, that a cognitive vulnerability-stress interaction does not reliably predict depression until this developmental period (e.g., Cole et al., 2008).

Perhaps some of the strongest support for the cognitive vulnerability hypothesis of both Beck's and hopelessness theories comes from the Cognitive Vulnerability to Depression (CVD) Project (Alloy et al., 2006c), a truly prospective study of first lifetime onset of depression. Alloy et al. (2006c) recruited undergraduates at hypothesized high-risk versus low-risk for depression based on scoring in the top versus bottom quartile of a large screening sample on both dysfunctional attitudes and negative inferential styles. They found that among students with no prior history of depression, the cognitive high-risk group was significantly (7 times) more likely to develop a first onset of major depressive disorder during 2.5 years of follow-up than was the cognitive low-risk group. Among students who did have a past depressive episode, the high-risk group also developed recurrences of major depression at significantly (3 times) higher rates than the low-risk group. Furthermore, the cognitive high-risk group developed a significantly greater number of depressive episodes, episodes of greater severity, and a more chronic course of depression than the cognitive low-risk group (Iacoviello, Alloy, Abramson, Whitehouse, & Hogan, 2006). In summary, although some studies do not support the cognitive vulnerability hypotheses of Beck's and hopelessness theories, the preponderance of evidence indicates that negative cognitive styles do increase vulnerability to depression.

Bipolar Disorder

Research on the role of cognitive styles as vulnerabilities for BSDs has grown in the last two decades. To date, some studies suggest that the positivity versus negativity of the cognitive styles of individuals with BSDs vary depending on their symptomatic state at assessment and whether explicit or implicit (non-face valid, less conscious) assessments are used (e.g., see Alloy et al., 2006b, for review). Generally, many studies have indicated that individuals with BSD in a depressive episode exhibit underlying cognitive styles at least as or more negative than those of unipolar depressed persons and more negative than those of healthy comparison individuals on explicit measures (see Alloy et al., 2006a, 2006b, for reviews; Batmaz et al., 2013). Depressed bipolar participants also exhibit negative cognitive biases on implicit tasks (Jabben et al., 2012, 2014; Molz Adams, Shapero, Pendergast, Alloy, & Abramson, 2014). Hypomanic BSD individuals often present positive cognitive styles on explicit measures, but continue to exhibit evidence of underlying negative cognitive styles on implicit assessments (see Alloy et al., 2006a, 2006b for reviews). For example, Lyon, Startup, and Bentall (1999) investigated the attributional styles of bipolar patients on both an explicit attribution questionnaire (the Attributional Style Questionnaire [ASQ]; Peterson et al., 1982) and a pragmatic inference task (PIT) that assessed attributions implicitly. The PIT included brief self-referent, hypothetical scenarios derived from the ASQ items, but disguised as a memory test for the facts in the scenarios. Participants were surprised by unexpected questions regarding the cause of the outcomes described in the PIT scenarios. Lyons et al. found that whereas bipolar depressed patients exhibited a negative attributional style on both the explicit ASQ and the implicit PIT, the bipolar manic patients showed a positive attributional bias on the explicit ASQ, but exhibited negative attributions like those of the depressed bipolar patients on the implicit PIT.

More recent studies have obtained findings congruent with an integration of the BAS/reward hypersensitivity theory with cognitive models of BSD. That is, euthymic individuals with BSDs exhibit dysfunctional attitudes and cognitive styles characterized by the high drive and incentive motivation associated with high BAS/reward sensitivity, but not by maladaptive dependency and attachment attitudes typically observed among unipolar depressed individuals (Alloy et al., 2009b; Goldberg, Gerstein, Wenze, Welker, & Beck, 2008; Lam, Wright, & Smith, 2004; Rosenfarb, Becker, Khan, & Mintz, 1998; Scott, Stanton, Garland, & Ferrier, 2000; Shapero et al., 2015; Wright, Lam, & Newsom-Davis, 2005; but see Batmaz et al., 2013, for an exception). For example, Alloy et al. (2009b) found that euthymic BSD individuals exhibited greater BAS-relevant dysfunctional attitudes of excessive perfectionism, high autonomy, and self-criticism, but not sociotropy, dependency, or high need for approval, compared to healthy control individuals. Similarly, Lam et al. (2004) observed that patients with bipolar disorder scored higher than unipolar depressed patients only on goal-attainment dysfunctional attitudes, and Johnson and colleagues (2012; Lozano & Johnson, 2001) reported that BSD individuals exhibit more ambitious goal-striving and higher achievement motivation than controls, controlling for current mood symptoms. Shapero et al. (2015) also observed that BSD participants exhibited more ambitious goal-striving and self-criticism than unipolar depressed participants. Indeed, Fulford, Johnson, Llabre, and Carver (2010) found that it is difficult for people with BSD to curb their ambitious goal-striving.

Some research has examined whether the cognitive styles of individuals with BSDs are stable and independent of mood state. In general, cross-sectional studies of euthymic or remitted BSD individuals, divide evenly between those that do and do not find evidence of negative cognitive styles in the euthymic state (see Alloy et al., 2006a, 2006b for reviews; Lex, Hautzinger, & Meyer, 2011). Likewise, longitudinal studies that assess cognitive patterns across mood phases of BSD within individuals also obtain mixed findings. On the one hand, Alloy, Reilly-Harrington, Fresco, Whitehouse, and Zechmeister (1999) found that dysfunctional attitudes and attributional styles were stable across cyclothymic individuals' mood swings. On the other hand, Ashworth et al. (1985) found that explicit measures of self-esteem returned to normal levels when previously manic or depressed bipolar patients remitted and Pavlickova et al. (2013) observed that explicit self-esteem was higher in manic than depressive states among bipolar patients.

Despite some findings that indicate explicit measures of cognitive style may not be stable across mood phases of BSDs, there is also some evidence that cognitive styles assessed during euthymic states predict bipolar mood symptoms and episodes prospectively, alone and in combination with relevant life events. Whereas some studies (e.g., Johnson & Fingerhut, 2004; Johnson, Meyer, Winett, & Small, 2000; Pavlickova et al., 2013) found that negative cognitions predicted subsequent depressive, but not manic, symptoms in bipolar I patients, Scott and Pope (2003) reported that low self-esteem predicted both manic and depressive relapse at twelve-month follow-up among bipolar patients. Moreover, studies that specifically examined BAS-relevant cognitive styles obtained greater support for cognitive vulnerability to bipolar symptoms and episodes. For example, Lozano and Johnson (2001) reported that cognitive styles involving high need for achievement predicted increases in manic symptoms over six months in bipolar I patients. In addition, Alloy et al. (2009b) found that the BAS-relevant styles of high autonomy and self-criticism measured at baseline predicted a greater likelihood of onset of hypomanic episodes over a 3.2-year follow-up among individuals with BSDs, controlling for past bipolar mood episodes and baseline mood symptoms. Moreover, Alloy et al. (2012a) observed that controlling for initial mood symptoms and family history of bipolar disorder, Time 1 ambitious goal-striving predicted first lifetime onset of BSD over a thirteen-month follow-up among adolescents with no prior history of BSD.

Prospective cognitive vulnerability-stress studies have examined whether cognitive styles featured as vulnerabilities in Beck's and hopelessness theories interact with congruent life events to predict bipolar symptoms. Consistent with hopelessness theory, in a sample of unipolar depressed and BSD participants, Alloy et al. (1999) found that a negative attributional style for negative events interacted with subsequently occurring negative events to predict increases in depressive symptoms and that a positive attributional style interacted with later positive events to predict increases in hypomanic symptoms. Dysfunctional attitudes combined with life events did not predict symptom changes. However, Reilly-Harrington, Alloy, Fresco, and Whitehouse (1999) found that controlling for initial symptoms, baseline negative attributional styles, dysfunctional attitudes, and negative self-schemas each interacted with later negative events to predict increases in both depressive and hypomanic symptoms in a BSD sample. Inasmuch as Reilly-Harrington et al.'s (1999) study included bipolar I and II participants who had experienced major depressive episodes, they may have been more responsive to negative life events than were the participants in Alloy et al.'s (1999) study, who had milder bipolar conditions (i.e., cyclothymia) and no history of major depression. Exploring Beck's constructs of sociotropy and autonomy, Hammen, Ellicott, and Gitlin (1992) reported that sociotropy interacted with negative interpersonal events to predict subsequent symptom severity in a bipolar I sample. (N.B., Hammen, Ellicott, Gitlin, & Jamison, 1989 also obtained a trend for this effect.) However, autonomy did not interact with negative achievement events to predict bipolar symptom severity in this study. Finally, Francis-Raniere, Alloy, and Abramson (2006) found that controlling for initial symptoms and the number of events experienced, baseline BAS-relevant cognitive styles of perfectionistic dysfunctional attitudes and autonomy and self-criticism predicted prospective increases in hypomanic symptoms in interaction with style-congruent positive events and prospective increases in depressive symptoms in interaction with style-congruent negative events.

In summary, based on the foregoing research reviewed, similar maladaptive cognitive styles may serve as vulnerabilities to unipolar depression and bipolar disorders, with the additional caveat that the cognitive styles that provide risk for BSDs involve distinctive BAS-relevant features. The dysfunctional attitudes, self-schemas, and inferential styles featured as vulnerabilities in Beck's and hopelessness theories appear to be associated with depression and BSD in children, adolescents, and adults; exhibit some independence from current mood state; and prospectively predict onsets and recurrences of mood symptoms and episodes alone and in combination with style-relevant life events.

CLINICAL APPLICATIONS OF THE COGNITIVE MODELS OF DEPRESSION AND BIPOLAR DISORDER

The cognitive models of depression and BSD, particularly Beck's model, have generated efficacious therapies for depression and BSDs (Beck, Rush, Shaw, & Emery, 1979). However, research on attributional or inferential style generated by the hopelessness theory also has led to the use of effective strategies for treating mood disorders (Rubenstein, Freed, Shapero, Fauber, & Alloy, 2016).

Unipolar Depression

Arising from the cognitive model of depression is perhaps the most prominent form of psychotherapy for depression, cognitive-behavioral therapy (CBT; Beck et al., 1979). The main goal of this therapy is to alter maladaptive automatic thoughts and negative self-schemas, thereby modifying individuals' biased interpretations of life events. In doing so, CBT is hypothesized to result in decreases in negative affect, maladaptive behaviors, and depressive symptomatology. Clients receiving CBT are expected to actively participate in therapy, working with the therapist to identify automatic thoughts, challenge cognitive biases (including those triggered by negative inferential styles), and alter behavioral patterns. CBT is one of the most widely implemented and heavily researched forms of therapy and was originally designed for treatment of unipolar depression. Between 1986 and 1993, over 120 controlled trials were added to the literature (Hollon & Beck, 1994).

Not only have the theoretical models on which CBT was built been shown to have robust research support, but also CBT itself has amassed significant research support as an efficacious treatment for depression. Two recent reviews of meta-analyses of CBT suggest that CBT is significantly more effective in treating unipolar depression than control conditions (e.g., wait list, no treatment) (Cuijpers et al., 2013; Hofmann, Asnaani, Vonk, Sawyer, & Fang, 2012). These reviews further indicated that there are mixed results regarding CBT's effectiveness compared to other active treatments (e.g., problem-solving therapy, interpersonal therapy, psychodynamic treatment), with some finding equal effectiveness and others revealing that CBT is superior to other treatments (Cuijpers et al., 2013; Hofmann et al., 2012). Reviews of meta-analyses comparing CBT to pharmacological treatment suggest that these treatment approaches are equally effective and that

CBT plus psychopharmacology is superior to psychopharmacology alone (Cuijpers et al., 2013; Hofmann et al. 2012).

Bipolar Disorder

Inasmuch as relapse rates for individuals with bipolar disorder who rely solely on medication remain relatively high, psychosocial interventions, including CBT modified for bipolar disorder, have been developed as adjunctive treatments for BSD (Miklowitz & Johnson, 2006). CBT has been shown to be an efficacious intervention for bipolar disorder that can significantly reduce depressive and hypomanic symptoms, increase the time between bipolar episodes, decrease the frequency of episode recurrences, and improve psychosocial functioning in a number of domains (Lam et al., 2003; Lam, Hayward, Watkins, Wright, & Sham 2005; Scott, Colom, & Vieta, 2007). Research suggests that hypomanic and depressive prodromes might be effective periods in which to target the BAS-relevant cognitive styles found to be predictive of bipolar mood symptoms and episodes (Lam et al., 2003). In particular, it may be possible to apply cognitive restructuring to the client's thoughts regarding goal-striving and attainment, such as identifying and challenging the beliefs that lead to excessive goal-setting and achievement motivation (Hamlat, O'Garro-Moore, Nusslock, & Alloy, 2016; Nusslock, Abramson, Harmon-Jones, Alloy, & Coan, 2009). Indeed, CBT focused on extreme goal-striving has been found to significantly reduce maladaptive perfectionistic and goal-striving attitudes as well as lower rates of both depressive and manic episode relapse (Lam et al., 2003). Another CBT-based approach for BSDs that has not yet been empirically supported is schema-focused therapy (SFT; Hawke, Provencher, & Parikh, 2013). SFT focuses on (1) education about early maladaptive schemas, (2) adaptive cognitive strategies such as reframing and evaluating coping responses, and (3) experiential techniques, such as imagery dialogues and psychodrama (Hawke et al., 2013).

Inasmuch as CBT for bipolar disorder as currently practiced has been found to reduce depression more than hypomania (e.g., Scott et al., 2006), Johnson and Fulford (2009) developed a preliminary treatment program focused on improving goal regulation for mania (the GOALS program). Drawing on CBT strategies as well as goal dysregulation research, the GOALS program involves four main modules designed to target goal-regulation variables shown to be related to BSDs: (1) excessive emotional reactivity to positive events; (2) ambitious goal-setting; (3) excessive increases in confidence after success, and (4) goal-pacing. Each module includes assessment of the client's status on the risk factor, motivational interviewing to promote motivation for change, and specific cognitive-behavioral strategies to address these issues. The GOALS program was found to significantly reduce manic symptoms in bipolar patients. Although further replication incorporating a control group, larger sample size, and follow-up data is needed, it is encouraging that treatment targets specified by a BAS-informed CBT approach were useful for reducing hypomanic symptoms.

CONCLUSIONS

Some research (e.g., Hankin, Abramson, Miller, & Haeffel, 2004) suggests that when the cognitive vulnerabilities featured in Beck's and hopelessness theories of depression are entered into a predictive model simultaneously, they are no longer significantly predictive of depression, calling into question the extent to which these models are examining unique constructs. However, there is mixed evidence regarding this potential overlap (Hankin, Lakdawalla, Carter, Abela, & Adams, 2007), and thus, future research should focus on determining the degree to which Beck's model and the hopelessness theory of depression measure similar constructs with the overarching goal of achieving theoretical parsimony. Furthermore, over the past decade, a growing body of literature has supported modified cognitive models of depression. The transactional cognitive vulnerability-stress model (e.g., Hankin & Abramson, 2001) suggests that the relationships between stressful life events, cognitive vulnerabilities, and depressive symptoms are bidirectional, as opposed to solely unidirectional, and research has supported this model (Calvete, Orue, & Hankin, 2013). Future research should continue to clarify the transactional relationships between these variables by rigorously examining the hypotheses of the stress generation model of depression (Hammen, 1991; for a review, see Liu, 2013).

Another exciting and important direction for future research is work that provides integration between cognitive and neurobiological models of mood disorders. Abramson et al. (2002) suggested that cognitive styles that predispose individuals to hopelessness, as specified in the hopelessness theory, should be related to biological vulnerabilities associated with deficits in BAS/reward system activity. And Nusslock et al. (2011) provided support for this perspective, suggesting that increased cognitive vulnerability and decreased relative left frontal asymmetry on EEG during the resting state (a neurophysiological measure of reduced BAS/reward system activity) may reflect common predictors of depression onset. And other growing evidence suggests that the cognitive styles associated with bipolar disorder also may be based in increased BAS/reward system activity (see Alloy et al., 2015 for review). Similarly, Disner, Beevers, Haigh, and Beck (2011) suggested an integration of Beck's cognitive model of depression with recent research on the neural mechanisms of depression. They hypothesized that the negative cognitive biases featured in Beck's theory may be facilitated by decreased top-down cognitive control from prefrontal cortical systems combined with enhanced activation of subcortical emotion processing brain regions.

Research that tests these cognitive-neural integrative models may be especially fruitful in leading to a new understanding of mood disorders and the development of novel interventions.

REFERENCES

Abela, J. R., & Sarin, S. (2002). Cognitive vulnerability to hopelessness depression: A chain is only as strong as its weakest link. *Cognitive Therapy and Research, 26,* 811–829.

Abela, J. R., & Scheffler, P. (2008). Conceptualizing cognitive vulnerability to depression in youth: A comparison of the weakest link and additive approaches. *International Journal of Cognitive Therapy, 1,* 333–351.

Abela, J. R., & Skitch, S. A. (2007). Dysfunctional attitudes, self-esteem, and hassles: Cognitive vulnerability to depression in children of affectively ill parents. *Behaviour Research and Therapy, 45,* 1127–1140.

Abela, J. R., Stolow, D., Zhang, M., & McWhinnie, C. M. (2012). Negative cognitive style and past history of major depressive episodes in university students. *Cognitive Therapy and Research, 36,* 219–227.

Abramson, L. Y., Alloy, L. B., Hankin, B. L., Haeffel, G. J., MacCoon, D. G., & Gibb, B. E. (2002). Cognitive vulnerability-stress models of depression in a self-regulatory and psychobiological context. In I. H. Gotlib & C. L. Hammen (Eds.), *Handbook of depression* (3rd ed., pp. 268–294). New York: Guilford Press.

Abramson, L. Y., Metalsky, G. I., & Alloy, L. B. (1989). Hopelessness depression: A theory-based subtype of depression. *Psychological Review, 96,* 358–372.

Alloy, L. B., & Abramson, L. Y. (2010). The role of the behavioral approach system (BAS) in bipolar spectrum disorders. *Current Directions in Psychological Science, 19,* 189–194.

Alloy, L. B., Abramson, L. Y., Hogan, M. E., Whitehouse, W. G., Rose, D. T., Robinson, M. S., . . . Lapkin, J. B. (2000). The Temple—Wisconsin Cognitive Vulnerability to Depression (CVD) Project: Lifetime history of Axis I psychopathology in individuals at high and low cognitive risk for depression. *Journal of Abnormal Psychology, 109,* 403–418.

Alloy, L. B., Abramson, L. Y., Keyser, J., Gerstein, R. K., & Sylvia, L. G. (2008). Negative cognitive style. In K. S. Dobson & D. Dozois (Eds.), *Risk factors for depression* (pp. 237–262). New York: Academic Press/Elsevier.

Alloy, L. B., Abramson, L. Y., Urosevic, S., Bender, R. E., & Wagner, C. A. (2009a). Longitudinal predictors of bipolar spectrum disorders: A behavioral approach system (BAS) perspective. *Clinical Psychology: Science and Practice, 16,* 206–226.

Alloy, L. B., Abramson, L. Y., Urosevic, S., Walshaw, P. D., Nusslock, R., & Nereen, A. M. (2005). The psychosocial context of bipolar disorder: Environmental, cognitive, and developmental risk factors. *Clinical Psychology Review, 25,* 1043–1075.

Alloy, L. B., Abramson, L. Y., Walshaw, P. D., Gerstein, R. K., Keyser, J. D., Whitehouse, W. G., . . . Harmon-Jones, E. (2009b). Behavioral approach system (BAS)—relevant cognitive styles and bipolar spectrum disorders: Concurrent and prospective associations. *Journal of Abnormal Psychology, 118*, 459–471.

Alloy, L. B., Abramson, L. Y., Walshaw, P. D., Keyser, J., & Gerstein, R. K. (2006a). A cognitive vulnerability-stress perspective on bipolar spectrum disorders in a normative adolescent brain, cognitive, and emotional development context. *Development and Psychopathology, 18*, 1055–1103.

Alloy, L. B., Abramson, L. Y., Walshaw, P. D., & Nereen, A. M. (2006b). Cognitive vulnerability to unipolar and bipolar mood disorders. *Journal of Social and Clinical Psychology, 25*, 726–754.

Alloy, L. B., Abramson, L. Y., Whitehouse, W. G., Hogan, M. E., Panzarella, C., & Rose, D. T. (2006c). Prospective incidence of first onsets and recurrences of depression in individuals at high and low cognitive risk for depression. *Journal of Abnormal Psychology, 115*, 145–156.

Alloy, L. B., Bender, R. E., Whitehouse, W. G., Wagner, C. A., Liu, R. T., Grant, D. A., . . . Abramson, L. Y. (2012a). High Behavioral Approach System (BAS) sensitivity, reward responsiveness, and goal-striving predict first onset of bipolar spectrum disorders: A prospective behavioral high-risk design. *Journal of Abnormal Psychology, 121*, 339–351.

Alloy, L. B., Black, S. K., Young, M. E., Goldstein, K. E., Shapero, B. G., Stange, J. P., . . . Abramson, L. Y. (2012b). Cognitive vulnerabilities and depression versus other psychopathology symptoms and diagnoses in early adolescence. *Journal of Clinical Child and Adolescent Psychology, 41*, 539–560.

Alloy, L. B., Nusslock, R., & Boland, E. M. (2015). The development and course of bipolar spectrum disorders: An integrated reward and circadian rhythm dysregulation model. *Annual Review of Clinical Psychology, 11*, 213–250.

Alloy, L. B., Reilly-Harrington, N., Fresco, D. M., Whitehouse, W. G., & Zechmeister, J. S. (1999). Cognitive styles and life events in subsyndromal unipolar and bipolar disorders: Stability and prospective prediction of depressive and hypomanic mood swings. *Journal of Cognitive Psychotherapy: An International Quarterly, 13*, 21–40.

Ashworth, C. M., Blackburn, I. M., & McPherson, F. M. (1985). The performance of depressed and manic patients on some repertory grid measures: A longitudinal study. *British Journal of Medical Psychology, 58*, 337–342.

Batmaz, S., Kaymak, S. U., Soygur, A. H., Ozalp, E., & Turkcapar, M. H. (2013). The distinction between unipolar and bipolar depression: A cognitive theory perspective. *Comprehensive Psychiatry, 54*, 740–749.

Beck, A. T. (1967). *Depression: Clinical, experimental, and theoretical aspects.* New York: Harper & Row.

Beck, A. T. (1976). *Cognitive therapy and the emotional disorders.* New York: International Universities Press.

Beck, A. T. (1987). Cognitive models of depression. *Journal of Cognitive Psychotherapy: An International Quarterly, 1*, 5–37.

Beck, A. T., Rush, A. J., Shaw, B. F., & Emery, G. (1979). *Cognitive therapy of depression.* New York: Guilford Press.

Calvete, E., Orue, I., & Hankin, B. L. (2013). Transactional relationships among cognitive vulnerabilities, stressors, and depressive symptoms in adolescence. *Journal of Abnormal Child Psychology, 41*, 399–410.

Clark, D. A., Beck, A. T., & Brown, G. K. (1992). Sociotropy, autonomy, and life event perceptions in dysphoric and nondysphoric individuals. *Cognitive Therapy and Research, 16,* 635–652.

Cole, D. A., Ciesla, J. A., Dallaire, D. H., Jacquez, F. M., Pineda, A. Q., LaGrange, B., . . . Felton, J. (2008). Emergence of attributional style and its relation to depressive symptoms. *Journal of Abnormal Psychology, 117,* 16–31.

Connolly, S. L., Abramson, L. Y., & Alloy, L. B. (2016). Information processing biases concurrently and prospectively predict depressive symptoms in adolescence: Evidence from a self-referent encoding task. *Cognition and Emotion, 30,* 550–560.

Cuijpers, P., Berking, M., Andersson, G., Quigley, L., Kleiboer, A., & Dobson, K. S. (2013). A meta-analysis of cognitive-behavioural therapy for adult depression, alone and in comparison with other treatments. *Canadian Journal of Psychiatry, 58,* 376–385.

Depue, R. A., & Iacono, W. G. (1989). Neurobehavioral aspects of affective disorders. *Annual Review of Psychology, 40,* 457–492.

Disner, S. G., Beevers, C. G., Haigh, E. A. P., & Beck A. T. (2011). Neural mechanisms of the cognitive model of depression. *Nature Reviews Neuroscience, 12,* 467–477.

Fairbrother, N., & Moretti, M. (1998). Sociotropy, autonomy, and self-discrepancy: Status in depressed, remitted depressed, and control participants. *Cognitive Therapy and Research, 22,* 279–297.

Francis-Raniere, E. L., Alloy, L. B., & Abramson, L. Y. (2006). Depressive personality styles and bipolar spectrum disorders: Prospective tests of the event congruency hypothesis. *Bipolar Disorders, 8,* 382–399.

Fresco, D. M., Alloy, L. B., & Reilly-Harrington, N. (2006). Association of attributional style for negative and positive events and the occurrence of life events with depression and anxiety. *Journal of Social and Clinical Psychology, 25,* 1140–1159.

Fresco, D. M., Sampson, W. S., Craighead, L. W., & Koons, A. N. (2001). The relationship of sociotropy and autonomy to symptoms of depression and anxiety. *Journal of Cognitive Psychotherapy, 15,* 17–31.

Fulford, D., Johnson, S. L., Llabre, M. M., & Carver, C. S. (2010). Pushing and coasting in dynamic goal pursuit: Coasting is attenuated in bipolar disorder. *Psychological Science, 21,* 1021–1027.

Goldberg, J. F., Gerstein, R. K., Wenze, S. J., Welker, T. M., & Beck, A. T. (2008). Dysfunctional attitudes and cognitive schemas in bipolar manic and unipolar depressed outpatients: Implications for cognitively based psychotherapeutics. *Journal of Nervous and Mental Disease, 196,* 207–210.

Gotlib, I. H., & Joormann, J. (2010). Cognition and depression: Current status and future directions. *Annual Review of Clinical Psychology, 27,* 285–312.

Gray, J. A. (1994). Three fundamental emotion systems. In P. Eckman & R. J. Davidson (Eds.), *The nature of emotion: Fundamental questions* (pp. 243–247). New York: Oxford University Press.

Haber, S. N., & Knutson, B. (2010). The reward circuit: Linking primate anatomy and human imaging. *Neuropsychopharmacology Review, 35,* 4–26.

Haeffel, G. J. (2010). Cognitive vulnerability to depressive symptoms in college students: A comparison of traditional, weakest-link, and flexibility operationalizations. *Cognitive Therapy and Research, 34,* 92–98.

Haeffel, G. J., Abramson, L. Y., Voelz, Z. R., Metalsky, G. I., Halberstadt, L., Dykman, B. M., . . . Alloy, L. B. (2005). Negative cognitive styles, dysfunctional attitudes, and the remitted depression paradigm: A search for the elusive cognitive vulnerability to depression factor among remitted depressives. *Emotion, 5,* 343–348.

Hamlat, E. J., O'Garro-Moore, J. K., Nusslock, R., & Alloy, L. B. (2016). Assessment and treatment of bipolar spectrum disorders in emerging adulthood: Perspective from the behavioral approach system hypersensitivity model. *Cognitive and Behavioral Practice, 23,* 289–299.

Hammen, C. (1991). Generation of stress in the course of unipolar depression. *Journal of Abnormal Psychology, 100,* 555–561.

Hammen, C., Ellicott, A., & Gitlin, M. (1992). Stressors and sociotropy/autonomy: A longitudinal study of their relationship to the course of bipolar disorder. *Cognitive Therapy and Research, 16,* 409–418.

Hammen, C., Ellicott, A., Gitlin, M., & Jamison, K. (1989). Sociotropy/autonomy and vulnerability to specific life events in patients with unipolar depression and bipolar disorders. *Journal of Abnormal Psychology, 98,* 154–160.

Hankin, B. L., & Abramson, L. Y. (2001). Development of gender differences in depression: An elaborated cognitive vulnerability–transactional stress theory. *Psychological Bulletin, 127,* 773–796.

Hankin, B. L., Abramson, L. Y., Miller, N., & Haeffel, G. J. (2004). Cognitive vulnerability-stress theories of depression: Examining affective specificity in the prediction of depression versus anxiety in three prospective studies. *Cognitive Therapy and Research, 28,* 309–345.

Hankin, B. L., Lakdawalla, Z., Carter, I. L., Abela, J. R., & Adams, P. (2007). Are neuroticism, cognitive vulnerabilities and self-esteem overlapping or distinct risks for depression?: Evidence from exploratory and confirmatory factor analyses. *Journal of Social and Clinical Psychology, 26,* 29–63.

Hankin, B. L., Wetter, E., Cheely, C., & Oppenheimer, C. W. (2008). Beck's cognitive theory of depression in adolescence: Specific prediction of depressive symptoms and reciprocal influences in a multi-wave prospective study. *International Journal of Cognitive Therapy, 1,* 313–332.

Hawke, L. D., Provencher, M. D., & Parikh, S. V. (2013). Schema therapy for bipolar disorder: A conceptual model and future directions. *Journal of Affective Disorders, 148,* 118–122.

Hofmann, S. G., Asnaani, A., Vonk, I. J., Sawyer, A. T., & Fang, A. (2012). The efficacy of cognitive behavioral therapy: A review of meta-analyses. *Cognitive Therapy and Research, 36,* 427–440.

Hollon, S. D., & Beck, A. T. (1994). Cognitive and cognitive-behavioral therapies. In A. E. Bergin & S. L. Garfield (Eds.), *Handbook of psychotherapy and behavior change* (4th ed., pp. 428–466). Oxford, UK: Wiley.

Husky, M. M., Mazure, C. M., Maciejewski, P. K., & Swendsen, J. D. (2007). A daily life comparison of sociotropy–autonomy and hopelessness theories of depression. *Cognitive Therapy and Research, 31,* 659–676.

Iacoviello, B. M., Alloy, L. B., Abramson, L. Y., & Grant, D. (2009). Cognitive-personality characteristics impact the course of depression: A prospective test of sociotropy, autonomy, and domain-specific life events. *Cognitive Therapy and Research, 33,* 187–198.

Iacoviello, B. M., Alloy, L. B., Abramson, L. Y., Whitehouse, W. G., & Hogan, M. E. (2006). The course of depression in individuals at high and low cognitive risk for depression: A prospective study. *Journal of Affective Disorders, 93,* 61–69.

Ingram, R. E., Miranda, J., & Segal, Z. V. (1998). *Cognitive vulnerability to depression.* New York: Guilford Press.

Jabben, N., Arts, B., Jongen, E. M., Smulders, F. T., van Os, J., & Krabbendam, L. (2012). Cognitive processes and attitudes in bipolar disorder: A study into personality, dysfunctional attitudes and attention bias in patients with bipolar disorder and their relatives. *Journal of Affective Disorders, 143,* 265–268.

Jabben, N., de Jong, P. J., Kupka, R. W., Glashouwer, K. A., Nolen, W. A., & Penninx, B. W. J. H. (2014). Implicit and explicit self-associations in bipolar disorder: A comparison with healthy controls and unipolar depressive disorder. *Psychiatry Research, 215,* 329–334.

Johnson, S. L., Edge, M. D., Holmes, M. K., & Carver, C. S. (2012). The behavioral activation system and mania. *Annual Review of Clinical Psychology, 8,* 243–267.

Johnson, S. L., & Fingerhut, R. (2004). Cognitive styles predict the course of bipolar depression, not mania. *Journal of Cognitive Psychotherapy: An International Quarterly, 18,* 149–162.

Johnson, S. L., & Fulford, D. (2009). Preventing mania: A preliminary examination of the GOALS program. *Behavior Therapy, 40,* 103–113.

Johnson, S. L., Meyer, B., Winett, C., & Small, J. (2000). Social support and self-esteem predict changes in bipolar depression but not mania. *Journal of Affective Disorders, 58,* 79–86.

Johnson, S. L., & Roberts, J. E. (1995). Life events and bipolar disorder: Implications from biological theories. *Psychological Bulletin, 117,* 434–449.

Joiner, T. E., Jr., Metalsky, G. I., Lew, A., & Klocek, J. (1999). Testing the causal mediation component of Beck's theory of depression: Evidence for specific mediation. *Cognitive Therapy and Research, 23,* 401–412.

Just, N., Abramson, L. Y., & Alloy, L. B. (2001). Remitted depression studies as tests of the cognitive vulnerability hypotheses of depression onset: A critique and conceptual analysis. *Clinical Psychology Review, 21,* 63–83.

Lam, D., Hayward, P., Watkins, E. R., Wright, K., & Sham, P. (2005). Relapse prevention in patients with bipolar disorder: Cognitive therapy outcome after 2 years. *American Journal of Psychiatry, 162,* 324–329.

Lam, D., Watkins, E. R., Hayward, P., Bright, J., Wright, K., Kerr, N., . . . Sham, P. (2003). A randomized controlled study of cognitive therapy for relapse prevention for bipolar affective disorder: Outcome of the first year. *Archives of General Psychiatry, 60,* 145–152.

Lam, D., Wright, K., & Smith, N. (2004). Dysfunctional assumptions in bipolar disorder. *Journal of Affective Disorders, 79,* 193–199.

Lee, A., & Hankin, B. L. (2009). Insecure attachment, dysfunctional attitudes, and low self-esteem predicting prospective symptoms of depression and anxiety during adolescence. *Journal of Clinical Child and Adolescent Psychology, 38,* 219–231.

Lex, C., Hautzinger, M., & Meyer, T. D. (2011). Cognitive styles in hypomanic episodes of bipolar I disorder. *Bipolar Disorders, 13,* 355–364.

Liu, R. T. (2013). Stress generation: Future directions and clinical implications. *Clinical Psychology Review, 33,* 406–416.

Liu, R. T., Kleiman, E. M., Nestor, B. A., & Cheek, S. M. (2015). The hopelessness theory of depression: A quarter century in review. *Clinical Psychology: Science and Practice, 22,* 345–365.

Lozano, B. E., & Johnson, S. L. (2001). Can personality traits predict increases in manic and depressive symptoms? *Journal of Affective Disorders, 63,* 103–111.

Lyon, H. M., Startup, M., & Bentall, R. P. (1999). Social cognition and the manic defense: Attributions, selective attention, and self-schema in bipolar affective disorder. *Journal of Abnormal Psychology, 10,* 273–282.

Miklowitz, D. J., & Johnson, S. L. (2006). The psychopathology and treatment of bipolar disorder. *Annual Review of Clinical Psychology, 2,* 199–235.

Molz Adams, A., Shapero, B. G., Pendergast, L. H., Alloy, L. B., & Abramson, L. Y. (2014). Self-referent information processing in individuals with bipolar spectrum disorders. *Journal of Affective Disorders, 152,* 483–490.

Monroe, S. M., & Harkness, K. L. (2005). Life stress, the "kindling" hypothesis, and the recurrence of depression: Considerations from a life stress perspective. *Psychological Review, 112,* 417–445.

Nusslock, R., Abramson, L. Y., Harmon-Jones, E., Alloy, L. B., & Coan, J. A. (2009). Psychosocial interventions for bipolar disorder: Perspective from the Behavioral Approach System (BAS) dysregulation theory. *Clinical Psychology: Science and Practice, 16,* 449–469.

Nusslock, R., Shackman, A. J., Harmon-Jones, E., Alloy, L. B., Coan, J. A., & Abramson, L. Y. (2011). Cognitive vulnerability and frontal brain asymmetry: Common predictors of first prospective depressive episode. *Journal of Abnormal Psychology, 120,* 497–503.

Olinger, L. J., Kuiper, N. A., & Shaw, B. F. (1987). Dysfunctional attitudes and stressful life events: An interactive model of depression. *Cognitive Therapy and Research, 11,* 25–40.

Pavlickova, H., Varese, F., Turnbull, O., Scott, J., Morriss, R., Kinderman, P., . . . Bentall, R. P. (2013). Symptoms-specific self-referential cognitive processes in bipolar disorder: A longitudinal analysis. *Psychological Medicine, 43,* 1895–1907.

Persons, J. B., & Miranda, J. (1992). Cognitive theories of vulnerability to depression: Reconciling negative evidence. *Cognitive Therapy and Research, 16,* 485–502.

Peterson, C., Semmel, A., Von Baeyer, C., Abramson, L., Metalsky, G. I., & Seligman, M. E. P. (1982). The Attributional Style Questionnaire. *Cognitive Therapy and Research, 3,* 287–300.

Reilly, L. C., Ciesla, J. A., Felton, J. W., Weitlauf, A. S., & Anderson, N. L. (2012). Cognitive vulnerability to depression: A comparison of the weakest link, keystone and additive models. *Cognition and Emotion, 26,* 521–533.

Reilly-Harrington, N. A., Alloy, L. B., Fresco, D. M., & Whitehouse, W. G. (1999). Cognitive styles and life events interact to predict bipolar and unipolar symptomatology. *Journal of Abnormal Psychology, 108,* 567–578.

Romens, S. E., Abramson, L. Y., & Alloy, L. B. (2009). High and low cognitive risk for depression: Stability from late adolescence to early adulthood. *Cognitive Therapy and Research, 33,* 480–498.

Rosenfarb, I. S., Becker, J., Khan, A., & Mintz, J. (1998). Dependency and self-criticism in bipolar and unipolar depressed women. *British Journal of Clinical Psychology, 37,* 409–414.

Rubenstein, L. M., Freed, R. D., Shapero, B. G., Fauber, R. L., & Alloy, L. B. (2016). Cognitive attributions in depression: Bridging the gap between research and clinical practice. *Journal of Psychotherapy Integration, 26,* 103–115.

Scott, J., Colom, F., & Vieta, E. (2007). A meta-analysis of relapse rates with adjunctive psychological therapies compared to usual psychiatric treatment for bipolar disorders. *International Journal of Neuropsychopharmacology, 10,* 123–129.

Scott, J., Paykel, E., Morriss, R., Bentall, R., Kinderman, P., Johnson, T., . . . Hayhurst, H. (2006). Cognitive-behavioural therapy for severe and recurrent bipolar disorders: Randomised controlled trial. *British Journal of Psychiatry, 188,* 313–320.

Scott, J., & Pope, M. (2003). Cognitive styles in individuals with bipolar disorders. *Psychological Medicine, 33,* 1081–1088.

Scott, J., Stanton, B., Garland, A., & Ferrier, I. N. (2000). Cognitive vulnerability in patients with bipolar disorder. *Psychological Medicine, 30,* 467–472.

Seligman, M. E. P. (1975). *Helplessness: On depression, development, and death.* San Francisco: Freeman.

Shapero, B. G., Stange, J. P., Goldstein, K. E., Black, C. L., Molz, A. R., Hamlat, E. J., . . . Alloy, L. B. (2015). Cognitive styles in mood disorders: Discriminative ability of unipolar and bipolar cognitive profiles. *International Journal of Cognitive Therapy, 8,* 35–60.

Urosevic, S., Abramson, L. Y., Harmon-Jones, E., & Alloy, L. B. (2008). Dysregulation of the Behavioral Approach System (BAS) in bipolar spectrum disorders: Review of theory and evidence. *Clinical Psychology Review, 28,* 1188–1205.

Wisco, B. E., & Nolen-Hoeksema, S. (2008). Ruminative response style. In K. S. Dobson & D. J. Dozois (Eds.), *Risk factors in depression* (pp. 221–236). New York: Academic Press/Elsevier.

Wright, K., Lam, D., & Newsom-Davis, I. (2005). Induced mood change and dysfunctional attitudes in remitted bipolar I affective disorder. *Journal of Abnormal Psychology, 114,* 689–696.

Xiao, J., Qiu, Y., He, Y., Cui, L., Auerbach, R. P., McWhinnie, C. M., . . . Yao, S. (2016). "Weakest link" as a cognitive vulnerability within the hopelessness theory of depression in Chinese university students. *Stress and Health, 32,* 20–27.

Zuroff, D. C., Igreja, I., & Mongrain, M. (1990). Dysfunctional attitudes, dependency, and self-criticism as predictors of depressive mood states: A 12-month longitudinal study. *Cognitive Therapy and Research, 14,* 315–326.

CHAPTER 8

Cognitive Mediation of Symptom Change in Cognitive-Behavioral Therapy

A Review of the Evidence

Stefan G. Hofmann
Joseph K. Carpenter
Joshua Curtiss

Since Aaron T. Beck (1967) first identified the importance of maladaptive cognitions in individuals with depression, the cognitive model has become central to understanding the development and maintenance of numerous forms of psychopathology. The model states that dysfunctional cognitive schemas, or internal representations of stimuli, ideas, or experiences, can lead to biases in information processing and negative beliefs about the self and the world (Beck & Haigh, 2014). These cognitive biases and negative beliefs can cause a number of maladaptive behaviors and affective states that underlie psychological disorders. The cognitive model has been the basis for a wide array of cognitive-behavioral therapies (CBTs) that seek to modify maladaptive beliefs in order to treat psychological disorders by (Hofmann, Asmundson, & Beck, 2013). The theory of change underlying CBT, known as the cognitive mediation hypothesis, is that changes in beliefs or schemas about the self, others, or the world should account for the effect of treatment on symptom change (Clark & Beck,

2010). While CBT has consistently been shown to be highly efficacious (Hofmann, Asnaani, Vonk, Sawyer, & Fang, 2012; Hofmann & Smits, 2008), an explicit examination of the evidence for the cognitive mediation hypothesis is also needed. Examining whether cognitive change is in fact responsible for symptom improvement is important first because it helps to test and refine the cognitive model. Furthermore, testing the extent to which change in *different* belief domains accounts for changes in symptoms provides important information about which mechanisms are most relevant, thereby identifying the most promising targets for future treatment development (Kazdin, 2007).

CRITERIA FOR MEDIATION

Several important points should be considered when assessing the evidence for the cognitive mediation hypothesis. First, cognitive mediation does not require that explicit cognitive techniques be used (Hofmann, 2008a). Cognitive change can occur in response to a number of techniques, including behavioral approaches such as exposure therapy, which has even been suggested to be a form of cognitive intervention targeting beliefs related to the expectancy of harm (Hofmann, 2008b). Thus, evidence for cognitive mediation should be examined in a broad array of CBT treatments. Second, meaningful assessment of cognitive mediation requires proper identification and measurement of the beliefs and attitudes relevant to the condition being treated. While cognitive theory speaks generally to the importance of negative and threat-related appraisals, the specific target of these thoughts can vary by disorder. For instance, panic disorder is thought to be maintained by catastrophic thoughts about the potential harm of physical sensations of anxiety (Clark, 1986), whereas social anxiety disorder is characterized by fears of negative evaluation leading to social rejection (Clark & Wells, 1995; Hofmann, 2007). Even within a single disorder, different types of appraisals can be investigated. For instance, the impact of changes in appraisals regarding both the probability of negative outcomes and the cost of negative outcomes has been tested in social anxiety disorder (SAD; Smits, Rosenfield, McDonald, & Telch, 2006). Thus, cognitions should not be viewed as a single category; rather, careful attention should be paid to the types of cognitions being assessed and tested as potential mediators of symptom change.

Finally, assessing the evidence for cognitive mediation necessitates an operational definition for how mediation can be established. As described by Kraemer and colleagues (2001), mediation requires that (1) the mediator (e.g., cognitive change) be correlated with the independent variable (e.g., treatment), (2) the mediator partially or fully account for the effect of treatment on the outcome, and (3) the change in the mediator occur prior to change in the outcome. This last criterion, demonstrating temporal precedence, is particularly important as a way to demonstrate that changes in the mediator cause changes in the dependent variable, and are not simply correlated with the outcome (Kraemer, Wilson, Fairburn, & Agras, 2002). Doing so requires assessments at multiple time points throughout treatment, so that cognitive changes at an earlier point in treatment can be shown to account for subsequent symptom changes, while controlling for prior levels of symptom change (Cole & Maxwell, 2003)

Based on recommendations by Kazdin (2007), Smits, Julian, Rosenfield, and Powers (2012) outline several additional criteria that need to be met to establish cognitive mediation. First, rather than solely demonstrating that treatment is correlated with cognitive change, they emphasize that research should demonstrate that CBT *causes* changes in cognitions. This can be done by comparing the effect of CBT on cognitions in comparison to another treatment group within the context of a randomized trial. Importantly, the strength of such causal evidence is determined by the quality of the comparison group. Trials comparing CBT to a wait list control cannot rule out the possibility that changes in cognitions are due to nonspecific factors related to therapy like therapist contact or expectancies for change, so placebo controls or viable alternative treatments provide the strongest evidence.

Second, evidence for specificity of the impact of cognitive change on symptom change should be demonstrated. Because third variables may be responsible for mediational effects, it is important to test other plausible mediators. This could include variables such as depression or indices of extinction learning, or in the case of cognitive change, it may involve testing different types of cognitions to identify which belief domain is most important for symptom improvement. For instance, changes in beliefs about the catastrophic consequences of a panic attack and beliefs about one's ability to cope with panic have been simultaneously tested as mediators of symptom change in the treatment of panic disorder, as discussed later in this chapter (Fentz et al., 2013; Gallagher et al., 2013). Finally, reverse mediation, or the impact of symptom change on subsequent cognitive change, should also be investigated to establish whether this relationship is uni- or bidirectional.

While very few studies address all of these criteria, assessing the cumulative evidence for each across the existing literature can provide an estimate of how strongly current research supports the cognitive mediation hypothesis. The remainder of this chapter will be devoted to reviewing the evidence for these criteria in panic disorder (PD), social anxiety disorder (SAD), posttraumatic stress disorder (PTSD) obsessive–compulsive disorder (OCD), generalized anxiety disorder (GAD), and major depressive disorder (MDD), as these are emotional disorders for which the most research has been conducted. In addition, a discussion of the relevant domains of cognitions that have been theorized to mediate symptom change will be presented.

PANIC DISORDER

Theories on mechanisms of cognitive change in PD have proposed two related but distinct domains of beliefs (Casey, Oei, & Newcombe, 2004). Clark's (1986) cognitive model of panic proposes that catastrophic interpretations of the danger of certain bodily sensations are central to the disorder. According to this model, CBT for PD works to provide evidence to disconfirm such appraisals of danger, which reduces the intensity of the anxiety and panic response (Clark, 1999). Barlow's (2002) anxiety control theory, in contrast, proposes that an individual's perceived inability to cope with anxiety-related bodily sensations plays an important role in the development and maintenance of PD. Accordingly, Casey and colleagues (2004) proposed that the development of panic self-efficacy, or the belief that one can effectively cope with such bodily sensations, is a central cognitive mechanism of change.

A number of studies have tested cognitive change as a mediator of panic symptoms during treatment of PD. Specifically, Hofmann and colleagues (2007) and Smits, Powers, Cho, and Telch (2004) both found that pre–post changes in catastrophic cognitions mediated PD symptom change over the course of CBT. Moreover, the study by Hofmann et al. (2007) demonstrated such mediation to be present among patients in a CBT condition and not in a medication-only condition. In addition, Casey, Newcombe, and Oei (2005) tested pre–post changes in both catastrophic cognitions and self-efficacy beliefs as mediators of treatment outcome simultaneously and found that both significantly accounted for the impact of CBT on treatment outcome. In examining whether CBT leads to cognitive change, Fentz and colleagues (2014) identified nine randomized controlled trials comparing the effect of CBT on both catastrophic and panic self-efficacy beliefs to a wait list control. Meta-analytic results produced a between-groups effect size of Cohen's d = 1.46 for self-efficacy beliefs and Cohen's d = 1.25 for catastrophic beliefs. Notably, however, no studies were identified that showed superior cognitive change in CBT compared to an active treatment or placebo control.

A number of studies have provided rigorous tests of mediation that examine whether cognitive change accounts for *subsequent* change in panic symptoms. Teachman, Marker, and Clerkin (2010) demonstrated that changes in catastrophic misinterpretations during the course of CBT predicted subsequent changes in panic severity, panic attack frequency, distress, and avoidance behavior, whereas the reverse was not true. Fentz and colleagues (2013) examined changes in both catastrophic and self-efficacy beliefs within CBT treatment sessions and found that only changes in panic self-efficacy predicted panic symptoms the following week. The reverse was also true, however, suggesting a bidirectional relationship between panic self-efficacy and anxiety levels. In contrast, Gallagher and colleagues (2013) found that when examining intra-individual changes in cognitions between sessions, both catastrophic and self-efficacy beliefs simultaneously predicted subsequent changes in panic symptoms. In addition, results suggested that changes in catastrophic cognitions were greater early on in treatment, while self-efficacy beliefs changed more in the latter stages of treatment. It may be, then, that changes in beliefs about the ability to cope with panic symptoms occur most readily once the consequences of a panic attack are no longer seen as dangerous.

Together, these results generally show support for the cognitive mediation hypothesis in PD, and it seems that changes in both self-efficacy beliefs and catastrophic appraisals are important for reductions in panic symptoms. Demonstration that CBT leads to greater cognitive change than other plausible treatments, however, is lacking. In addition, no study to date has examined changes in other plausible mediators (e.g., depression, inhibitory learning) simultaneously with cognitions, leaving the possibility that other variables related to cognitive change are responsible for symptom change.

SOCIAL ANXIETY DISORDER

Cognitive models of SAD highlight how socially anxious individuals perceive there to be a high likelihood that they will behave in an inept or unacceptable manner in social situations, and also exaggerate the negative consequences of perceived social blunders (Clark & Wells, 1995; Hofmann, 2007). These biases, often referred to as the *cost bias* and *probability bias,* maintain social anxiety by leading to a hypervigilance to potential negative evaluation from others, and the subsequent use of safety behaviors or overt avoidance of social situations. CBT for SAD aims to demonstrate to patients that their predictions about the likelihood and cost of harm are exaggerated, thereby modifying such beliefs and leading to a reduction of fear in social situations (Hofmann, 2007). While cost and probability biases are viewed as central, other beliefs or appraisals are theorized to be relevant to the maintenance and treatment of SAD, including excessively high standards for social performance and negative beliefs about the self as strange, unattractive, or inadequate (Clark & Wells, 1995).

A number of treatment studies have shown that CBT leads to improvements in probability and cost biases, as well as other cognitive variables (Hofmann, 2004; Rapee, Gaston, & Abbott, 2009; Taylor & Alden, 2008). Rapee and colleagues (2009), for instance, found that an enhanced form of CBT that included social performance feedback and attention retraining led to greater reductions in cost of negative evaluation and negative views of one's skills and appearance compared to standard CBT and a stress management control. This is important because it demonstrates that the addition of techniques explicitly designed to target cognitive appraisals had specific effects on theoretically predicted belief domains compared to control conditions. Furthermore, changes in these cognitive variables were responsible for differences between the treatments on changes in social anxiety severity. Hofmann (2004) also examined changes in social cost estimates from pre- to posttreatment and found that such changes mediated reductions in social anxiety in CBT with and without explicit cognitive interventions. When examining changes in cost bias and probability bias simultaneously, however, Smits et al. (2006) found that only probability bias reductions accounted for symptom change and that changes in cost bias appeared to be a result of social anxiety symptom reduction.

Only two studies thus far have investigated the temporal precedence of cognitive change and symptom change in SAD. Calamaras, Tully, Tone, Price, and Anderson (2015) found results consistent with Smits et al. (2006) regarding the relative importance of probability bias compared to cost bias. When examining whether changes in cognitive variables from pre- to posttreatment accounted for changes in social anxiety symptoms, both probability and cost biases were found to be significant mediators. However when simultaneously examining whether changes in these biases from pre- to midtreatment predicted treatment outcome, only probability bias remained significant. The second study examining temporal precedence of cognitive change in social anxiety treatment was conducted by Hoffart, Borge, Sexton, and Clark (2009), and assessed weekly changes in social anxiety and a number of cognitive variables among patients receiving residential cognitive or interpersonal therapy. Results showed that four primary factors predicted subsequent changes in social anxiety, regardless of treatment received: changes in self-focus, estimated probability and cost of negative social events, and perceived acceptance by others. With the exception of perceived acceptance, anxiety reductions in turn predicted changes in the cognitive variables, suggesting a reciprocal relationship between cognitive and symptom change. Such a result shows that changes in beliefs and symptoms are mutually reinforcing. Patients who feel less socially anxious may find it easier to overcome their self-focused attention and biased beliefs about threat. Such changes in turn make it easier to feel less socially anxious.

In summary, there is substantial evidence that changes in cognitions related to the cost and probability of negative social outcomes account for symptom change in SAD, with some suggestion that probability biases are more important. However, more studies examining temporal precedence with closely spaced assessments (i.e., weekly) are needed.

GENERALIZED ANXIETY DISORDER

Contemporary conceptualizations of GAD posit that excessive and uncontrollable worry is a consequence of metacognitive beliefs (Wells, 1999, 2009) and contrast avoidance mechanisms (Newman & Llera, 2011). Furthermore, research supports worry as the core cognitive feature underlying GAD (Curtiss & Klemanski, 2015). In accord with the metacognitive model of GAD, two distinct cognitive mechanisms maintain prolonged worry: positive metacognitive beliefs and negative metacognitive beliefs. The positive class of metacognitive beliefs refers to underlying beliefs that worrying is a good problem-solving strategy that facilitates one's sense of preparedness. The negative class includes negative beliefs about the uncontrollability of worry and about its harmful or dangerous consequences. Although positive metacognitive beliefs might prompt an initial worry cycle, negative metacognitive beliefs about control and harm maintain clinical levels of anxiety over time. The metacognitive model hypothesizes that anxiety results from difficulty in controlling thinking rather than negative appraisals of the self and world. This model can be contrasted with the schema model of anxiety, which posits that underlying beliefs and assumptions about danger confer vulnerability to pathological anxiety (Beck & Haigh, 2014). Thus, the metacognitive model emphasizes beliefs about thoughts as opposed to beliefs about things (Wells, 2015).

The contrast avoidance model of GAD posits that individuals with GAD are particularly sensitive to abrupt changes from positive to negative emotions (Newman, Llera, Erickson, Przeworski, & Castonguay, 2013). To avoid negative emotional contrasts, individuals with GAD engage in worry to create a sustained period of emotional distress, thereby minimizing the emotional impact of negative life events. Research suggests that prior worrying makes individuals feel better able to cope with future stressors (Llera & Newman, 2010). The negative affect created by worry enables individuals to tolerate negative life events because they are able to avoid an abrupt contrast from a positive emotion to a negative emotion. In addition, intolerance of uncertainty (i.e., a dispositional tendency to fear future uncertainty) has been conceptualized as a relevant core belief contributing to worry in GAD (Dugas, Gagnon, Ladouceur, & Freeston, 1998).

Although several studies have demonstrated that CBT ameliorates worry symptoms and alters metacognitive beliefs throughout the course of treatment (Covin, Ouimet, Seeds, & Dozois, 2008; Wells & King, 2006; Wells et al., 2010; van der Heiden, Melchior, & de Stigter, 2012), only a small number of studies have investigated whether worry or metacognitive beliefs mediate treatment change. Donegan and Dugas (2012) examined whether reductions in worry mediated reductions in somatic anxiety among individuals with GAD who were randomly assigned to CBT or applied relaxation (AR). The authors demonstrated that reductions in worry accounted for subsequent change in somatic anxiety to a greater extent in CBT than in AR, which suggests that worry may be a cognitive mechanism that is more specifically targeted by CBT than other active interventions. A reverse mediation model revealed that change in somatic anxiety also accounts for change in worry, providing evidence of bidirectionality. Bomyea and colleagues (2015) found a unidirectional relationship between intolerance of uncertainty and worry over the course of treatment, such that changes in intolerance of uncertainty accounted for subsequent changes in worry, whereas the reverse relationship was not found. Another study by McEvoy, Erceg-Hurn, Anderson, Campbell, and Nathan (2015) examined whether changes in repetitive negative thinking, a transdiagnostic construct that reflects such processes as worry and rumination, mediated the effect of metacognitive beliefs on symptom reduction in CBT. Using pre- to postchange scores, the authors found evidence that repetitive negative thinking mediated the effect of negative metacognitions, but not that of positive metacognitions, on symptom reduction.

Overall, these studies provide some initial support that worry-related processes and intolerance of uncertainty might be cognitive mechanisms of change in CBT; however, no evidence exists suggesting that metacognitive beliefs or contrast avoidance mechanisms mediate treatment change. These constructs have been primarily studied in the context of basic psychopathology research. Furthermore, only two studies attempted to statistically address temporal precedence (Donegan & Dugas, 2012; Bomyea et al., 2015), and alternative cognitive mechanisms have yet to be examined. It would be beneficial for future research to investigate other cognitive mechanisms that are theoretically relevant (e.g., metacognitions) with sufficiently rigorous analytic techniques that better establish temporal precedence of the mediator.

POSTTRAUMATIC STRESS DISORDER

The predominant theory for understanding the development, maintenance, and effective treatment of PTSD is emotional processing theory (EPT; Foa, Huppert, & Cahill, 2006; Foa & Kozak, 1986), which emphasizes negative cognitions about the self (e.g., "I am a weak person"), others (e.g., "people can't be trusted"), and the world ("the world is a dangerous place") as being central to PTSD. Ehlers and Clark (2000) elaborate on this model by arguing that such cognitions have the effect of creating a sense of current threat as a result of past trauma. For instance, individuals who develop PTSD might believe that the fact that the trauma happened means that they are not currently safe or that because they are experiencing emotional numbing symptoms, they will never be able to relate to people again. These beliefs about the existence of a current threat also lead to a number of maladaptive behavioral and cognitive ways of coping. For example, individuals with PTSD often believe that they will have a nervous breakdown if they think about or go to the site of the trauma; therefore, they avoid such trauma reminders. In addition, assimilated beliefs such as denial and self-blame are often implicated in PTSD (Resick & Schnicke, 1992; Resick, Williams, Suvak, Monson, & Gradus, 2012). Effective treatment for PTSD occurs when such beliefs are disconfirmed through revisiting the trauma memory and/or cognitive challenging procedures, allowing patients to rebuild beliefs about the safety of the world and their own sense of worth.

A number of studies have demonstrated that CBT for PTSD leads to decreases in negative cognitions. Foa and Rausch (2004) found that CBT consisting of prolonged exposure therapy was associated with reductions in negative beliefs about the self, world, and others, and that such changes were correlated with symptom improvement. No differences in these results were found for patients who received just prolonged exposure compared to those who received prolonged exposure plus cognitive restructuring. Similar changes in negative cognitions, as indicated by patient narratives about the impact of trauma on their lives before and after treatment, were seen in a study on cognitive processing therapy (Sobel, Resick, & Rabalais, 2009). Again, these changes in cognitions were correlated with symptom reductions. Furthermore, a study on children and adolescents with PTSD found that CBT led to significant reductions in trauma-related cognitions compared to a wait list control, and such reductions partially mediated the effect of treatment on PTSD symptom improvement (Smith et al., 2007).

More recently, several studies have examined the temporal precedence of cognitive change relative to PTSD symptom change. Kleim and colleagues (2013) showed that week-to-week changes in negative trauma-related appraisals accounted for subsequent reductions in symptom scores over the course of cognitive therapy for PTSD, whereas the reverse effect of symptom change on appraisals was not found. Similarly, Zalta and colleagues (2014) found that changes in session-to-session PTSD-related cognitions drove subsequent changes in PTSD and depression among a sample of assault survivors receiving prolonged prolonged exposure (PE) therapy. Reverse mediation in this study was not statistically significant. Finally, McLean, Yeh, Rosenfield, and Foa (2015) also replicated these results with PE among adolescent sexual abuse survivors, finding that changes in trauma-related cognitions accounted for subsequent PTSD symptom change. Of note, similar results were seen among adolescents who received client-centered therapy in this study, though mediation effects were significantly larger in PE.

These consistent results provide substantial evidence for the cognitive mediation hypothesis in PTSD treatment, and the evidence suggests that such results hold for both behaviorally and cognitively focused treatments. However, alternative mediators have not been tested to establish specificity of the negative cognitions as a mediator of symptom change. In addition, few studies have compared cognitive change in CBT with a non-CBT treatment, and one study that did so (McLean, Su, & Foa, 2015) also found cognitive mediation to be present in an alternative treatment.

OBSESSIVE–COMPULSIVE DISORDER

Cognitive theories of OCD emphasize beliefs related to (1) inflated responsibility and overestimation of threat, (2) overimportance of thoughts and importance of controlling one's thoughts, and (3) intolerance of uncertainty and perfectionism as playing a fundamental role in the development and maintenance of the disorder (OCCWG, 2005). Modifying these belief systems is seen as central to the reduction of OCD symptoms from a cognitive therapy perspective (Wilhelm & Steketee, 2006). Emotional processing theory (EPT; Foa et al., 2006; Foa & Kozak, 1986), which underlies behaviorally focused treatment of OCD, emphasizes a related but distinct set of beliefs. Specifically, EPT states that beliefs related to a patient's obsessions about the probability of harm (e.g., I will definitely get sick if I touch that doorknob), the cost of harm (e.g., being sick will ruin everything), and the persistence of anxiety (e.g., I will feel anxious forever if I don't wash my hands) should be modified in order for symptom reduction to occur.

Several studies have shown that CBT for OCD leads to a reduction in obsessive beliefs (Anholt et al., 2010; Solem, Håland, Vogel, Hansen, & Wells, 2009) and that such changes are associated with OCD symptom improvement (Adams, Riemann, Wetterneck, & Cisler, 2012; Emmelkamp, van Oppen, & van Balkom, 2002; Whittal, Thordarson, & McLean, 2005). While these studies encompass both behavioral and cognitive treatments, they did not compare CBT's impact on obsessive beliefs in comparison to other treatments in order to assess the effect of CBT specifically (as opposed to treatment generally) on cognitive change.

Several recent studies have specifically addressed the question of mediation, with varying results. Wilhelm, Berman, Keshaviah, Schwartz, and Steketee (2015) found that changes in obsessive beliefs about perfectionism and certainty predicted subsequent OCD symptom change over the course of cognitive therapy. In a study by Woody, Whittal, and McLean (2011), however, weekly change in obsessive symptoms was found to mediate subsequent change in cognitions (i.e., reverse mediation), but the reverse was not found. Olatunji et al. (2013) similarly found unexpected results when examining whether cognitive changes accounted for subsequent OCD improvements. Specifically, when simultaneously examining changes in depression and obsessive beliefs as mediators, only reductions in depression significantly predicted subsequent OCD improvement. These null results of the impact of cognitive change were replicated by Su, Carpenter, Zandberg, Simpson, and Foa (2016). Of note, both Olatunji et al. (2013) and Su et al. (2016) found that when testing whether changes in cognitions accounted for concurrent changes in OCD symptoms, significant mediational effects were found. When examining temporal precedence of cognitions as a mediator of subsequent symptom improvement, however, such effects were reduced to nonsignificance, highlighting the risk of relying on pre–post changes in cognitions and symptoms.

Together these results show limited support for the cognitive mediation hypothesis in OCD. Notably, the studies by Woody et al. (2011), Olatunji et al. (2013), and Su et al. (2016) each examined varying types of obsessive beliefs (e.g., beliefs about responsibility, appraisals of personal significance of obsessions, intolerance of uncertainty, among others) within different forms of CBT (i.e., cognitive therapy and exposure and response prevention [EX/RP]). Thus, null findings with regard to cognitive change and reduction in OCD symptoms do not appear to be exclusive to certain belief types or therapies.

MAJOR DEPRESSIVE DISORDER

The seminal cognitive model of MDD emphasizes that negative beliefs about the self, world, and future (e.g., "No one likes me," "I am a failure") underlie the disorder (Beck, 1967; Clark & Beck, 2010; Hofmann, et al., 2013). These beliefs form schemas that cause information processing to be biased toward negative self-referential information, thus perpetuating low mood and automatic negative thinking. In the recent formulation of the cognitive model (i.e., the generic cognitive model), Beck and Haigh (2014) consider cognitive beliefs and schemas in the context of *modes*. Modes refer to a network of cognitive, affective, motivational, and behavioral systems that orchestrate goal-oriented behavior. Beck and Haigh (2014) postulate that modes actuate behavior by invoking cognitive schemas that contain a set of beliefs relevant to the goal. For example, the *self-expansive* mode is concerned with the enhancement of personal resources or value of an individual. A number of cognitive schemas and beliefs (e.g., "If I accomplish this goal, then I will be happy and of value") are associated with the self-expansive mode. Aberrations in the self-expansive mode and recurrent negative life events, in which valued life-goals are thwarted, can contribute to the development of MDD. CBT techniques such as cognitive restructuring are designed to help patients challenge the accuracy of such maladaptive schemas, and generate more positive and realistic alternative beliefs (Clark & Beck, 2010).

Although a number of studies have suggested that CBT ameliorates maladaptive cognitions, there is also evidence that pharmacotherapy does so as well, which could indicate that changes in cognition are not a treatment-specific outcome (Driessen & Hollon, 2010). Examination of temporal patterns of change and mediational pathways revealed that early changes in cognition precede changes in depression symptoms in CBT but not pharmacotherapy (DeRubeis et al., 1990). Teasdale and colleagues (2001) found evidence that a particular type of maladaptive cognition (i.e., dichotomous thinking style) mediated the treatment efficacy of CBT. Furthermore, another study demonstrated that changes in negative automatic thoughts function as a mediator of CBT in reducing depressive symptoms among adolescents with MDD (Kaufman, Rohde, Seeley, Clark, & Stice, 2005).

Warmerdam, van Straten, Jongsma, Twisk, and Cuijpers (2010) investigated a multiple mediation model using multilevel modeling to determine which mediators accounted for symptom improvement. The results indicated that changes in worrying, perceptions of control, and negative problem orientation all mediated treatment improvement in CBT and problem-solving therapy. This suggests that no single cognitive mechanism accounts for the reduction of depressive symptoms in MDD and also that these mechanisms may not be unique to a single treatment. Indeed, additional research has replicated findings that the same cognitive mechanisms underlie different interventions. A study by Forman et al. (2012) demonstrated that changes in cognitive defusion and dysfunctional thinking mediated reductions in depressive symptoms in both CBT and acceptance and commitment therapy (ACT).

Collectively, these studies afford support for the cognitive mediation hypothesis in MDD; however, there is limited evidence of temporal precedence such that changes in cognitions precede changes in depressive symptoms. In a review of the causal relationship between cognitive change and depressive symptom change, Lorenzo-Luaces, German, and DeRubeis (2015) concluded that the direction of causality has not been well established. Thus, more substantial evidence for the cognitive mediation hypothesis will necessitate further investigation of the directionality of the relationship between cognition change and symptom reduction, as well as consideration of alternative mechanisms.

CONCLUSIONS

This chapter reviewed the evidence for the hypothesis that changes in cognitions are a driving mechanism of symptom change in CBT for anxiety and depression. Following criteria put forth by Kraemer et al. (2001) and expanded by Smits and colleagues (2012), research was examined for evidence of (1) statistical mediation of cognitions on symptom change, (2) the effect of CBT on cognitive change, (3) temporal precedence of cognitive change on symptom change, and (4) specificity of cognitive change on symptoms. Based on the first three criteria, substantial support of cognitive mediation was found for PD, SAD, and PTSD. For GAD and MDD, initial evidence exists but is less conclusive, whereas for OCD the evidence is weakest.

A notable gap in the literature for nearly all disorders was research testing the specificity of cognitive change treatment outcomes when controlling for other plausible mediators aside from cognitive change. Relatedly, greater clarity regarding the types of cognitions most important for symptom change is an important direction for future research. For instance, in OCD, it is possible that the weak evidence for cognitive mediation is the result of not having properly identified the most relevant cognitions. Similarly, in GAD and MDD, there was less consistency in the types of cognitive measures and belief domains investigated. Finally, few studies tested whether cognitive mediation was greater for CBT than alternative treatments. This leaves open the possibility that changes in beliefs and their subsequent impact on symptoms are a result of general features of psychological treatments, rather than a feature unique to CBT. In spite of these gaps in the literature, cognitive theories of symptom change in anxiety and depression have received substantial support. This promising area for future research is of great theoretical and clinical importance.

REFERENCES

Adams, T. J., Riemann, B. C., Wetterneck, C. T., & Cisler, J. M. (2012). Obsessive beliefs predict cognitive behavior therapy outcome for obsessive compulsive disorder. *Cognitive Behaviour Therapy, 41,* 203–211.

Anholt, G. A., van Oppen, P., Cath, D. C., Emmelkamp, P. G., Smit, J. H., & van Balkom, A. M. (2010). Sensitivity to change of the Obsessive Beliefs Questionnaire. *Clinical Psychology and Psychotherapy, 17,* 154–159.

Barlow, D. H. (2002). *Anxiety and its disorders: The nature and treatment of anxiety and panic.* New York: Guilford Press.

Beck, A. T. (1967). *Depression: Causes and treatment.* Philadelphia: University of Pennsylvania Press.

Beck, A. T., & Haigh, E. A. (2014). Advances in cognitive theory and therapy: The generic cognitive model. *Annual Review of Clinical Psychology, 10,* 1–24.

Bomyea, J., Ramsawh, H., Ball, T. M., Taylor, C. T., Paulus, M. P., Lang, A. J., & Stein, M. B. (2015). Intolerance of uncertainty as a mediator of reductions in worry in a cognitive behavioral treatment program for generalized anxiety disorder. *Journal of Anxiety Disorders, 33,* 90–94.

Calamaras, M. R., Tully, E. C., Tone, E. B., Price, M., & Anderson, P. L. (2015). Evaluating changes in judgmental biases as mechanisms of cognitive-behavioral therapy for social anxiety disorder. *Behaviour Research and Therapy, 71,* 139–149.

Casey, L. M., Newcombe, P. A., & Oei, T. P. (2005). Cognitive mediation of panic severity: The role of catastrophic misinterpretation of bodily sensations and panic self-efficacy. *Cognitive Therapy and Research, 29,* 187–200.

Casey, L. M., Oei, T. P., & Newcombe, P. A. (2004). An integrated cognitive model of panic disorder: The role of positive and negative cognitions. *Clinical Psychology Review, 24,* 529–555.

Clark, D. A., & Beck, A. T. (2010). Cognitive theory and therapy of anxiety and depression: Convergence with neurobiological findings. *Trends in Cognitive Sciences, 14,* 418–424.

Clark, D. M. (1986). A cognitive approach to panic. *Behaviour Research and Therapy, 24,* 461–470.

Clark, D. M. (1999). Anxiety disorders: Why they persist and how to treat them. *Behaviour Research and Therapy, 37,* S5–S27.

Clark, D. M., & Wells, A. (1995). A cognitive model of social phobia. In R. G. Heimberg, M. R. Liebowitz, D. A. Hope, F. R. Schneier, R. G. Heimberg, M. R. Liebowitz, . . . F. R. Schneier (Eds.), *Social phobia: Diagnosis, assessment, and treatment* (pp. 69–93). New York: Guilford Press.

Cole, D. A., & Maxwell, S. E. (2003). Testing mediational models with longitudinal data: Questions and tips in the use of structural equation modeling. *Journal of Abnormal Psychology, 112,* 558–577.

Covin, R., Ouimet, A. J., Seeds, P. M., & Dozois, D. J. (2008). A meta-analysis of CBT for pathological worry among clients with GAD. *Journal of Anxiety Disorders, 22,* 108–116.

Curtiss, J., & Klemanski, D. H. (2015). Identifying individuals with generalized anxiety disorder: A receiver operator characteristic analysis of theoretically relevant measures. *Behaviour Change, 32,* 255–272.

DeRubeis, R. J., Evans, M. D., Hollon, S. D., Garvey, M. J., Grove, W. M., & Tuason, V. B. (1990). How does cognitive therapy work? Cognitive change and symptom change in cognitive therapy and pharmacotherapy for depression. *Journal of Consulting and Clinical Psychology, 58,* 862–869.

Donegan, E., & Dugas, M. J. (2012). Generalized anxiety disorder: A comparison of symptom change in adults receiving cognitive-behavioral therapy or applied relaxation. *Journal of Consulting and Clinical Psychology, 80,* 490–496.

Driessen, E., & Hollon, S. D. (2010). Cognitive behavioral therapy for mood disorders: Efficacy, moderators and mediators. *Psychiatric Clinics of North America, 33,* 537–555.

Dugas, M. J., Gagnon, F., Ladouceur, R., & Freeston, M. H. (1998). Generalized anxiety disorder: A preliminary test of a conceptual model. *Behaviour Research and Therapy, 36,* 215–226.

Ehlers, A., & Clark, D. M. (2000). A cognitive model of posttraumatic stress disorder. *Behaviour Research and Therapy, 38,* 319–345.

Emmelkamp, P. G., van Oppen, P., & van Balkom, A. M. (2002). Cognitive changes in patients with obsessive compulsive rituals treated with exposure in vivo and response prevention. In R. O. Frost, G. Steketee, R. O. Frost, & G. Steketee (Eds.) , *Cognitive approaches to obsessions and compulsions: Theory, assessment, and treatment* (pp. 391–401). Amsterdam, Netherlands: Pergamon/Elsevier Science.

Fentz, H. N., Arendt, M., O'Toole, M. S., Hoffart, A., & Hougaard, E. (2014). The mediational role of panic self-efficacy in cognitive behavioral therapy for panic disorder: A systematic review and meta-analysis. *Behaviour Research and Therapy, 60,* 23–33.

Fentz, H. N., Hoffart, A., Jensen, M. B., Arendt, M., O'Toole, M. S., Rosenberg, N. K., & Hougaard, E. (2013). Mechanisms of change in cognitive behaviour therapy for panic disorder: The role of panic self-efficacy and catastrophic misinterpretations. *Behaviour Research and Therapy, 51,* 579–587.

Foa, E. B., Huppert, J. D., & Cahill, S. P. (2006). Emotional processing theory: An update. In B. O. Rothbaum & B. O. Rothbaum (Eds.), *Pathological anxiety: Emotional processing in etiology and treatment* (pp. 3–24). New York: Guilford Press.

Foa, E. B., & Kozak, M. J. (1986). Emotional processing of fear: Exposure to corrective information. *Psychological Bulletin, 99,* 20–35.

Foa, E. B., & Rauch, S. A. (2004). Cognitive changes during prolonged exposure versus prolonged exposure plus cognitive restructuring in female assault survivors with posttraumatic stress disorder. *Journal of Consulting and Clinical Psychology, 72,* 879.

Forman, E. M., Chapman, J. E., Herbert, J. D., Goetter, E. M., Yuen, E. K., & Moitra, E. (2012). Using session-by-session measurement to compare mechanisms of action for acceptance and commitment therapy and cognitive therapy. *Behavior Therapy, 43,* 341–354.

Gallagher, M. W., Payne, L. A., White, K. S., Shear, K. M., Woods, S. W., Gorman, J. M., & Barlow, D. H. (2013). Mechanisms of change in cognitive behavioral therapy for panic disorder: The unique effects of self-efficacy and anxiety sensitivity. *Behaviour Research and Therapy, 51,* 767–777.

Hoffart, A., Borge, F. M., Sexton, H., & Clark, D. M. (2009). Change processes in residential cognitive and interpersonal psychotherapy for social phobia: A process-outcome study. *Behavior Therapy, 40,* 10–22.

Hofmann, S. G. (2004). Cognitive mediation of treatment change in social phobia. *Journal of Consulting and Clinical Psychology, 72,* 392–399.

Hofmann, S. G. (2007). Cognitive factors that maintain social anxiety disorder: A comprehensive model and its treatment implications. *Cognitive Behaviour Therapy, 36,* 193–209.

Hofmann, S. G. (2008a). Common misconceptions about cognitive mediation of treatment change: A commentary to Longmore and Worrell (2007). *Clinical Psychology Review, 28,* 67–70.

Hofmann, S. G. (2008b). Cognitive processes during fear acquisition and extinction in animals and humans: Implications for exposure therapy of anxiety disorders. *Clinical Psychology Review, 28,* 199–210.

Hofmann, S. G., Asmundson, G. J., & Beck, A. T. (2013). The science of cognitive therapy. *Behavior Therapy, 44,* 199–212.

Hofmann, S. G., Asnaani, A., Vonk, I. J., Sawyer, A. T., & Fang, A. (2012). The efficacy of cognitive behavioral therapy: A review of meta-analyses. *Cognitive Therapy and Research, 36,* 427–440.

Hofmann, S. G., Meuret, A. E., Rosenfield, D., Suvak, M. K., Barlow, D. H., Gorman, J. M., . . . Woods, S. W. (2007). Preliminary evidence for cognitive mediation during cognitive-behavioral therapy of panic disorder. *Journal of Consulting and Clinical Psychology, 75,* 374–379.

Hofmann, S. G., & Smits, J. A. (2008). Cognitive-behavioral therapy for adult anxiety disorders: A meta-analysis of randomized placebo-controlled trials. *Journal of Clinical Psychiatry, 69,* 621–632.

Kaufman, N. K., Rohde, P., Seeley, J. R., Clarke, G. N., & Stice, E. (2005). Potential mediators of cognitive-behavioral therapy for adolescents with comorbid major depression and conduct disorder. *Journal of Consulting and Clinical Psychology, 73,* 38–46.

Kazdin, A. E. (2007). Mediators and mechanisms of change in psychotherapy research. *Annual Review of Clinical Psychology, 3,* 1–27.

Kleim, B., Grey, N., Wild, J., Nussbeck, F. W., Stott, R., Hackmann, A., . . . Ehlers, A. (2013). Cognitive change predicts symptom reduction with cognitive therapy for posttraumatic stress disorder. *Journal of Consulting and Clinical Psychology, 81,* 383–393.

Kraemer, H. C., Stice, E., Kazdin, A., Offord, D., & Kupfer, D. (2001). How do risk factors work together? Mediators, moderators, and independent, overlapping, and proxy risk factors. *American Journal of Psychiatry, 158,* 848–856.

Kraemer, H. C., Wilson, G. T., Fairburn, C. G., & Agras, W. S. (2002). Mediators and moderators of treatment effects in randomized clinical trials. *Archives of General Psychiatry, 59,* 877–883.

Llera, S. J., & Newman, M. G. (2010). Effects of worry on physiological and subjective reactivity to emotional stimuli in generalized anxiety disorder and nonanxious control participants. *Emotion, 10,* 640–650.

Lorenzo-Luaces, L., German, R. E., & DeRubeis, R. J. (2015). It's complicated: The relation between cognitive change procedures, cognitive change, and symptom change in cognitive therapy for depression. *Clinical Psychology Review, 41,* 3–15.

McEvoy, P. M., Erceg-Hurn, D. M., Anderson, R. A., Campbell, B. N., & Nathan, P. R. (2015). Mechanisms of change during group metacognitive therapy for repetitive negative thinking in primary and non-primary generalized anxiety disorder. *Journal of Anxiety Disorders, 35,* 19–26.

McLean, C. P., Su, Y., & Foa, E. B. (2015). Mechanisms of symptom reduction in a combined treatment for comorbid posttraumatic stress disorder and alcohol dependence. *Journal of Consulting and Clinical Psychology, 83,* 655–661.

McLean, C. P., Yeh, R., Rosenfield, D., & Foa, E. B. (2015). Changes in negative cognitions mediate PTSD symptom reductions during client-centered therapy and prolonged exposure for adolescents. *Behaviour Research and Therapy, 68,* 64–69.

Newman, M. G., & Llera, S. J. (2011). A novel theory of experiential avoidance in generalized anxiety disorder: A review and synthesis of research supporting a contrast avoidance model of worry. *Clinical Psychology Review, 31,* 371–382.

Newman, M. G., Llera, S. J., Erickson, T. M., Przeworski, A., & Castonguay, L. G. (2013). Worry and generalized anxiety disorder: A review and theoretical synthesis of evidence on nature, etiology, mechanisms, and treatment. *Annual Review of Clinical Psychology, 9,* 275–297.

Obsessive Compulsive Cognitions Working Group (OCCWG). (2005). Psychometric validation of the Obsessive Belief Questionnaire and Interpretation of Intrusions Inventory—Part 2: Factor analyses and testing of a brief version. *Behaviour Research and Therapy, 43,* 1527–1542.

Olatunji, B. O., Rosenfield, D., Tart, C. D., Cottraux, J., Powers, M. B., & Smits, J. A. (2013). Behavioral versus cognitive treatment of obsessive–compulsive disorder: An examination of outcome and mediators of change. *Journal of Consulting and Clinical Psychology, 81,* 415–428.

Rapee, R. M., Gaston, J. E., & Abbott, M. J. (2009). Testing the efficacy of theoretically derived improvements in the treatment of social phobia. *Journal of Consulting and Clinical Psychology, 77,* 317–327.

Resick, P. A., & Schnicke, M. K. (1992). Cognitive processing therapy for sexual assault victims. *Journal of Consulting and Clinical Psychology, 60,* 748–756.

Resick, P. A., Williams, L. F., Suvak, M. K., Monson, C. M., & Gradus, J. L. (2012). Long-term outcomes of cognitive-behavioral treatments for posttraumatic stress disorder among female rape survivors. *Journal of Consulting and Clinical Psychology, 80,* 201–210.

Smith, P., Yule, W., Perrin, S., Tranah, T., Dalgleish, T., & Clark, D. M. (2007). Cognitive-behavioral therapy for PTSD in children and adolescents: A preliminary randomized controlled trial. *Journal of the American Academy of Child and Adolescent Psychiatry, 46,* 1051–1061.

Smits, J. A., Julian, K., Rosenfield, D., & Powers, M. B. (2012). Threat reappraisal as a mediator of symptom change in cognitive-behavioral treatment of anxiety disorders: A systematic review. *Journal of Consulting and Clinical Psychology, 80,* 624–635.

Smits, J. A., Powers, M. B., Cho, Y., & Telch, M. J. (2004). Mechanism of change in cognitive-behavioral treatment of panic disorder: Evidence for the fear of fear mediational hypothesis. *Journal of Consulting and Clinical Psychology, 72,* 646–652.

Smits, J. A., Rosenfield, D., McDonald, R., & Telch, M. J. (2006). Cognitive mechanisms of social anxiety reduction: An examination of specificity and temporality. *Journal of Consulting and Clinical Psychology, 74,* 1203–1212.

Sobel, A. A., Resick, P. A., & Rabalais, A. E. (2009). The effect of cognitive processing therapy on cognitions: Impact statement coding. *Journal of Traumatic Stress, 22,* 205–211.

Solem, S., Håland, Å. T., Vogel, P. A., Hansen, B., & Wells, A. (2009). Change in metacognitions predicts outcome in obsessive–compulsive disorder patients undergoing treatment with exposure and response prevention. *Behaviour Research and Therapy, 47,* 301–307.

Su, Y., Carpenter, J. K., Zandberg, L. J., Simpson, H. B., & Foa, E. B. (2016). Cognitive mediation of exposure and ritual prevention outcome in obsessive compulsive disorder. *Behavior Therapy, 47,* 474–486.

Taylor, C. T., & Alden, L. E. (2008). Self-related and interpersonal judgment biases in social anxiety disorder: Changes during treatment and relationship to outcome. *International Journal of Cognitive Therapy, 1,* 125–137.

Teachman, B. A., Marker, C. D., & Clerkin, E. M. (2010). Catastrophic misinterpretations as a predictor of symptom change during treatment for panic disorder. *Journal of Consulting and Clinical Psychology, 78,* 964–973.

Teasdale, J. D., Scott, J., Moore, R. G., Hayhurst, H., Pope, M., & Paykel, E. S. (2001). How does cognitive therapy prevent relapse in residual depression? Evidence from a controlled trial. *Journal of Consulting and Clinical Psychology, 69,* 347–357.

van der Heiden, C., Melchior, K., & de Stigter, E. (2013). The effectiveness of group metacognitive therapy for generalised anxiety disorder: A pilot study. *Journal of Contemporary Psychotherapy, 43,* 151–157.

van der Heiden, C., Muris, P., & van der Molen, H. T. (2012). Randomized controlled trial on the effectiveness of metacognitive therapy and intolerance-of-uncertainty therapy for generalized anxiety disorder. *Behaviour Research and Therapy, 50,* 100–109.

Warmerdam, L., van Straten, A., Jongsma, J., Twisk, J., & Cuijpers, P. (2010). Online cognitive behavioral therapy and problem-solving therapy for depressive symptoms: Exploring mechanisms of change. *Journal of Behavior Therapy and Experimental Psychiatry, 41,* 64–70.

Wells, A. (1999). A metacognitive model and therapy for generalized anxiety disorder. *Clinical Psychology and Psychotherapy, 6,* 86–95.

Wells, A. (2009). *Metacognitive therapy for anxiety and depression.* New York: Guilford Press.

Wells, A. (2015). Cognitive and metacognitive therapy case formulation in anxiety disorders. In N. Tarrier & J. Johnson (Eds.), *Case formulation in cognitive behavioral therapy: The treatment of challenging and complex cases* (pp. 90–118). New York: Routledge.

Wells, A., & King, P. (2006). Metacognitive therapy for generalized anxiety disorder: An open trial. *Journal of Behavior Therapy and Experimental Psychiatry, 37,* 206–212.

Wells, A., Welford, M., King, P., Papageorgiou, C., Wisely, J., & Mendel, E. (2010). A pilot randomized trial of metacognitive therapy vs. applied relaxation in the treatment of adults with generalized anxiety disorder. *Behaviour Research and Therapy, 48,* 429–434.

Whittal, M. L., Thordarson, D. S., & McLean, P. D. (2005). Treatment of obsessive–compulsive disorder: Cognitive behavior therapy vs. exposure and response prevention. *Behaviour Research and Therapy, 43,* 1559–1576.

Wilhelm, S., Berman, N. C., Keshaviah, A., Schwartz, R. A., & Steketee, G. (2015). Mechanisms of change in cognitive therapy for obsessive compulsive disorder: Role of maladaptive beliefs and schemas. *Behaviour Research and Therapy, 65,* 5–10.

Wilhelm, S., & Steketee, G. (2006). *Cognitive therapy for obsessive-compulsive disorder: A guide for professionals.* Oakland, CA: New Harbinger Publications.

Woody, S. R., Whittal, M. L., & McLean, P. D. (2011). Mechanisms of symptom reduction intreatment for obsessions. *Journal of Consulting and Clinical Psychology, 79,* 653–664.

Zalta, A. K., Gillihan, S. J., Fisher, A. J., Mintz, J., McLean, C. P., Yehuda, R., & Foa, E. B. (2014). Change in negative cognitions associated with PTSD predicts symptom reduction in prolonged exposure. *Journal of Consulting and Clinical Psychology, 82,* 171–175.

CHAPTER 9

Mental Imagery in Cognitive Therapy

Research and Examples of Imagery-Focused Emotion, Cognition, and Behavior Change

Fritz Renner
Emily A. Holmes

INTRODUCTION: IMAGERY IN PSYCHOPATHOLOGY—FROM BECK'S EARLY DAYS TO A RESURGENCE OF SCIENTIFIC RESEARCH

Beck defined cognitive therapy as a "set of operations focused on a patient's cognitions (verbal or pictorial) and on the premises, assumptions, and attitudes underlying these cognitions" (A. T. Beck, 1970, p. 347). Despite Beck's recognition that dysfunctional cognitions can take the form of mental images (i.e., "pictorial" cognitions) as well as verbal thoughts, until recently mental imagery and its clinical applications within a CBT framework were relatively underresearched. In this chapter, we aim to define what is meant by mental imagery in a clinical context, using examples from our group; discuss research establishing the strong relation between mental imagery and emotions; review recent developments in imagery-focused CBT; and consider future research directions for CBT treatment innovation using imagery.

Mental imagery is a perceptual-like experience in the absence of sensory input, which is often described as "seeing with the mind's eye; hearing with the mind's ear and so on" (Kosslyn, Ganis, & Thompson, 2001). Perceptual information recalled from memory gives rise to mental imagery, allowing us to reexperience the past and preexperience the future. Mental imagery can be voluntary (i.e., be conjured up deliberately) or involuntary (i.e., spring to mind unbidden) and can occur in all sensory modalities from vision to hearing. In the context of psychopathology, mental imagery has most extensively been studied in the visual domain.

Intrusive imagery occurs across a range of mental disorders and was described early on by Beck. For example, Beck described a student with "anxiety neurosis" suffering from intrusive visual imagery of "several people telling her they hate her; then they leave, she is alone" (A. T. Beck, Laude, & Bohnert, 1974, p. 322). Table 9.1 provides a selected overview of different areas of psychopathology in which intrusive imagery occurs and examples of imagery content from our group. Although it is now clear that mental imagery plays an important role across a range of mental disorders (Holmes, Blackwell, Burnett Heyes, Renner, & Raes, 2016; Holmes &

TABLE 9.1. Examples of Intrusive Images across Psychopathologies

Psychopathology	Example of image content	Reference
Agoraphobia	"On a tube train and it stops. Trying not to show fear, but being terrified. Looking at other people's shoes and feet. Having inner fear. Train stopping. Carriages closing in around. Seeing myself and how I look. Things closing in on me."	Day, Holmes, & Hackmann (2004, p. 423)
Depression	" . . . scenes of past childhood physical or sexual assault and images of humiliation (e.g., being bullied at school), failure (e.g., being sacked from work), and overwhelming sadness (e.g., losing a loved one)."	Holmes, Blackwell, et al. (2016, p. 254)
Mania in bipolar disorder	"Ideas for children's picture book. Publishing it and becoming a huge overnight success."	Ivins, Di Simplicio, Close, Goodwin, & Holmes (2014, p. 237)
PTSD	"Mugger put knife to my neck."	Holmes, Grey, & Young (2005, p. 9)
Suicidality	"My family identifying my body, which has gun-shot wounds. My face is ashen-coloured."	Hales, Deeprose, Goodwin, & Holmes (2011, p. 656)

Mathews, 2010), its therapeutic application is ripe for further development and innovation.

In his early work, Beck described the potential therapeutic benefit of exploring clients' images (dream images): By "moving from the verbal to the visual, we have automatic thoughts—spontaneous daydreams—drug induced hallucinations—dreams" (A. T Beck, 2002, p. 27). Despite these early ideas of the role of mental images in psychopathology and its treatment, CBT models have typically focused on verbal processes such as negative automatic (verbal) thoughts and rumination rather than the therapeutic application of mental imagery. This may be for a variety of reasons, from therapists' reluctance to probe mental imagery with patients (Bell, Mackie, & Bennett-Levy, 2014) to the ease of teaching and training on verbal methods, negative automatic thoughts diaries and so forth.

In the last decade, the advancement of new research methods to study internal processes such as mental imagery has led to a resurgence of interest in mental imagery. One area of science in which advancements in methodology have contributed to a better understanding of mental imagery is neuroscience. Brain-imaging studies have shown that the brain structures that underlie mental imagery resemble the same structures of those that underlie actual perception (Kosslyn et al., 2001; Pearson, Naselaris, Holmes, & Kosslyn, 2015). For example, visual mental imagery relies on the same areas in the visual cortex than actual visual perception (Kosslyn et al., 2001). Similarly, motor imagery relies on many of the same brain areas that are involved in actual movement control (Kosslyn et al., 2001). Consistent and robust findings from the neuroimaging literature like this have led to the conclusion that mental imagery can indeed be considered as weak perception, that is, a mental representation resembling features of actual sensory perception (Pearson et al., 2015). For example, visual features of visual imagery such as brightness of the image have a similar effect on pupil constriction as does the brightness of an image that is actually perceived from an external stimulus (Laeng & Sulutvedt, 2013). Given that mental imagery relies on the same brain areas as actual perception, thereby mimicking real-life perceptual events, it is likely that imagery can have a powerful impact on our emotions and behavior just as actual perception does.

RESEARCH INVESTIGATING MENTAL IMAGERY, EMOTION, AND BEHAVIOR

Mental Imagery and Emotions

Does mental imagery have a special impact on emotion? Although it has long been assumed that mental imagery can have an "emotion-enhancing" effect, until recently relatively little empirical evidence was available to support this idea. Early ideas about the role of imagery in emotion within a psychotherapy context were formulated by Beck, who described several case-examples of situations in which imagery-based cognitions drive negative emotions: For example, there is a situation in which "the report of an automobile accident stimulates a pictorial image in which the patient himself is the victim. . . . The image then leads to anxiety" or there is a student who "discovered that his fear of leaving his dormitory at night was triggered by visual fantasies of being attacked" (A. T. Beck, 1970, p. 348).

Early experimental work on the role of imagery in emotion conducted by Peter J. Lang (1979) confirmed the validity of these clinical case-examples by showing that the mental imagery of emotional content elicits emotional responses at neurophysiological and subjective levels (for a recent review of Lang's work on emotional imagery, see Ji, Burnett Heyes, MacLeod, & Holmes, 2016). Despite this pioneering early work, it was only recently that a series of behavioral experiments have comprehensively studied the relationship between imagery and emotions and compared imagery-processing modes with verbal processing of the same material. This research program has greatly enhanced our understanding of the impact of mental imagery on emotion and has shown that mental imagery can have an "emotion-enhancing" effect. We will briefly review a selected sample of these studies here. For further reviews, see, for example, Holmes and Mathews (2010) and Pictet and Holmes (2013).

Experimental studies directly contrasting the processing of emotional information in a mental imagery versus verbal mode have confirmed that mental imagery of emotional content elicits stronger emotion than verbal processing of the same content (Holmes, Lang, & Shah, 2009; Holmes & Mathews, 2005; Holmes, Mathews, Dalgleish, & Mackintosh, 2006). For example, in Experiment I in Holmes and Mathews (2005), participants were instructed to imagine unpleasant events (imagery condition) or to listen to the same materials while focusing on the words and their meaning (verbal condition). Imagery of the unpleasant events resulted in more self-reported anxiety than did verbal processing of the same material (Holmes & Mathews, 2005). In line with this finding are results showing that emotional memories have more perceptual features than nonemotional memories (Arntz, de Groot, & Kindt, 2005). The special relationship between mental imagery and emotion has also been demonstrated in the context of psychopathology. For example, in social phobia, it has been shown that holding a negative self-image in mind, compared to a less negative self-image, evokes greater anxiety (self-reported and observer-reported) (Hirsch, Clark, Mathews, & Williams, 2003).

Importantly, this "emotional amplifier" effect of mental imagery also works for *positive* emotions (e.g., Holmes et al., 2006). These effects of positive mental imagery seem to persist in the short term and protect against mood deterioration following a negative mood induction, an effect that has been described as a "*cognitive vaccine*" for depressed mood (Holmes et al.,

2009). Positive future imagery has also been shown to reinstate positive affect/mood following a negative mood induction, compared to imagery of a typical day (Renner, Schwarz, Peters, & Huibers, 2014). The "emotional amplifier" effect of mental imagery also extended to an evaluative conditioning paradigm in which ambiguous pictures are paired with words that can make them positive or negative (Holmes, Mathews, Mackintosh, & Dalgleish, 2008). Demonstrating that the "emotional amplifier" effect of mental imagery can be established with different experimental paradigms speaks to the robustness of this effect.

Studies investigating the relationship between mental imagery and emotion have advanced our understanding of the phenomenology of imagery across a range of mental disorders and led to the development of clinical applications targeting imagery directly or indirectly to change cognitive and emotional dysfunctional processes across a range of mental disorders (discussed later in the Clinical Applications section). In summary, there is now compelling evidence that mental imagery not only has a powerful impact on emotional processing, but a more powerful impact than does verbal thought. These findings should be harnessed to improve cognitive-behavioral therapy (CBT) and develop new applications of the cognitive model.

Mental Imagery and Behavior

One area of functioning that has not been explored substantially in relation to mental imagery and mental health is *behavior*. In this section, we present a selected overview of studies on the relation between mental imagery of behavioral activities across a range of adaptive and maladaptive behaviors. Findings from these studies could have implications for the use of imagery interventions to target behavioral aspects of psychopathology. A number of studies in nonclinical samples have shown that engaging in mental imagery of a future behavior can influence actual behavior across a range of behaviors. For example, Chan and Cameron (2012) compared the effects of four different imagery interventions involving the repeated imagery of engaging in physical activities on intentions to engage in physical activities and actual frequency of subsequent physical activities. The authors found that particularly approach-related mental imagery (imagery of achieving a desired goal such as being a physically active person) led to increased intentions to be physically active and increased physical activity levels. Other studies have focused on imagery interventions to increase consumption of healthy food (Knäuper et al., 2011), voting behavior (Libby, Shaeffer, Eibach, & Slemmer, 2007), sleeping behavior (Loft & Cameron, 2013), or dental health-related behaviors (Uskul & Kikutani, 2014) and found that imagery interventions have the potential to increase engagement in the targeted behaviors. These studies suggest that mental imagery might also have a "motivational amplifier" effect by increasing engagement in behavioral activities.

Does the processing mode (imagery vs. verbal) matter when the aim is to increase engagement in target activities? Studies on the relation between mental imagery and emotions, reviewed earlier, have shown that the processing mode (mental imagery vs. verbal processing) is critical in enhancing either positive or negative emotions (e.g., Holmes et al., 2009; Holmes & Mathews, 2005; Holmes et al., 2006). Similarly, when the goal is to influence future behavioral activities, studies contrasting mental imagery with verbal processing have demonstrated that mental imagery has a stronger impact on behavior. For example, the mental imagery of experiencing the benefits of a cable TV service compared to reading about (verbal processing) the benefits of the same service led participants to subscribe to the service more often (Gregory, Cialdini, & Carpenter, 1982).

What can we learn from the studies reviewed here for helping us understand psychopathology and enhance its treatment? These studies suggest that mental imagery of engaging in behavioral activities can have a "motivational amplifier" effect by increasing engagement in the imagined activities. Increased engagement in specific behavioral activities is an important treatment goal across a range of psychological disorders. Findings from these studies could therefore be applied to psychopathology where the aim is to increase behavioral engagement.

CLINICAL APPLICATIONS

Basic laboratory- based research on the relation between mental imagery and emotion has informed clinical applications across a range of different forms of psychopathology. These imagery interventions can be roughly divided into two categories: (1) imagery interventions used in cognitive therapy as traditionally delivered with a therapist, and (2) imagery interventions used in recent "therapist-free" (computerized) imagery-based applications directly targeting specific processes underlying psychopathology with, for example, technology. Here we provide a brief overview of both the more traditional role of imagery interventions used in cognitive therapy and recent branches as well as imagery interventions as used in recent developments targeting dysfunctional emotional and cognitive processes directly using computerized training programs.

Mental Imagery and the Cognitive Model

As discussed, Beck described the importance of *identifying* and *modifying* imagery (A. T. Beck, 1970; A. T. Beck & Emery, 1985; Singer, 2006). This has led to a variety of imagery-related developments within CBT and recent CBT-related approaches. Hackmann, Bennett-Levy, and Holmes (2011) provide a detailed clinical guide of imagery techniques in cognitive therapy. Here we review some recent developments in CBT for imagery assessment and imagery modification using examples from our group as illustrations.

Identifying Imagery: Imagery Assessment

Given the powerful impact of mental imagery on emotions, it can be useful to assess mental imagery across different forms of psychopathology. That is, we should specifically probe for imagery-based cognitions in addition to assessment of verbal thoughts due to their clinical utility. Different methods can be used to assess mental imagery, ranging from pen-and-paper measures of imagery experience to qualitative methods such as interviews (for a review, see Hales et al., 2015).

Mental imagery is a core component of cognitive therapy. Patients may experience negative automatic thoughts as mental images (A. T. Beck & Emery, 1985), and techniques to identify "imaginal" automatic thoughts in cognitive therapy have been described (J. S. Beck, 1995). This includes educating patients about imagery and trying to elicit spontaneous images or inducing images in session (J. S. Beck, 1995). For example, some patients might report difficulties in identifying images, or they might be reluctant to engage in imagery in the case of distressing images. In these instances, it can be useful, for example, to induce less distressing imagery first to help the patient increase his or her awareness of what is meant by mental imagery (J. S. Beck, 1995). The importance of assessment and formulation of problematic imagery has also been highlighted for social phobia and PTSD (Clark & Wells, 1995; Ehlers & Clark, 2000). We suggest, and going back to Beck's early writing, that assessment of imagery should be a standard part of all clinical assessment across the spectrum of mental disorders (Hales et al., 2015) including PTSD, social phobia, depression, agoraphobia, OCD, bipolar disorder, psychosis, and so forth. Following this approach, assessment of imagery-based cognitions involves several steps, including an imagery micro-formulation (see Figure 9.1) guiding assessment and "mapping out" the imagery content.

Modifying Imagery: Imagery Techniques in CBT

Following detailed assessment of problematic imagery, imagery-based techniques can be used to intervene with the problematic imagery. Techniques to identify and modify imagery are a core part of cognitive therapy and are often used to reduce distress associated with the imagery. Examples include guiding patients through imagery and introducing coping strategies in the imagined scene or reimagining distressing images and changing the

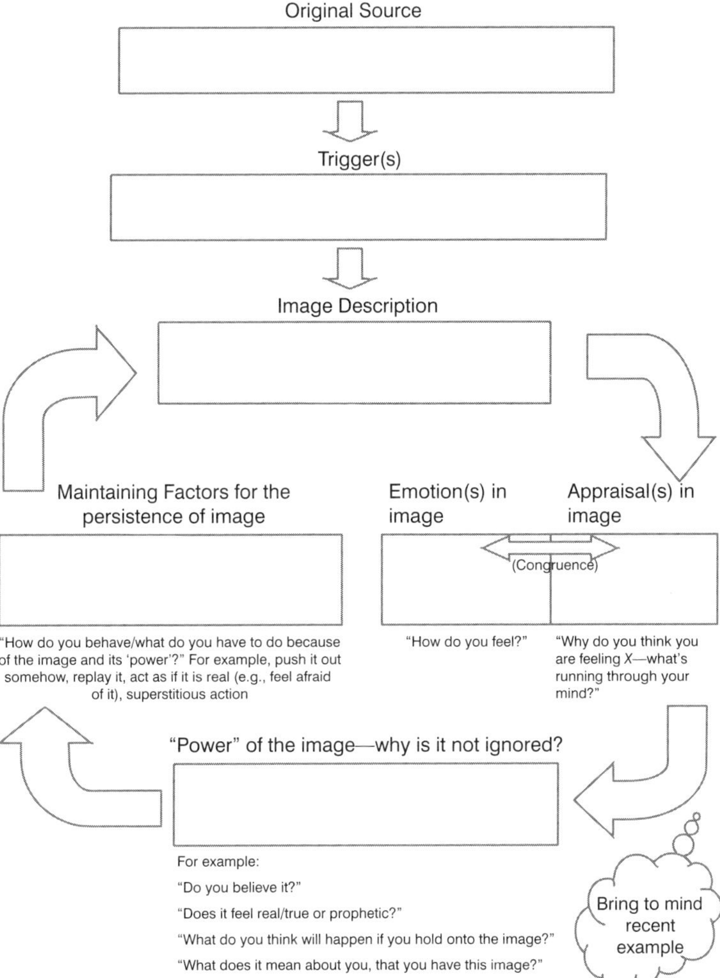

FIGURE 9.1. Imagery micro-formulation: a template that can be used collaboratively with clients across a wide spectrum of possible disorders.

(negative) ending of the image by replacing it either with a realistic positive ending or with a "magical" positive image (J. S. Beck, 1995). Many of the CBT techniques that are used with verbal cognitions can also be used to address imagery-based cognitions. For example, using Socratic questioning, evidence for and against imagery content can be used in the same way as it would be used for verbal dysfunctional thoughts (J. S. Beck, 1995). For example, what do you know now that you didn't know then (i.e., the time you are having the image / the time the event in the image originally occurred); what would you advise a friend who was imagining something similar? (Padesky, 1993). Imagery-based cognitions might also be tested out via behavioral experiments in the same way as verbal cognitions—for example, testing out the question of whether mental images are real. If you imagine something (specify in detail), does it then become true? Other examples of imagery applications in CBT include systematic desensitization and imaginal exposure, for example, by repeatedly imagining approaching a feared object (e.g., spider) until anxiety decreases.

Interestingly, mental imagery also plays a prominent role in modern branches of CBT such as schema therapy (Young, Klosko, & Weishaar, 2003), where imagery rescripting is used to transform emotional experiences associated with early traumatic experiences, for example, by rescripting the negative outcome of traumatic experiences with more adaptive outcomes. This imagery-focused approach has been shown to be effective in the treatment of personality disorders (Jacob & Arntz, 2013), and evidence for treating chronic forms of depression is emerging (Malogiannis et al., 2014; Renner, Arntz, Leeuw, & Huibers, 2013; Renner, Arntz, Peeters, Lobbestael, & Huibers, 2016). Imagery rescripting has also been shown to be effective as a stand-alone intervention across a range of psychological disorders , such as PTSD, simple phobia, and depression(for a review, see Arntz, 2012).

Another example of where an imagery focus in cognitive therapy has contributed to treatment innovation is in the psychological treatment of bipolar disorder. People with bipolar disorder show high rates of emotional mental imagery (Hales, Deeprose, Goodwin, & Holmes, 2011; Holmes et al., 2011; Ivins, Di Simplicio, Close, Goodwin, & Holmes, 2014) The Mood Action Psychology Program (MAPP) is an imagery-based cognitive therapy protocol consisting of an imagery assessment phase, an active treatment phase in which techniques such as imagery rescripting are used to dampen the emotional impact of intrusive imagery, and a consolidation phase focused on learning and recall of treatment techniques. In a recent case-series, eleven of fourteen patients with bipolar disorder had improved mood stability following treatment with MAPP (Holmes, Bonsall, et al., 2016).

In summary, imagery-based techniques to assess and modify dysfunctional cognitions in the context of CBT were traditionally part of CBT and still play a prominent role in modern branches of CBT. While some imagery-based techniques are established components of cognitive-behavioral treatments, the effectiveness of some of the more recent developments needs to be further tested in randomized controlled trials. At the same time, laboratory-based research on processes underlying psychopathology and the development of new imagery-based techniques to target these processes can contribute to the evolution of CBT by further informing potential clinical applications emerging from the cognitive model.

From the Lab to the Clinic: Cognitive Science Informed Emotional Imagery Techniques

Another route through which laboratory-based research has contributed to imagery-based treatment innovation is through the identification of mechanisms underlying current treatments and the development of innovative, direct ways to target them (Holmes, Craske, & Graybiel, 2014). Emotional mental imagery plays a role in different forms of psychopathology (for reviews, see Brewin, Gregory, Lipton, & Burgess, 2010; Holmes, Blackwell, et al., 2016; Holmes & Mathews, 2010): Vivid and intrusive images of traumatic events that pop to mind involuntarily are the hallmark symptom of PTSD. Individuals with depression may experience low levels of positive prospective imagery (Holmes & Coughtrey, 2008) and an excess of negative imagery-based memories (Patel et al., 2007). People with social phobia might experience imagery of the self being embarrassed in social situations, and imagery dysfunction has been reported for generalized anxiety disorder (Hirsch, Hayes, Mathews, Perman, & Borkovec, 2012). Other areas of psychopathology where imagery dysfunction plays a role is bipolar disorder (Ivins et al., 2014; Ng, Di Simplicio, & Holmes, 2015) and suicidality (Hales et al., 2011; Ng, Di Simplicio, McManus, Kennerley, & Holmes, 2015).

Based on the findings from laboratory-based experimental studies on the relationship between imagery and emotion, a number of interventions have been developed targeting various forms of imagery dysfunction via computerized training programs. Imagery interventions include interrupting the formation of unwanted intrusive imagery formation in trauma-related disorders such as PTSD (James et al., 2016). A full-review of these "therapist-free" (i.e., psychological interventions without a therapist) clinical applications is beyond the scope of this chapter, and here we focus on interventions that have been designed to increase positive imagery in the context of depression.

Focusing on the "C" in CBT: Imagery and Cognitive Biases

One example of an imagery-based training program to target cognitive biases is a procedure called cognitive bias modification (CBM). In one version of this program, participants are asked to form specific mental images of each of a series of auditory-presented ambiguous scenarios that resolve in a positive way. Following a general instruction in using mental imagery, participants listen to a set of scenarios that are initially ambiguous but then resolve in a positive way. An example of such a scenario is "You are sitting waiting to go into a job interview. As you go through, you feel a wave of *confidence*" (positive resolution in italics; Blackwell et al., 2015). Approximately one hundred scenes are imagined.

Variations of the general imagery CBM procedure just described have been tested as a potential intervention in individuals with depression (Blackwell & Holmes, 2010; T. J. Lang, Blackwell, Harmer, Davison, & Holmes, 2012; Torkan et al., 2014). Following these smaller studies, Blackwell et al. (2015) conducted a clinical trial in which they randomized 150 individuals with depression to either a four-week positive imagery CBM intervention or an active control intervention. The two interventions did not differ with regard to overall improvement in depressive symptoms (the primary outcome). However, post-hoc analyses revealed greater improvements specifically in *anhedonia* (i.e., a diminished interest or pleasure in activities) for those in the positive imagery CBM condition, compared to controls. This suggests that the positive imagery intervention might have effects on specific aspects of dysfunction in depression (Blackwell et al., 2015). The finding of greater improvements in anhedonia in the positive imagery CBM condition has since been replicated (Williams et al., 2015). Future developments in this area might involve further tailoring the interventions to specific areas of dysfunction such as anhedonia (Blackwell et al., 2015).

Focusing on the "B" in CBT: Imagery and Behavior

The imagery-based CBM intervention reviewed earlier has focused on dysfunctional *cognitions* (interpretation bias) and *emotional* aspects of psychopathology (lack of positive imagery). Another important aspect of dysfunction across a range of psychological disorders is *behavior*. In cognitive therapy, behavioral techniques such as behavioral experiments are used to challenge or test dysfunctional beliefs and assumptions. In addition, in the treatment of depression, behavioral activation might be used to help individuals engage in potentially rewarding experiences early on in treatment before cognitive interventions are used (Martell, Addis, & Jacobson, 2001; Rush & Beck, 1978). Mental imagery may help individuals increase engagement in specific behavioral activities (Holmes, Blackwell, et al., 2016; Renner, Ji, Pictet, Holmes, & Blackwell, 2017).

Studies investigating imagery behavior relationships come from diverse fields stretching from consumer psychology to social and clinical psychology. One potential clinical application might be by stimulating engagement in potentially rewarding experiences through mental imagery. This idea is not new: Lazarus (1968) noted that getting clients to imagine engaging in pleasurable activities in the future could lift their depression and that the clients for whom this technique works were those who "were able to picture vivid images" (Lazarus, 1968, p. 87). Although Beck in the 1960s was impressed by these ideas and pointed out ways in which his theory could be extended to visual thoughts such as imagery of pleasurable activities described above (Letters from Beck to Lazarus 1967 cited in Rosner, 2002, p. 15), imagery of potentially behavioral activities with the aim of increasing engagement in those activities is not currently a treatment technique used in cognitive-behavioral therapies. As we will argue, an imagery focus on the behavioral aspects of psychopathology is highly complementary with CBT and its behavioral variant, Behavioral Activation (Martell et al., 2001; Martell, Dimidjian, & Herman-Dunn, 2010). Thus, one way forward in this field could be to focus on the "B" in CBT and explore applications of mental imagery for behavioral aspects of psychopathology and its treatment within a CBT context.

One approach in this direction is functional imagery training (Kavanagh, Andrade, & May, 2005). This training is an imagery-based motivational intervention, based on the elaborated intrusion theory of desire (Kavanagh et al., 2005), delivered in a client-centered counseling format. Functional imagery training has been found to reduce snacking by focusing on positive goals, thereby both increasing the motivation to snack less and by reducing snacking behavior (Andrade, Khalil, Dickson, May, & Kavanagh, 2016).

Another approach is to focus on positive imagery in response to ambiguous training scenarios. In the context of psychopathology, few studies have investigated the relation between the mental imagery of behaviors and engagement in behavioral activities. One study showed that dysphoric participants who were instructed to generate positive imagery performed better on a behavioral task (catching fishes in a fishing game) than those who were instructed to generate negative or both positive and negative imagery (Pictet, Coughtrey, Mathews, & Holmes, 2011).

In another study that used data from a randomized controlled trial (Blackwell et al., 2015), it has been shown that participants with depression who engaged in repeated positive imagery of future events, reported increased behavioral activation at the end of the four-week intervention compared to an active nonimagery control condition (Renner, Ji, et al., 2017). Such findings suggest that the effects of mental imagery on behavior could be harnessed to develop clinical applications that promote engagement in adaptive behaviors across a range of mental health problems such as depression.

CONCLUSIONS

Beck's early recognition of the role of imagery in cognitive therapy is now becoming more integrated in CBT. Although from the very beginning cognitive therapy has recognized the importance of mental imagery in psychopathology and its treatment, until recently mental imagery and its clinical applications within a CBT framework have been underresearched. With methodological advancement of the study of internal processes such as imagery (e.g., modern brain-imaging techniques), a return of interest in mental imagery and its clinical applications has occurred in the last decades. This has led to modern imagery-focused adaptions of cognitive therapy that add new treatment techniques to the CBT toolbox. A parallel development is the idea that specific mechanisms underlying different forms of psychopathology can be targeted directly through imagery-based training programs. Although both of these innovative developments need further empirical testing, it is clear that mental imagery can play a prominent and diverse role in modern innovations in cognitive therapy.

While it is now clear that mental imagery plays an important role across a wide range of mental disorders (Brewin et al., 2010; Holmes, Blackwell, et al., 2016; Holmes & Mathews, 2010), its therapeutic application is ripe for further development and innovation. One potentially important area that has been underresearched in this context is the development of imagery procedures to support engagement in adaptive behaviors. Such an approach is highly compatible with the focus on behavioral techniques used in CBT. By combining basic research in mental imagery with its clinical application, future research in this field will open up possibilities for clinical applications targeting behavioral aspects of psychopathology either in a traditional therapy setting or via computerized training programs as adjunct to traditional cognitive therapy.

ACKNOWLEDGMENTS

F. Renner is supported by a Marie Sklodowska-Curie individual Fellowship from the European Union. E. A. Holmes is supported by the Karolinskan Institutet (Stockholm, Sweden) and the Lupine Foundation. We are grateful for comments on this chapter from our colleague Simon Blackwell.

REFERENCES

Andrade, J., Khalil, M., Dickson, J., May, J., & Kavanagh, D. J. (2016). Functional imagery training to reduce snacking: Testing a novel motivational intervention based on elaborated intrusion theory. *Appetite, 100*, 256–262.

Arntz, A. (2012). Imagery rescripting as a therapeutic technique: Review of clinical trials, basic studies, and research agenda. *Journal of Experimental Psychopathology, 3*, 121–126.

Arntz, A., de Groot, C., & Kindt, M. (2005). Emotional memory is perceptual. *Journal of Behavior Therapy and Experimental Psychiatry, 36*(1), 19–34.

Beck, A. T. (1970). Cognitive therapy: Nature and relation to behavior therapy. *Behavior Therapy, 1*(2), 184–200.

Beck, A. T. (2002). Cognitive patterns in dreams and daydreams. *Journal of Cognitive Psychotherapy, 16*(1), 23–28.

Beck, A. T., & Emery, G. (1985). *Anxiety disorders and phobias: A cognitive perspective.* New York: Basic Books.

Beck, A. T., Laude, R., & Bohnert, M. (1974). Ideational components of anxiety neurosis. *Archives of General Psychiatry, 31*(3), 319–325.

Beck, J. S. (1995). *Cognitive therapy: Basics and beyond.* New York: Guilford Press.

Bell, T., Mackie, L., & Bennett-Levy, J. (2014). "Venturing towards the dark side": The use of imagery interventions by recently qualified cognitive-behavioural therapists. *Clinical Psychology and Psychotherapy, 22*(6), 591–603.

Blackwell, S. E., Browning, M., Mathews, A., Pictet, A., Welch, J., Davies, J., . . . Holmes, E. A. (2015). Positive imagery-based cognitive bias modification as a web-based treatment tool for depressed adults: A randomized controlled trial. *Clinical Psychological Science, 3*(1), 91–111.

Blackwell, S. E., & Holmes, E. A. (2010). Modifying interpretation and imagination in clinical depression: A single case series using cognitive bias modification. *Applied Cognitive Psychology, 24*(3), 338–350.

Brewin, C. R., Gregory, J. D., Lipton, M., & Burgess, N. (2010). Intrusive images in psychological disorders: Chararcteristics, neural mechanisms, and treatment implications. *Psychological Review, 117*(1), 210–232.

Chan, C. K. Y., & Cameron, L. D. (2012). Promoting physical activity with goal-oriented mental imagery: A randomized controlled trial. *Journal of Behavioral Medicine, 35*(3), 347–363.

Clark, D. M., & Wells, A. (1995). A cognitive model of social phobia. In R. G. Heimberg, M. Liebowitz, D. Hope, & F. Schneier (Eds.), *Social phobia: Diagnosis, assement and treatment* (pp. 69–93). New York: Guilford Press.

Day, S. J., Holmes, E. A., & Hackmann, A. (2004). Occurrence of imagery and its link with early memories in agoraphobia. *Memory, 12*(4), 416–427.

Ehlers, A., & Clark, D. M. (2000). A cognitive model of posttraumatic stress disorder. *Behaviour Research and Therapy, 38*(4), 319–345.

Gregory, W. L., Cialdini, R. B., & Carpenter, K. M. (1982). Self-relevant scenarios as mediators of likelihood Estimates and Compliance—Does imagining make it so. *Journal of Personality and Social Psychology, 43*(1), 89–99.

Hackmann, A., Bennett-Levy, J., & Holmes, E. A. (2011). *Oxford guide to imagery in cognitive therapy.* Oxford, UK: Oxford University Press.

Hales, S. A., Blackwell, S. E., Di Simplicio, M., Iyadurai, L., Young, K., & Holmes, E. A. (2015). Imagery-based cognitive-behavioral assessment. In G. P. Brown & D. A. Clark (Eds.), *Assessment in cognitive therapy* (pp. 69–93). New York: Guilford Press.

Hales, S. A., Deeprose, C., Goodwin, G. M., & Holmes, E. A. (2011). Cognitions in bipolar disorder versus unipolar depression: Imagining suicide. *Bipolar Disorders, 13*(7–8), 651–661.

Hirsch, C. R., Clark, D. M., Mathews, A., & Williams, R. (2003). Self-images play a causal role in social phobia. *Behaviour Research and Therapy, 41*(8), 909–921.

Hirsch, C. R., Hayes, S., Mathews, A., Perman, G., & Borkovec, T. (2012). The extent and nature of imagery during worry and positive thinking in generalized anxiety disorder. *Journal of Abnormal Psychology, 121*(1), 238–243.

Holmes, E. A., Blackwell, S. E., Burnett Heyes, S., Renner, F., & Raes, F. (2016). Mental imagery in depression: Phenomenology, potential mechanisms, and treatment implications. *Annual Review of Clinical Psychology, 12,* 249–280.

Holmes, E. A., Bonsall, M. B., Hales, S. A., Mitchell, H., Renner, F., Blackwell, S. E., . . . Di Simplicio, M. (2016). Applications of time-series analysis to mood fluctuations in bipolar disorder to promote treatment innovation: A case series. *Translational Psychiatry, 6,* e720.

Holmes, E. A., & Coughtrey, A. E. (2008). *Fishing for happiness: Positive cognitive bias modification and mental imagery in dysphoria.* Paper presented at the British Association of Behavioural and Cognitive Psychotherapies 36th Annual Conference, Edinburgh, UK.

Holmes, E. A., Craske, M. G., & Graybiel, A. M. (2014). Psychological treatments: A call for mental-health science. Clinicians and neuroscientists must work together to understand and improve psychological treatments [Comment]. *Nature, 511*(7509), 287–289.

Holmes, E. A., Deeprose, C., Fairburn, C. G., Wallace-Hadrill, S. M. A., Bonsall, M. B., . . . Goodwin, G. M. (2011). Mood stability versus mood instability in bipolar disorder: A possible role for emotional mental imagery. *Behaviour Research and Therapy, 49*(10), 707–713.

Holmes, E. A., Grey, N., & Young, K. A. D. (2005). Intrusive images and "hotspots" of trauma memories in posttraumatic stress disorder. *Journal of Behavior Therapy and Experimental Psychiatry, 36*(1), 3–17.

Holmes, E. A., Lang, T. J., & Shah, D. M. (2009). Developing interpretation bias modification as a "cognitive vaccine" for depressed mood—Imagining positive events makes you feel better than thinking about them verbally. *Journal of Abnormal Psychology, 118*(1), 76–88.

Holmes, E. A., & Mathews, A. (2005). Mental imagery and emotion: A special relationship? *Emotion, 5*(4), 489–497.

Holmes, E. A., & Mathews, A. (2010). Mental imagery in emotion and emotional disorders. *Clinical Psychology Review, 30*(3), 349–362.

Holmes, E. A., Mathews, A., Dalgleish, T., & Mackintosh, B. (2006). Positive interpretation training: Effects of mental imagery versus verbal training on positive mood. *Behavior Therapy, 37*(3), 237–247.

Holmes, E. A., Mathews, A., Mackintosh, B., & Dalgleish, T. (2008). The causal effect of mental imagery on emotion assessed using picture-word cues. *Emotion, 8*(3), 395–409.

Ivins, A., Di Simplicio, M., Close, H., Goodwin, G. M., & Holmes, E. A. (2014). Mental imagery in bipolar affective disorder versus unipolar depression: Investigating cognitions at times of "positive" mood. *Journal of Affective Disorders, 166,* 234–242.

Jacob, G. A., & Arntz, A. (2013). Schema therapy for personality disorders—A review. *International Journal of Cognitive Therapy, 6*(2), 171–185.

James, E. L., Lau-Zhu, A., Visser, R., Clark, I. A., Hagenaars, M. A., & Holmes, E. A. (2016). The trauma film paradigm as an experimental psychopathology model of psychological trauma: Intrusive memories and beyond. *Clinical Psychology Review, 47,* 106–142.

Ji, J. L., Burnett Heyes, S., MacLeod, C., & Holmes, E. A. (2016). Emotional mental imagery as simulation of reality: Fear and beyond: A tribute to Peter Lang. *Behavior Therapy, 47*(5), 702–719.

Kavanagh, D. J., Andrade, J., & May, J. (2005). Imaginary relish and exquisite torture: The elaborated intrusion theory of desire. *Psychological Review, 112*(2), 446–467.

Knäuper, B., McCollam, A., Rosen-Brown, A., Lacaille, J., Kelso, E., & Roseman, M. (2011). Fruitful plans: Adding targeted mental imagery to implementation intentions increases fruit consumption. *Psychological Health, 26*(5), 601–617.

Kosslyn, S. M., Ganis, G., & Thompson, W. L. (2001). Neural foundations of imagery. *Nature Reviews Neuroscience, 2*(9), 635–642.

Laeng, B., & Sulutvedt, U. (2013). The eye pupil adjusts to imaginary light. *Psychological Science, 25*(1), 188–197.

Lang, P. J. (1979). A bio-informational theory of emotional imagery. *Psychophysiology, 16*(6), 495–512.

Lang, T. J., Blackwell, S. E., Harmer, C. J., Davison, P., & Holmes, E. A. (2012). Cognitive bias modification using mental imagery for depression: Developing a novel computerized intervention to change negative thinking styles. *European Journal of Personality, 26*(2), 145–157.

Lazarus, A. A. (1968). Learning theory and the treatment of depression. *Behavioral Research Therapy, 6*(1), 83–89.

Libby, L. K., Shaeffer, E. M., Eibach, R. P., & Slemmer, J. A. (2007). Picture yourself at the polls: Visual perspective in mental imagery affects self-perception and behavior. *Psychological Science, 18*(3), 199–203.

Loft, M. H., & Cameron, L. D. (2013). Using mental imagery to deliver self-regulation techniques to improve sleep behaviors. *Annals of Behavioral Medicine, 46*(3), 260–272.

Malogiannis, I. A., Arntz, A., Spyropoulou, A., Tsartsara, E., Aggeli, A., Karveli, S., . . . Zervas, I. (2014). Schema therapy for patients with chronic depression: A single case series study. *Journal of Behavior Therapy and Experimental Psychiatry, 45*(3), 319–329.

Martell, C. R., Addis, M. E., & Jacobson, N. S. (2001). *Depression in context: Strategies for guided action.* New York: Norton Press.

Martell, C. R., Dimidjian, S., & Herman-Dunn, R. (2010). *Behavioral activation for depression: A clinician's guide.* New York: Guilford Press.

Ng, R. M. K., Di Simplicio, M., & Holmes, E. A. (2015). Mental imagery and bipolar disorders: Introducing scope for psychological treatment development? [Editorial]. *International Journal of Social Psychiatry, 1*(4), 110–113.

Ng, R. M. K., Di Simplicio, M., McManus, F., Kennerley, H., & Holmes, E. A. (2015). "Flash-forwards" and suicidality: A prospective investigation of mental imagery, entrapment and defeat in a cohort from the Hong Kong Mental Morbidity Survey. *Depression and Anxiety, 246,* 453–460.

Padesky, C. A. (1993). Socratic questioning: Changing minds or guiding discovery? Keynote address presented at the 1993 European Congress of Behaviour and Cognitive Therapies, London. Retrieved from *www.padesky.com/clinical-corner/publications.*

Patel, T., Brewin, C. R., Wheatley, J., Wells, A., Fisher, P., & Myers, S. (2007). Intrusive images and memories in major depression. *Behaviour Research and Therapy, 45*(11), 2573–2580.

Pearson, J., Naselaris, T., Holmes, E. A., & Kosslyn, S. M. (2015). Mental imagery:

Functional mechanisms and clinical applications. *Trends in Cognitive Sciences, 19*(10), 590–602.

Pictet, A., Coughtrey, A. E., Mathews, A., & Holmes, E. A. (2011). Fishing for happiness: The effects of positive imagery on interpretation bias and a behavioral task. *Behaviour Research and Therapy, 49*(12), 885–891.

Pictet, A., & Holmes, E. A. (2013). The powerful impact of mental imagery in changing emotion. In B. Rimé, B. Mesquita, & D. Hermans (Eds.), *Changing emotions* (p. 256). London: Psychology Press.

Renner, F., Arntz, A., Leeuw, I., & Huibers, M. (2013). Treatment for chronic depression using schema therapy. *Clinical Psychology: Science and Practice, 20*(2), 166–180.

Renner, F., Arntz, A., Peeters, F. P. M. L., Lobbestael, J., & Huibers, M. J. H. (2016). Schema therapy for chronic depression: Results of a multiple single case series. *Journal of Behavior Therapy and Experimental Psychiatry, 51,* 66–73.

Renner, F., Ji, J. L., Pictet, A., Holmes, E. A., & Blackwell, S. E. (2017). Effects of engaging in repeated mental imagery of future positive events on behavioural activation in individuals with major depressive disorder. *Cognitive Therapy and Research, 41*(3), 369–380.

Renner, F., Schwarz, P., Peters, M. L., & Huibers, M. J. H. (2014). Effects of a best-possible-self mental imagery exercise on mood and dysfunctional attitudes. *Psychiatry Research, 215,* 105–110.

Rosner, R. I. (2002). Aaron T. Beck's dream theory in context: An introduction to his 1971 article on cognitive patterns in dreams and daydreams. *Journal of Cognitive Psychotherapy, 16*(1), 7–22.

Rush, A. J., & Beck, A. T. (1978). Cognitive therapy of depression and suicide. *American Journal of Psychotherapy, 32*(2), 201–219.

Singer, J. L. (2006). *Imagery applications in cognitive-behavioral therapies.* Washington, DC: American Psychological Association.

Torkan, H., Blackwell, S. E., Holmes, E. A., Kalantari, M., Neshat-Doost, H. T., Maroufi, M., . . . Talebi, H. (2014). Positive imagery cognitive bias modification in treatment-seeking patients with major depression in Iran: A pilot study. *Cognitive Therapy and Research, 38,* 132–145.

Uskul, A. K., & Kikutani, M. (2014). Concerns about losing face moderate the effect of visual perspective on health-related intentions and behaviors. *Journal of Experimental Social Psychology, 55,* 201–209.

Williams, A. D., O'Moore, K., Blackwell, S. E., Smith, J., Holmes, E. A., & Andrews, G. (2015). Positive imagery cognitive bias modification (CBM) and Internet-based cognitive behavioural therapy (iCBT): A randomized controlled trial. *Journal of Affective Disorders, 178,* 131–141.

Young, J. E., Klosko, J. S., & Weishaar, M. E. (2003). *Schema therapy: A practitioner's guide.* New York: Guilford Press.

CHAPTER 10

Mindfulness-Based Cognitive Therapy

Treatment Development from a Common Cognitive Therapy Core

Zindel V. Segal
Amanda M. Ferguson

Even with a number of efficacious pharmacological and psychotherapeutic treatments for depression, it remains the leading cause of disability worldwide for both men and women (World Health Organization, 2008). Global prevalence rates for major depressive disorder (MDD) range from 3 to 13% (Gelenberg, 2010; Richards, 2011), and lifetime risk of MDD in the United States is estimated at 17 to 19% (Kessler et al., 1994). Mindfulness-based cognitive therapy (MBCT; Segal, Williams, & Teasdale, 2013) was developed to address the challenges associated with effectively treating chronic depression.

One of the problems associated with treating depression is its inherently chronic and recurrent nature. Individuals who have recovered from a major depressive episode are 40–50% more likely to have a second episode, and for those with two or more episodes, relapse rates are as high as 60–70% (Judd, 1997; Solomon et al., 2000). Indeed, MDD is often experienced in multiple phases (i.e., acute phase, treatment response, episode relapse, episode recurrent; Frank et al., 1991). Contemporary approaches, working from this classification, have demonstrated the utility of sequential treatment algorithms in which effective management of MMD is tied to treatment interventions that are specific to each phase. An interesting corollary of this approach is that interventions used to attain treatment response and remission may not resemble those put in place to sustain recovery (Guidi, Tomba, & Fava, 2015). At present, antidepressant medication (ADM) and psychotherapy (e.g., cognitive-behavioral therapy [CBT]) have proven to be the most effective treatments for the acute phase of depressive illness, each demonstrating approximately 40–50% recovery rates (Hollon et al., 2006). Until recently, the most widely supported approach for prevention of relapse/recurrence in formerly depressed patients has been maintenance antidepressant medication (mADM; Geddes et al., 2003). Cognitive therapy (CT) for depression delivered during the acute phase has also demonstrated protective benefits in both adults and adolescents (Hollon et al., 2005; Garber et al., 2009) that endure beyond the point at which therapy is terminated.

PREVENTING RELAPSE IN FORMERLY DEPRESSED PATIENTS: CLUES FROM BECK'S COGNITIVE THERAPY

With trends indicating an increase in the use of antidepressants and a decrease in other therapeutics for the treatment of depression (Olfson & Marcus, 2010), patients in recovery were left with fewer options for maintaining wellness. While the best evidence pointed to mADM as providing protection against relapse/recurrence, the rates of compliance over long-term follow-up were low (Samples & Mojtabai, 2015). This may have been because antidepressants were associated with a high side-effect burden, that efficacy would wear off over time, and that women who were pregnant did not feel safe taking these medications. All these factors left a large number of formerly depressed patients potentially "uncovered" during a period when their risk of relapse/recurrence was still high. It was against this backdrop that Segal, Teasdale, and Williams (2002) sought to develop a maintenance version of CT that could offer a psychotherapeutic alternative to mADM.

Treatment development was informed by Beck's model of cognitive vulnerability and the experimental literature on mood-related cognitive changes in remitted depressed patients (Beck, 1976; Segal, Williams, Teasdale, & Gemar, 1996; Teasdale, Segal, & Williams, 1995). Beck's model postulated that depressogenic thinking patterns could be retriggered in recovered patients when they experienced transient setbacks or dysphoric moods and it was these "latent" schemas that, if unaddressed, determined the risk of episode return. Indeed, experimental tests of Beck's formulation have shown that for recovered depressed patients, mild dysphoria activates thinking patterns similar to those previously present in episode, whereas never depressed control subjects do not change their thinking style when tested in either euthymic or dysphoric mood (Ingram, Atchley, & Segal, 2011). There is now good evidence that the thinking patterns evident during dysphoric mood among formerly depressed individuals not only intensify the dysphoric state by escalating self-perpetuating cycles of ruminative cognitive-affective processing (Teasdale, 1988), but also increase significantly the risk of relapse. Cognitive reactivity linked to sad moods is also found in patients with a history of depression but not in never depressed control participants, and formerly depressed individuals demonstrate mood-linked cognitive reactivity following remission achieved through either antidepressant pharmacotherapy or cognitive therapy (Gemar, Segal, Sagrati, & Kennedy, 2001). Most importantly, Segal et al. (2006) reported that patients showing increased mood-linked cognitive reactivity had a 69% relapse rate compared to those with minimal or decreased reactivity, who relapsed at rates of 30% and 32%, respectively, over an 18-month follow-up (Segal et al., 2006). These data illustrate the strong relationship between mood-linked changes in cognitive processing among formerly depressed patients and subsequent relapse.

In line with this theoretical understanding, Segal, Williams, and Teasdale (2013) sought to develop an intervention that teaches individuals how to preempt the establishment of such dysfunctional processing cycles by fostering metacognitive skills. Metacognitive skills refer to an awareness of and ability to understand and influence cognitive processing, and play a pivotal role in adaptive emotion regulation (Teasdale et al., 2002). Specifically, it was proposed that risk of relapse and recurrence would be reduced if patients who have recovered from episodes of major depression could learn, first, to be more aware of negative thoughts and feelings at times of potential relapse/recurrence, and, second, to respond to those thoughts and feelings in ways that allow them to disengage from ruminative depressive processing, such as overgeneral memories and thinking styles (Nolen-Hoeksema & Morrow, 1991; Williams, Teasdale, Segal, & Soulsby, 2000). MBCT was designed to achieve these aims (Segal, Williams, & Teasdale, 2002; Teasdale et al., 1995).

Segal et al. (2013) were aided in their efforts to develop an intervention that teaches metacognitive skills by the fact that one of the mechanisms through which CT achieves its therapeutic effects is known as "decentering." According to Ingram and Hollon (1986), CT enhances one's ability to take a distanced and disidentified view of depressive thoughts, which can help patients understand that thoughts do not necessarily reflect truth or reality (i.e., thoughts are not facts). In standard CT, decentering is viewed as a means toward the ultimate end of cognitive restructuring or changing the degree of belief in a thought (Beck, Rush, Shaw, & Emery, 1979). This is an important distinction because patients in CT are working with negative thinking or hot thoughts that are very dominant or "loud." But what about patients who are in remission? This group may not be working with thoughts of the same intensity, yet they would still need a way to practice decentering skills.

While it is true that a "decentered" perspective, which allows individuals to witness thoughts in a nonjudgmental and nonreactive fashion, is an outgrowth of cognitive-behavioral therapies, it is also a capacity that is engendered through traditional contemplative practices such as mindfulness meditation. Jon Kabat-Zinn's (1990) mindfulness-based stress reduction (MBSR) program provided an empirically supported framework of an intervention wherein a decentered relationship with thoughts, feelings, and body sensations (including pain) was promoted through various mindfulness meditation practices. A central strategy in MBSR is to help patients develop a different relationship to their thoughts, rather than work to modify the degree of belief in the thought's content. Drawing on this model and the existing theory and research on depressive relapse, Segal, Williams, and Teasdale (2013) designed MBCT, an integrated program combining cognitive therapy and mindfulness meditation.

CLINICAL APPLICATION

Key Principles

The MBCT program combines elements of MBSR and standard CT techniques for relapse prevention. Techniques drawn from MBSR include formal meditation, the body scan, mindful stretching, and mindfulness of breath, body, and sounds. Everyday mindfulness skills are also taught, such as mindful eating, and monitoring sensations and emotions during pleasant and unpleasant experiences. Together, these exercises teach the ability to mindfully approach daily activities that might otherwise be completed on "automatic pilot." The CT components of the MBCT program include psychoeducation about automatic thoughts and depressive thinking patterns, including the importance of questioning automatic thoughts and recognizing the ways in which thoughts can be affected by situations and moods. Individuals are also encouraged to identify individuals who can provide emotional support, as well as activities over which they feel a sense of mastery or pleasure. In addition to these techniques, the MBCT program teaches the "three-minute breathing space." This brief meditation exercise is designed to facilitate present-moment awareness during times of emotional challenge, and is offered as a strategy for dealing with everyday stress (Segal et al., 2013). Fundamental to the MBCT program is its group-based inquiry process. Meta-awareness of reactions and patterns discovered during meditative practices is facilitated through Socratic questioning and joint exploration of the thoughts, emotions, and sensations that arise during the practice. Taken together, the skills taught in the MBCT program are designed to help the individual differentiate depression from the self, while creating a "relapse toolkit" to be used during times of low mood.

Approaching Present-Moment Experience with Acceptance

The first half of the MBCT program is focused on developing an attitude in which individuals approach present-moment experiences in a nonjudgmental, accepting way. A common teaching in formal meditation is learning to use the breath as an attentional anchor, serving as a focal point to which the meditator can orient and reorient as needed. By training attention, the practice of formal meditation facilitates the ability to observe the moment-by-moment structure and content of one's internal experience. Individuals are taught to parse the experiences that arise during meditation into identifiable body sensations, feelings, and thoughts. This process of deconstruction is then specifically applied to depression through CT (e.g., via exercises that emphasize how reactions to a given situation can be affected by interpretation). Importantly, the theme of approaching experience with nonjudgment is emphasized throughout the program. This attitude adds a layer of protection against ruminative thinking, since it encourages individuals to simply notice their experience and move on to the next. Together, these strategies cultivate the understanding that thoughts and feelings are not facts but momentary events in human experience.

Expanding Awareness of Depression-Related Experience

MBCT aims to increase early detection of signs of depressive relapse. Midway through the program, psychoeducation specific to depression is introduced. The types of negative thinking associated with depression are explored, as is the nature of depressive symptoms. Ultimately, individuals are encouraged to identify their unique "relapse signature" and set in place an action plan for use when experiencing low mood. For example, some individuals may notice that they are waking up earlier in the morning than is usual or turning down social invitations and preferring to stay home by themselves. These changes would be highlighted in Session 4 where, if they were deemed harbingers of a relapse, patients could recognize them sooner as possible symptoms and take action to prevent them from building momentum toward a full depressive episode.

Promoting Flexible and Deliberate Responses at Times of Risk for Relapse

The second half of the MBCT program is focused on teaching flexible, deliberate responses during times of potential relapse. In Session 5, "letting be" as a strategy to deal with difficult experiences is explicitly introduced.

This strategy invites individuals to move away from the need to "fix" problems. The "fixing" mindset reinforces the attitude that problems are an enemy to be eliminated. Conversely, rather than attempting to change the content of one's thoughts or problems, MBCT seeks to change the ways in which an individual relates to his or her problems.

Assessment and Eligibility

MBCT was specifically designed and evaluated for the prevention of relapse to depression. Given the demands of the MBCT program (e.g., in terms of patience, time commitment), individual eligibility should be determined in an initial assessment interview. First, depression status and symptom severity should be measured (e.g., via the Structured Clinical Interview for Diagnosis for DSM-IV [SCID-IV] and Hamilton Rating Scale for Depression [HRSD]; First, Spitzer, Gibbon, & Williams, 1996; Hamilton, 1960). Second, the extent to which an individual is able to persist through the demands of the program must be determined. For example, individuals who are actively suicidal or are currently abusing substances should not be accepted into the program. Finally, following treatment, assessment (e.g., via the SCID-IV, HRSD) is necessary to ensure that participants are not experiencing a return of depressive symptoms.

Instructor Qualification

MBCT instructors must understand the integration of mindfulness meditation and CT techniques, which requires particular training and skills. Segal et al. (2013) suggest a number of qualifications for MBCT instructors. First, some recognized training in psychotherapy, or as a mental health professional, is recommended. Second, instructors should have training in cognitive therapy and experience conducting group sessions of CT. Third, instructors must participate in an intensive, week-long, MBCT teacher development course, so that the fundamental components of the therapy are understood in context. Finally, and perhaps most importantly, instructors of MBCT should have an ongoing meditation practice. Personal experience with meditation is necessary to adequately address the questions and difficulties often faced by new meditators. Importantly, instructors should model "being present" during sessions—they should embody the ways in which individuals can pay attention to experience in the moment.

Session Structure

MBCT consists of eight sessions, with each session focusing on a different core theme (see Table 10.1). Session 1 is devoted to introductions and a review of the administrative issues (e.g., confidentiality). A mindful eating exercise is introduced, as are the body scan and a short breathing meditation. The remaining sessions follow a consistent format. The sessions begin with a meditation exercise (e.g., body scan, sitting meditation) to facilitate the transition from daily life to present-moment awareness. Participants discuss their experiences with the meditation following the exercise. The previous week's homework is also discussed, and new homework is assigned at the end of the session.

Similarities and Differences with CT

MBCT, like CT, focuses on the importance of recognizing symptoms of depression as they develop. For example, individuals are taught to identify the experience of automatic negative thoughts and to monitor their thoughts and feelings during unpleasant events. These strategies can help an individual stay aware in the moment and ultimately allow for the identification of deteriorating mood. Similarly, as in CT, individuals are taught to create an action plan for self-care during times of stress and negative mood.

TABLE 10.1. Description of Session Theme and Associated CT Concept

MBCT Session	MBCT Core Theme	Possible overlap with CT
1	Awareness and Automatic Pilot	Automatic thoughts and automatic processing
2	Living in Our Heads	ABC model of situation-thought-feeling
3	Gathering the Scattered Mind	Building awareness through the first three columns of the thought record
4	Recognizing the Territory of Aversion	Becoming familiar with depressive symptoms and thought patterns
5	Allowing/Letting Be	Using these skills during situations that carry an emotional charge
6	Thoughts Are Not Facts	Treating thoughts as ideas or hypotheses
7	How Can I Best Take Care of Myself?	Behavioral routines and constructing a relapse prevention plan
8	Maintaining and Extending New Learning	Emphasizing continued practice of therapy skills once the program has ended

An additional similarity exists in the domain of homework. Both interventions stress the importance of experiential learning outside of the therapy hour or group. CT is somewhat further down the road of being able to empirically demonstrate a relationship between homework and outcome (e.g., Conklin & Strunk, 2015), whereas in MBCT, this issue is still being investigated. There are studies documenting clinical gains associated with the practice frequency of mindfulness meditation (Crane et al., 2014), but some studies have also failed to find this relationship (MacCoon et al., 2012).

The fundamental difference between CT and MBCT is the relative locus of change. The mechanism underlying CT is change-based—the targets of therapy are the negative thoughts themselves, and the goal is to change the contents of those thoughts. MBCT uses an acceptance-based approach in which negative thoughts need not be changed, but simply acknowledged and accepted. This approach utilizes decentering and "letting be" so that negative thoughts can be noticed and accepted as simple events occurring in the mind. Further differences between MBCT and CT include CT's method of purposefully exposing individuals to problematic situations. In MBCT, individuals are invited to address their experience naturally, as it unfolds during the session.

EMPIRICAL SUPPORT FOR MBCT

Early trials of MBCT established it as an effective prophylactic treatment for depressive relapse (Ma & Teasdale, 2004; Teasdale et al., 2000). In the initial multicenter trial by Teasdale et al. (2000), individuals were randomized into either MBCT or treatment as usual (TAU) conditions (N = 145). Participants were in remission from depression but had a history of at least two previous episodes. Those in the TAU condition were instructed to seek support from their physician or community sources as they normally would. Those in the MBCT condition participated in eight weekly group sessions, plus four follow-up sessions scheduled at one-, two-, three- and four-month intervals. Both groups were followed for a total of 60 weeks. Severity of depressive symptoms and relapse were evaluated with the Structured Clinical Interview for Diagnosis (SCID; Spitzer, Williams, Gibbon, & First, 1990), and the primary outcome measure was whether and when participants experienced relapse (i.e., met criteria for a major depressive episode according to the DSM). In each condition, participants were stratified according to the number of previous episodes (two versus three or more) they had experienced. Results revealed a significantly different pattern of relapse for those with a history of only two previous episodes compared to those with three or more. For the former group (two or fewer past episodes), there were no differences between MBCT and TAU in terms of relapse rates at 15 months. However, in the sample of individuals with three or more previous episodes (77% of the overall sample), there was a significant benefit of MBCT for those who had completed at least four treatment sessions. Relapse was observed in only 37% of the MBCT group, while those in the TAU condition had a relapse rate of 66%. Importantly, this difference remained significant when analyses were repeated on the intent-to-treat (ITT) sample. These findings were replicated in a smaller single-site trial (*N* = 75; Ma & Teasdale, 2004). It is still unclear what the cardinal differences are between these two groups, other than recognizing that they may come from populations with different risk profiles and that the more vulnerable patients showed greater treatment gains. What is still unclear is the extent to which this vulnerability is driven by psychological factors such as higher rumination, childhood maltreatment (Williams et al., 2014), and/or genetic and neurobiological factors associated with mood disorders in general.

More recently, Segal et al. (2010) conducted a randomized controlled trial (RCT) comparing MBCT to mADM and a placebo medication. Participants in this trial had been on an algorithmically determined antidepressant treatment regimen for the previous eight months. Of the original sample (*N* = 165), eighty-four individuals achieved remission and were assigned to one of the study conditions. Participants were further categorized according to the "stability" of their remission states during the acute phase of treatment for depression, as determined by symptom elevations on the HRSD (Hamilton, 1960). Unstable remitters (51% of the sample), compared to stable remitters (49% of the sample), were those who experienced "symptom flurries," or occasional, transient symptom elevations on the HRSD. Stable remitters (49% of the sample) had no such elevations. For stable remitters, ITT analyses demonstrated no difference in relapse rates across treatments. For unstable remitters, ITT results revealed comparable rates of relapse in the MBCT condition (28%) and the mADM condition (27%), but a much higher rate in the placebo condition (71%). The authors concluded that the MBCT provided protective benefits for remitted individuals consistent with those conferred by maintenance pharmacotherapy, and that these treatments were particularly effective for individuals with a history of unstable remission.

Several independent trials have found further support for the efficacy of MBCT in preventing relapse. Beneficial outcomes such as longer periods of wellness between episodes of depression, reduced residual depressive symptoms, and lowered rates of relapse (in the range of 50%) have been observed in MBCT treatment groups (Bondolfi et al., 2010; Geschwind, Peeters, Drukker, Van Os, & Wichers, 2011; Godfrin & van Heeringen, 2010; Kuyken et al., 2008; Kuyken et al., 2010).

A recent meta-analysis examined the efficacy of MBCT in preventing relapse to depression when compared with active treatments including

TAU (Kuyken et al., 2016). The authors examined individual patient-level data for nine randomized controlled trials (*N* = 1329) conducted by different research groups and using a range of European and North American participants. Compared with those in a non-MBCT treatment, individuals who completed MBCT had a significantly reduced risk of depressive relapse within a 60-week follow-up period (hazard ratio: 0.69 [0.58, 0.82]). When compared to ADM treatment only (*N* = 637), MBCT reduced the risk of relapse (hazard ratio: 0.77 [0.60, 0.98]). Importantly, the treatment effect of MBCT on risk of relapse was larger in participants who reported more severe depression at baseline, as compared with non-MBCT conditions. Consistent with the findings of Teasdale and colleagues (2000), these results suggest that MBCT may be particularly helpful for individuals with higher levels of residual depressive symptoms.

While MBCT was specifically designed for individuals in remission for depression, it has been applied to the treatment of several other disorders with hypothetically similar underlying mechanisms. For example, it can be argued that anxiety and pain disorders are maintained by rumination, avoidance, and hypervigilance to body sensations, all of which are targeted by MBCT. A recent RCT (*N* = 182) compared a modified version of MBCT with CBT-based psychoeducation and TAU in the treatment of generalized anxiety disorder (GAD; Wong et al., 2016; see also Evans et al., 2008). Modifications to the MBCT protocol (specifically the CT components therein) were made so as to make the intervention more suitable for people with anxiety disorders (e.g., discussing automatic thoughts related to anxiety; developing an action plan to prevent relapse to anxiety). Results revealed the significant benefit of both the MBCT and psychoeducational treatments when compared with TAU in symptom reduction (i.e., anxiety level, worry). Similar results have been demonstrated for the treatment of health anxiety/hypochondriasis (McManus, Surawy, Muse, Vazquez-Montes, & Williams, 2012) and perinatal depression (Dimidjian et al., 2016). For example, in a recent RCT (*N* = 74) that compared MBCT for hypochondriasis to TAU, participants who completed MBCT were significantly less likely to meet the criteria for the diagnosis of hypochondriasis than those in the TAU condition (McManus et al., 2012). This was true immediately following treatment (50.0% vs. 78.9%) and at one-year follow-up (36.1% vs. 76.3%). The authors concluded that MBCT was an acceptable and beneficial treatment for patients with health anxiety.

While MBCT has considerable empirical support, it faces several practical challenges to dissemination. At the very least, physical access to a trained practitioner is required. In rural areas, or for those with inflexible schedules and obligations, access may be an important impediment to treatment. Beyond physical access, service costs and waiting lists may be prohibitive for those interested in treatment (Wang, Simon, & Kessler, 2003). Web-based treatments can offer an alternative that addresses several of these challenges (e.g., Clarke et al., 2005; Proudfoot et al., 2004; Warmerdam, van Straten, Jongsma, Twisk, & Cuijpers, 2010). Recently, MBCT has been adapted for dissemination online. Mindful Mood Balance (MMB; Dimidjian et al., 2014) was developed to incorporate the content of in-person MBCT into an eight-session, self-guided online program. MMB closely follows the session structure of MBCT but utilizes a variety of learning modalities (e.g., video, audio). To simulate the group-based inquiry component of MBCT, videos of selected portions of an in-person MBCT group are provided. A qualitative study of MMB has yielded positive results. In their exit interview, participants reported that they had developed affect regulation skills and identified several advantages to the online format of MMB, including flexibility, reduced cost, and time commitment (Boggs et al., 2014).

CONCLUSIONS

It is interesting to consider that Segal, Williams, and Teasdale were all trained as cognitive therapists and clinical scientists before they ventured into treatment development. The influence of their CT "roots" can be seen in MBCT's theoretical background and their views of how patients can learn to disengage from depressogenic patterns of thinking. Beck's early work outlining both the cognitive theory of depression and his subsequent views on vulnerability and schematic processing were influential in forming a theoretical bridge linking contemplative practices such as mindfulness meditation with a traditional therapy format such as CT.

MBCT was developed to prevent depression relapse among individuals with recurrent depression. Research from numerous randomized control trials support the efficacy of MBCT, and preliminary research evidences novel extensions of MBCT. A primary goal of MBCT is to teach participants to identify vulnerability-inducing habits of thinking with the goal of relating to them through a metacognitive, present-moment orientation. MBCT is firmly rooted in the view of mindfulness as a form of attentional training that first requires familiarity with the automatic or mindless modes of cognitive processing before consistent practice can acquaint patients with new modes that provide flexibility in the midst of possible relapse triggers and, more widely, with life's ever-present challenges and opportunities.

REFERENCES

Beck, A. T., Rush, A. J., Shaw, B. F., & Emery, G. (1979). *Cognitive therapy of depression*. New York: Guilford Press.

Boggs, J. M., Beck, A., Felder, J. N., Dimidjian, S., Metcalf, C. A., & Segal, Z. V.

(2014). Web-based intervention in mindfulness meditation for reducing residual depressive symptoms and relapse prophylaxis: A qualitative study. *Journal of Medical Internet Research, 16*(3), 1–12.

Bondolfi, G., Jermann, F., der Linden, M. Van, Gex-Fabry, M., Bizzini, L., Rouget, B. W., . . . Bertschy, G. (2010). Depression relapse prophylaxis with mindfulness-based cognitive therapy: Replication and extension in the Swiss health care system. *Journal of Affective Disorders, 122*(3), 224–231.

Casacalenda, N., Perry, J. C., & Looper, K. (2002). Remission in major depressive disorder: A comparison of pharmacotherapy, psychotherapy, and control conditions. *American Journal of Psychiatry, 159*(8), 1354–1360.

Clarke, G., Eubanks, D., Reid, C. K., O'Connor, E., DeBar, L. L., Lynch, F., . . . Gullion, C. (2005). Overcoming depression on the Internet (ODIN)(2): A randomized trial of a self-help depression skills program with reminders. *Journal of Medical Internet Research, 7*(2), e16.

Conklin, L. R., & Strunk, D. R. (2015). A session-to-session examination of homework engagement in cognitive therapy for depression: Do patients experience immediate benefits? *Behaviour Research and Therapy, 72*, 56–62.

Crane, C., Crane, R. S., Eames, C., Fennell, M. J., Silverton, S., Williams, J. M. G., . . . Barnhofer, T. (2014). The effects of amount of home meditation practice in mindfulness based cognitive therapy on hazard of relapse to depression in the Staying Well after Depression Trial. *Behaviour Research and Therapy, 63*, 17–24.

Dimidjian, S., Beck, A., Felder, J. N., Boggs, J. M., Gallop, R., & Segal, Z. V. (2014). Web-based mindfulness-based cognitive therapy for reducing residual depressive symptoms: An open trial and quasi-experimental comparison to propensity score matched controls. *Behaviour Research and Therapy, 63*, 83–89.

Dimidjian, S., Goodman, S. H., Felder, J. N., Gallop, R., Brown, A. P., & Beck, A. (2016). Staying well during pregnancy and the postpartum: A pilot randomized trial of mindfulness-based cognitive therapy for the prevention of depressive relapse/recurrence. *Journal of Consulting and Clinical Psychology, 84*(2), 134–145.

Evans, S., Ferrando, S., Findler, M., Stowell, C., Smart, C., & Haglin, D. (2008). Mindfulness-based cognitive therapy for generalized anxiety disorder. *Journal of Anxiety Disorders, 22*(4), 716–721.

Farb, N. A. S., Anderson, A. K., Bloch, R. T., & Segal, Z. V. (2011). Mood-linked responses in medical prefrontal cortex predict relapse in patients with recurrent unipolar depression. *Biological Psychiatry*. [E-pub ahead of print]

Fava, G. A., Rafanelli, C., Grandi, S., Canestrari, R., & Morphy, M. A. (1998). Six-year outcome for cognitive behavioral treatment of residual symptoms in major depression. *American Journal of Psychiatry, 155*(10), 1443–1445.

First, M. B., Spitzer, R. L., Gibbon, M., & Williams, J. B. W. (1996). *Structured Clinical Interview for DSM-IV Axis I Disorders, Clinician Version (SCID-CV)*. Washington, DC: American Psychiatric Press.

Frank, E., Prien, R. F., Jarrett, R. B., Keller, M. B., Kupfer, D. J., Lavori, P. W., . . . Weissman, M. M. (1991). Conceptualization and rationale for consensus definitions of terms in major depressive disorder: Remission, recovery, relapse, and recurrence. *Archives of General Psychiatry, 48*(9), 851–855.

Geddes, J. R., Carney, S. M., Davies, C., Furukawa, T. A., Kupfer, D. J., Frank, E., . . . Goodwin, G. M. (2003). Relapse prevention with antidepressant drug treatment in depressive disorders: A systematic review. *The Lancet, 361*(9358), 653–661.

Gelenberg, A. J. (2010). The prevalence and impact of depression. *Journal of Clinical Psychiatry, 71*(3), 1–478.

Gemar, M. C., Segal, Z. V., Sagrati, S., & Kennedy, S. J. (2001). Mood-induced changes on the Implicit Association Test in recovered depressed patients. *Journal of Abnormal Psychology, 110*(2), 282.

Geschwind, N., Peeters, F., Drukker, M., Van Os, J., & Wichers, M. (2011). Mindfulness training increases momentary positive emotions and reward experience in adults vulnerable to depression: A randomized controlled trial. *Journal of Consulting and Clinical Psychology, 79*(5), 618–628.

Godfrin, K. A., & van Heeringen, C. (2010). The effects of mindfulness-based cognitive therapy on recurrence of depressive episodes, mental health and quality of life: A randomized controlled study. *Behaviour Research and Therapy, 48*(8), 738–746.

Guidi, J., Tomba, E., & Fava, G. A. (2015). The sequential integration of pharmacotherapy and psychotherapy in the treatment of major depressive disorder: A meta-analysis of the sequential model and a critical review of the literature. *American Journal of Psychiatry, 173*(2), 128–137.

Hamilton, M. (1960). A rating scale for depression. *Journal of Neurology, Neurosurgery and Psychiatry, 23*, 56–62.

Hammen, C. (1991). Generation of stress in the course of unipolar depression. *Journal of Abnormal Psychology, 100*, 555–561.

Hollon, S. D., DeRubeis, R. J., Shelton, R. C., Amsterdam, J. D., Salomon, R. M., O'Reardon, J. P., . . . Gallop, R. (2005). Prevention of relapse following cognitive therapy vs. medications in moderate to severe depression. *Archives of General Psychiatry, 62*, 417–422.

Hollon, S. D., Stewart, M. O., & Strunk, D. (2006). Enduring effects for cognitive behavior therapy in the treatment of depression and anxiety. *Annual Review of Psychology, 57*, 285–315.

Ingram, R. E., & Hollon, S. D. (1986). Cognitive therapy of depression from an information processing perspective. In R. E. Ingram (Ed.), *Information processing approaches to clinical psychology* (pp. 259–281). San Diego, CA: Academic Press.

Judd, L. J. (1997). The clinical course of unipolar major depressive disorders. *Archives of General Psychiatry, 54*(11), 989–991.

Kabat-Zinn, J. (1990). *Full catastrophe living: Using the wisdom of your mind to face stress, pain and illness*. New York: Dell.

Kendler, K. S., Thornton, L. M., & Gardner, C. O. (2000). Stressful life events and previous episodes in the etiology of major depression in women: An evaluation of the "kindling" hypothesis. *American Journal of Psychiatry, 157*, 1243–1251.

Kendler, K. S., Thornton, L. M., & Gardner, C. O. (2001). Genetic risk, number of previous episodes, and stressful life events in predicting onset of depression. *American Journal of Psychiatry, 158*, 582–586.

Kessler, R. C., McGonagle, K. A., Zhao, S., Nelson, C. B., Hughes, M., Eshleman,

S., . . . Kendler, K. S. (1994). Lifetime and 12-month prevalence of DSM-III-R psychiatric disorders in the United States: Results from the National Comorbidity Survey. *Archives of General Psychiatry, 51*(1), 8–19.

Kuyken, W., Byford, S., Taylor, R. S., Watkins, E., Holden, E., White, K., . . . Teasdale, J. D. (2008). Mindfulness-based cognitive therapy to prevent relapse in recurrent depression. *Journal of Consulting and Clinical Psychology, 76*(6), 966–978.

Kuyken, W., Warren, F. C., Taylor, R. S., Whalley, B., Crane, C., Bondolfi, G., . . . Segal, Z. (2016). Efficacy of mindfulness-based cognitive therapy in prevention of depressive relapse: An individual patient data meta-analysis from randomized trials. *JAMA Psychiatry, 73*(6), 565–574.

Kuyken, W., Watkins, E., Holden, E., White, K., Taylor, R. S., Byford, S., . . . Dalgleish, T. (2010). How does mindfulness-based cognitive therapy work? *Behaviour Research and Therapy, 48*(11), 1105–1112.

Lau, M. A., Segal, Z. V., & Williams, J. M. G. (2004). Teasdale's differential activation hypothesis: Implications for mechanisms of depressive relapse and suicidal behaviour. *Behaviour Research and Therapy, 42*(9), 1001–1017.

Lewinsohn, P. M., Allen, N. B., Seeley, J. R., & Gotlib, I. H. (1999). First onset versus recurrence of depression: Differential processes of psychosocial risk. *Journal of Abnormal Psychology, 108*, 483–489.

Lovas, D. A., & Barsky, A. J. (2010). Mindfulness-based cognitive therapy for hypochondriasis, or severe health anxiety: A pilot study. *Journal of Anxiety Disorders, 24*(8), 931–935.

Ma, S. H., & Teasdale, J. D. (2004). Mindfulness-based cognitive therapy for depression: Replication and exploration of differential relapse prevention effects. *Journal of Consulting and Clinical Psychology, 72*(1), 31–40.

MacCoon, D. G., Imel, Z. E., Rosenkranz, M. A., Sheftel, J. G., Weng, H. Y., Sullivan, J. C., . . . Lutz, A. (2012). The validation of an active control intervention for mindfulness based stress reduction (MBSR). *Behaviour Research and Therapy, 50*(1), 3–12.

McManus, F., Surawy, C., Muse, K., Vazquez-Montes, M., & Williams, J. M. G. (2012). A randomized clinical trial of mindfulness-based cognitive therapy versus unrestricted services for health anxiety (hypochondriasis). *Journal of Consulting and Clinical Psychology, 80*(5), 817–828.

Nolen-Hoeksema, S. (1991). Responses to depression and their effects on the duration of depressive episodes. *Journal of Abnormal Psychology, 100*(4), 569–582.

Nolen-Hoeksema, S., & Morrow, J. (1991). A prospective study of depression and posttraumatic stress symptoms after a natural disaster: The 1989 Loma Prieta Earthquake. *Journal of Personality and Social Psychology, 61*(1), 115.

Paykel, E. S., Scott, J., Teasdale, J. D., Johnson, A. L., Garland, A., Moore, R., . . . Pope, M. (1999). Prevention of relapse in residual depression by cognitive therapy: A controlled trial. *Archives of General Psychiatry, 56*(9), 829–835.

Proudfoot, J., Ryden, C., Everitt, B., Shapiro, D. A., Goldberg, D., Mann, A., . . . Gray, J. A. (2004). Clinical efficacy of computerised cognitive-behavioural therapy for anxiety and depression in primary care: Randomised controlled trial. *British Journal of Psychiatry, 185*(1), 46–54.

Richards, D. (2011). Prevalence and clinical course of depression: A review. *Clinical Psychology Review, 31*(7), 1117–1125.

Segal, Z. V., Bieling, P., Young, T., MacQueen, G., Cooke, R., Martin, L., . . . Levitan, R. D. (2010). Antidepressant monotherapy vs. sequential pharmacotherapy and mindfulness-based cognitive therapy, or placebo, for relapse prophylaxis in recurrent depression. *Archives of General Psychiatry, 67*(12), 1256–1264.

Segal, Z. V., & Dobson, K. S. (1992). Cognitive models of depression: Report from a consensus development conference. *Psychological Inquiry, 3,* 219–224.

Segal, Z. V., Gemar, M., & Williams, S. (1999). Differential cognitive response to a mood challenge following successful cognitive therapy or pharmacotherapy for unipolar depression. *Journal of Abnormal Psychology, 108,* 3–10.

Segal, Z. V., Kennedy, S., Gemar, M., Hood, K., Pederson, R., & Buis, T. (2006). Cognitive reactivity to sad mood provocation and the prediction of depressive relapse. *Archives of General Psychiatry, 63,* 749–755.

Segal, Z. V., Kennedy, S., Gemar, M., Sagrati, S., Hood, K., & Pedersen, R. (2003, October). *Using mood induction to activate depression relapse vulnerability following cognitive or pharmacological treatment.* Presentation at the Society for Research in Psychopathology, Toronto, Ontario, Canada.

Segal, Z. V., Williams, J. M. G., & Teasdale, J. D. (2013). *Mindfulness-based cognitive therapy for depression: A new approach for preventing relapse.* New York: Guilford Press.

Segal, Z. V., Williams, J. M. G., Teasdale, J. D., & Gemar, M. (1996). A cognitive science perspective on kindling and episode sensitization in recurrent affective disorder. *Psychological Medicine, 26,* 371–380.

Simons, A. D., Angell, K. L., Monroe, S. M., & Thase, M. E. (1993). Cognition and life stress in depression: Cognitive factors and the definition, rating, and generation of negative life events. *Journal of Abnormal Psychology, 102*(4), 584–591.

Solomon, D. A., Keller, M. B., Leon, A. C., Mueller, T. I., Lavori, P. W., Shea, M. T., . . . Endicott, J. (2000). Multiple recurrences of major depressive disorder. *American Journal of Psychiatry, 157*(2), 229–233.

Spitzer, R. L., Williams, J., Gibbon, M., & First M. B. (1990). *Structured Clinical Interview for DSM-III-R, Patient Edition/Non-Patient Edition (SCID-P/SCID-NP).* Washington, DC: American Psychiatric Press.

Surawy, C., McManus, F., Muse, K., & Williams, J. M. G. (2015). Mindfulness-based cognitive therapy (MBCT) for health anxiety (hypochondriasis): Rationale, implementation and case illustration. *Mindfulness, 6*(2), 382–392.

Teasdale, J. D. (1988). Cognitive vulnerability to persistent depression. *Cognition and Emotion, 2,* 247–274.

Teasdale, J. D., & Barnard, P. J. (1993). *Affect, cognition, and change.* Hillsdale, NJ: Erlbaum.

Teasdale, J. D., Moore, R. G., Hayhurst, H., Pope, M., Williams, S., & Segal, Z. V. (2002). Metacognitive awareness and prevention of relapse in depression: Empirical evidence. *Journal of Consulting and Clinical Psychology, 70*(2), 275.

Teasdale, J. D., Segal, Z., & Williams, J. M. G. (1995). How does cognitive therapy prevent depressive relapse and why should attentional control (mindfulness) training help? *Behaviour Research and Therapy, 33*(1), 25–39.

Teasdale, J. D., Segal, Z. V., Williams, J. M. G., Ridgeway, V. A., Soulsby, J. M., & Lau, M. A. (2000). Prevention of relapse/recurrence in major depression by mindfulness-based cognitive therapy. *Journal of Consulting and Clinical Psychology, 68*(4), 615–623.

Wang, P. S., Simon, G., & Kessler, R. C. (2003). The economic burden of depression and the cost-effectiveness of treatment. *International Journal of Methods in Psychiatric Research, 12*(1), 22–33.

Warmerdam, L., van Straten, A., Jongsma, J., Twisk, J., & Cuijpers, P. (2010). Online cognitive behavioral therapy and problem-solving therapy for depressive symptoms: Exploring mechanisms of change. *Journal of Behavior Therapy and Experimental Psychiatry, 41*(1), 64–70.

Weissman, A., & Beck, A. T. (1978, November). *The Dysfunctional Attitudes Scale.* Paper presented at the annual meeting of the Association for the Advancement of Behaviour Therapy, Chicago, IL.

Williams, J. M. G., Crane, C., Barnhofer, T., Brennan, K., Duggan, D. S., Fennell, M. J., . . . Shah, D. (2014). Mindfulness-based cognitive therapy for preventing relapse in recurrent depression: A randomized dismantling trial. *Journal of Consulting and Clinical Psychology, 82*(2), 275–286.

Williams, J. M. G., Teasdale, J. D., Segal, Z. V., & Soulsby, J. (2000). Mindfulness-based cognitive therapy reduces overgeneral autobiographical memory in formerly depressed patients. *Journal of Abnormal Psychology, 109*(1), 150–155.

Williams, M. J., McManus, F., Muse, K., & Williams, J. M. G. (2011). Mindfulness-based cognitive therapy for severe health anxiety (hypochondriasis): An interpretative phenomenological analysis of patients' experiences. *British Journal of Clinical Psychology, 50*(4), 379–397.

Wong, S. Y. S., Yip, B. H. K., Mak, W. W. S., Mercer, S., Cheung, E. Y. L., Ling, C. Y. M., . . . Lee, T. M. C. (2016). Mindfulness-based cognitive therapy v. group psychoeducation for people with generalised anxiety disorder: Randomised controlled trial. *British Journal of Psychiatry, 209*(1), 68–75.

World Health Organization. (2008). The global burden of disease 2004 update. Available at *www.who.int/healthinfo/global_burden_disease/GBD_report_2004update_full.pdf.*

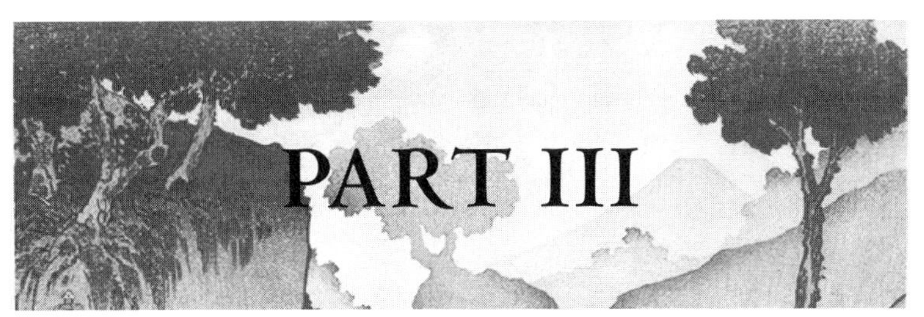

PART III

UNDERSTANDING AND TREATING PSYCHOLOGICAL DISORDERS

CHAPTER 11

Cognitive Therapy for Insomnia

Nicole B. Gumport
Allison G. Harvey

Insomnia is a chronic condition that involves difficulty getting to sleep or staying asleep even with satisfactory opportunity to sleep. The prevalence of insomnia in the United States is 33%, with 9% reporting insomnia on a regular nightly basis and 24% reporting that it occurs occasionally, especially during stressful life events (Ancoli-Israel & Roth, 1999). Insomnia is associated with daytime fatigue, greater medical service utilization, self-medication with alcohol or over-the-counter medication, greater functional impairment, greater work absenteeism, impaired concentration and memory, decreased enjoyment of interpersonal relationships, and increased risk of serious medical illness and traffic and work accidents (American Psychiatric Association, 2013; Drake, Pillai, & Roth, 2014; Pillai, Roth, & Drake, 2015). There is high comorbidity between insomnia and several psychological disorders, especially depression, anxiety, and substance abuse (Baglioni et al., 2011; Roth et al., 2006; Sarsour, Morin, Foley, Kalsekar, & Walsh, 2010). Insomnia is a risk factor for and may even be causal in the development of these disorders (Baglioni et al., 2011; Harvey, 2001).

This chapter describes and reviews the evidence in support of the cognitive model of insomnia and the treatments that have been derived based on the model.

OVERVIEW OF THE COGNITIVE MODEL OF INSOMNIA

The cognitive model of insomnia (Harvey, 2002) described in this chapter draws from cognitive models of other psychological disorders (Beck, 1976; Clark, 1997; Salkovskis, 1996); from previous theoretical and empirical work highlighting the importance of cognitive processes in insomnia (Borkovec, 1982; Espie, 2002; Morin, 1993; Perlis, Giles, Mendelson, Bootzin, & Wyatt, 1997); and from basic science literature in cognitive psychology (Dalgleish & Watts, 1990; Easterbrook, 1959). The cognitive model of insomnia focuses on the factors that operate at night and during the day that serve to maintain the presence of insomnia. This model focuses on five cognitive processes: worry and rumination, selective attention and monitoring, misperception of sleep and daytime deficits, unhelpful beliefs, and counterproductive safety behaviors (Harvey, 2002). The next sections review each component and briefly overview the accumulating evidence.

Worry and Rumination

Previous research has established that individuals with chronic insomnia worry while in bed about a range of topics, including difficulty falling asleep (Wicklow & Espie, 2000). It has been proposed that worry activates the sympathetic nervous system with its corresponding physiological arousal, which then hinders sleep onset (Espie, 2002; Harvey, 2002). Rumination is related to worry and also disrupts sleep. Rumination and worry are distinguishable temporally: while worry focuses on distress regarding future events, rumination involves thoughts of previous events or current symptoms (Carney, Harris, Moss, & Edinger, 2010; Kaplan, Talbot, & Harvey, 2009). Both worry and rumination contribute to heightened physiological arousal, which thereby inhibits sleep.

Based on research spanning several decades, we know that experimental manipulations designed to increase worry in good sleepers results in an increase in sleep-onset insomnia (Ansfield, Wegner, & Bowser, 1996; Gross & Borkovec, 1982) and that experimental manipulations designed to decrease worry in insomnia patients shortens sleep-onset insomnia (Haynes, Adams, & Franzen, 1981; Levey, Aldaz, Watts, & Coyle, 1991). A creative set of studies confirms and extends these findings.

Researchers have incorporated both constructs of pre-sleep worry and presleep rumination in a single experimental paradigm. Although not specifically focused on insomnia, Guastella and Moulds (2007) examined the relationship between rumination and sleep quality following a stressful midterm examination in an undergraduate sample. Individuals with high-trait and low-trait ruminative response styles were asked either to ruminate about the exam ("think about how you felt when you were taking the test today") or to distract ("think about clouds forming in the sky") prior to sleep. The following morning, participants filled out questionnaires on intrusive pre-sleep worry thoughts and overall sleep quality. A significant interaction was found, such that individuals with high-trait rumination who were asked to ruminate prior to sleep reported reduced sleep quality. Intrusive pre-sleep worry was increased in high-trait ruminators but was not increased by the experimental manipulation. In other words, no interaction between trait rumination and the "ruminate" and "distract" experimental conditions was found. Such results suggest that high-trait ruminators experience more pre-sleep worry and, if in a ruminative state, suffer from poorer sleep quality.

Building off these findings, a study examined the role of rumination in sleep quality utilizing an objective measure of sleep quality, actigraphy. Actigraphy is measured with the use of an actigraph, a wrist watch-like device that continuously measures movement and light. The findings from this study support those by Guastella and Moulds (2007) demonstrating that not only do trait ruminators have a subjective perception of delayed sleep onset, but also that their sleep quality is objectively worsened due to rumination (Zoccola, Dickerson, & Lam, 2009).

In recent years, research in the area of repetitive thought processes, an umbrella term that encompasses both worry and rumination, has begun to parse the roles of pre-sleep intrusive worry and pre-sleep ruminative thought in insomnia. Using a cross-sectional design, researchers assessed measures of insomnia, rumination, and worry in a clinical sample. A large sample of adults (N = 210) were assessed for levels of worry via the Penn State Worry Questionnaire (PSWQ; Meyer, Miller, Metzger, & Borkovec, 1990), levels of rumination via the Symptom-Focused Rumination Scale (SYM), which is a subscale of the Rumination Style Questionnaire (Nolen-Hoeksema, 1991), and subjective sleep quality via a two-week long sleep diary. The results indicated a main effect of rumination but no main effect of worry. High ruminators were more likely to have lower sleep efficiency, lower sleep quality, and more frequent wakening after sleep onset compared to low ruminators. These researchers next conducted a factor analysis and found three distinct factors—(1) all of the PSWQ high-worry items, (2) the rumination items from the SYM, and (3) the PSWQ low-worry items. The results were interpreted as indicating that worry and rumination may be separate constructs in the maintenance of insomnia (Carney, Harris, et al., 2010).

Providing further evidence for the separate, but interacting, roles of worry and rumination, Takano, Iijima, and Tanno (2012) conducted a prospective analysis in a large undergraduate sample. They found that rumination significantly predicted subjective sleep quality, even when parsing out depression, anxiety, and stress, whereas worry did not independently predict subjective sleep quality. Their findings also suggest that worry moderates the relationship between rumination and subjective sleep quality: for people with higher levels of worry, rumination was an even stronger predictor of sleep quality, whereas rumination did not predict sleep quality in individuals with low levels of worry. However, this study examined sleep quality more broadly and was not restricted to individuals diagnosed with insomnia, although the results are consistent with research in clinical insomnia populations.

Carney, Harris, Falco, and Edinger's (2013) recent development of a measure to assess rumination in insomnia further supports the role of rumination in maintaining insomnia. Specifically, these researchers developed a measure to assess rumination about insomnia-specific symptoms. They found that insomnia-specific rumination was correlated with insomnia severity. However, they did not find a relationship between generally self-focused rumination, which is common in depression, and insomnia severity. The results from this study continue to support the prominent role of rumination in insomnia.

In sum, the accumulating evidence from multiple studies and multiple mechanisms clearly supports the maintaining roles of rumination and worry in insomnia. The field is just beginning to examine the two processes as separate constructs within insomnia, demarcating this as a good area for future research and providing implications for improving cognitive treatments for insomnia.

Selective Attention and Monitoring

The role of attentional processes has been noted in several cognitive models of insomnia (Espie, 2002; Harvey, 2002). Experimental evidence suggests that when individuals are anxious, they attend to a narrower range of environmental stimuli, resulting in their attention becoming preferentially focused on potential threats. The potential threats are sleep-related within the context of insomnia. These sleep-related threats can be internal, such as unpleasant bodily sensations, or external, such as unpleasant environmental conditions. Because physiological arousal heightens one's ability to detect, monitor for, and attend to bodily sensations, symptoms of arousal create further possibilities for worry and rumination, which then results in an escalating cycle (Harvey, 2002; Rasskazova, Zavalko, Tkhostov, & Dorohov, 2014).

Generally, the research on attentional processes in insomnia has fallen into two categories: computerized information-processing tasks (which examine reaction times in order to make inferences regarding attentional processes; for a review, see Harris et al., 2015) and studies that have employed subjective measures (e.g., interviews and questionnaires). Several studies have used the Stroop task to examine attentional bias for sleep-related words in insomnia. In earlier research, one study did not find evidence for a sleep-related attentional bias in patients with primary insomnia (Lundh, Froding, Gyllenhammar, Broman, & Hetta, 1997), while another study did find that a group who suffered from persistent insomnia did demonstrate a sleep-related insomnia bias (Taylor, Espie, & White, 2003). Another study compared an insomnia group with a healthy control group and a sleep expert group. The sleep expert group, composed of staff from a sleep disorders clinic who had been working in sleep disorder research for several years, was included in order to control for "frequency of concept usage." The insomnia group demonstrated a sleep-related attentional bias, compared to the control group and the sleep expert group. This finding indicated that the bias likely originates not merely from an enhanced sleep focus but from emotional and cognitive involvement with sleep-related stimuli (Spiegelhalder, Espie, Nissen, & Riemann, 2008). An additional study with sleep-deprived healthy participants did not produce a sleep-related attention bias, suggesting that the attentional bias in patients with insomnia is unlikely to be primarily explained by the effect of sleepiness (Sagaspe et al., 2006). More recently, researchers did not find that poor sleepers have an attentional bias toward sleep-related words compared to neutral words. However, they observed that poor sleepers had hindered performance on sleep-related words compared to threat words unrelated to sleep (e.g., panic), which suggests that the attention bias found in insomnia is related to sleep, not just anxiety (Barclay & Ellis, 2013).

Another information-processing task that has been used to examine attention biases in insomnia is the flicker paradigm (Rensink, O'Regan, & Clark, 1996). The flicker paradigm for inducing change blindness (Rensink, 2002) involves the presentation of a visual scene with both bedroom environment and neutral objects. The scene "flickers" back and forth between the two scenes, with one object changing. This process continues until the participant identifies the change. Attentional bias is inferred based on change-detection latency. Two insomnia studies have utilized this methodology. In the first study, participants with primary insomnia exhibited a sleep-related attentional bias (i.e., they detected the sleep-related object change more quickly than the nonsleep object) while good sleepers did not (Jones, Macphee, Broomfield, Jones, & Espie, 2005). In the second, individuals with insomnia exhibited a sleep-related attentional bias relative to both good sleepers and individuals with delayed sleep phase syndrome (Marchetti, Biello, Broomfield, Macmahon, & Espie, 2006).

The dot probe (MacLeod, Mathews, & Tata, 1986) comprises a third information-processing task to assess attentional bias. Two stimuli—one sleep-related word and one neutral—are presented on a screen briefly (e.g., 500 ms) following the presentation of a fixation cross. The words then disappear and a dot appears in the location of one of the stimuli. Participants' reaction time to the dot is indicative of an attentional bias (if the participant is faster to respond to the dot when it appears where the sleep-related word previously appeared). Using this paradigm, several research groups have found a sleep-related attentional bias in the primary insomnia group relative to good sleepers (Jansson-Fröjmark, Bermås, & Kjellén, 2012; MacMahon, Broomfield, & Espie, 2006; Spiegelhalder et al., 2010) and individuals with delayed sleep phase (MacMahon et al., 2006).

Woods, Marchetti, Biello, and Espie (2009) utilized a modified Posner paradigm (Broomfield, Gumley, & Espie, 2005; Posner & Petersen, 1990) to assess attentional bias in insomnia. This paradigm involves a picture of a clock appearing briefly (250 ms) on either the right side or left side of the screen following the presentation of a fixation cross. The picture then disappears, and a horizontal or vertical target appears on either the same side (valid trial) or the other side of the screen (invalid trial) on which the clocks were presented. Participants' faster reaction time to the stimulus on a valid trial is indicative of attentional engagement, whereas slower reaction time to the invalid trials is indicative of difficulty with attention disengagement to the sleep-related stimulus. These researchers found that participants with insomnia were slower to disengage from the sleep-related cue relative to the normal sleepers, although there were no differences between the insomnia group and the normal sleepers on the valid trials.

Eye-tracking methodology has also started to be employed in attention research in insomnia in order to elucidate the timeline of attention allocation. Participants are asked to stare at a screen with a target word and a distractor comprised of fake words. Participants are then told to ignore the distractor fake words and are presented with sleep-positive words, sleep-negative words, and neutral words. Compared to healthy controls, participants with insomnia were less attentive to any words regardless of how sleep focused they were and took longer to differentiate between target and distractor words (Woods, Scheepers, Ross, Espie, & Biello, 2013).

A complementary line of research has examined the role of attentional biases using varied methodology (e.g., diary, interview, questionnaire, experimental manipulation). For example, an experimental manipulation demonstrated that a form of monitoring—clock-monitoring—resulted in more pre-sleep worry and longer sleep-onset latency (Tang, Schmidt, & Harvey, 2007). An interview study provided evidence for an association between monitoring and increased negative thoughts and use of safety behaviors at night and during the day in patients with insomnia (Semler & Harvey, 2004). Together, these studies add to the evidence that, compared to good sleepers, individuals with insomnia are more prone to selectively attend to, or monitor for, external and internal sleep-related threats. Moreover, they suggest that monitoring has adverse consequences for sleep (Tang & Harvey, 2004) and contributes to a vicious cycle of cognitive processes (Semler & Harvey, 2004).

Two experimental studies provide support for the role of attentional processes—and in particular, monitoring—as a cognitive mechanism in insomnia. In the first study, participants with insomnia were randomly assigned to either a monitoring group or a no-monitoring group. Upon waking in the morning, the monitoring group was instructed to monitor body sensations throughout the day while the other group was instructed to distract from body sensations. Results indicated that the monitoring group reported more negative thoughts, safety behaviors, and daytime sleepiness (Semler & Harvey, 2007). A second study examined the association between coping disposition (e.g., tendency to monitor) and insomnia. Results indicated that individuals with primary insomnia were more likely to use monitoring as a coping strategy (Voss, Kolling, & Heidenreich, 2006).

In sum, across a variety of methodologies, accumulating evidence suggests that attentional biases are present in insomnia. Such attentional biases not only contribute to insomnia but can also exacerbate perceived daytime impairment.

Misperception

Several research studies focusing on insomnia have found discrepancies between objective reports of sleep (e.g., polysomnography, actigraphy) and an individual's subjective perception of sleep (Chambers, 1993; Harvey & Tang, 2012; Mercer, Bootzin, & Lack, 2002). Although some may argue that traditional methods of sleep measurement may not be sensitive enough, as we describe elsewhere (Kaplan et al., 2009), it is also possible that individuals become more anxious about their perceived sleep difficulties. This vigilance and focus on the sleep state in individuals with insomnia may result in their overestimating the amount of time awake and underestimating the amount of time asleep. Notably, these two accounts of sleep state misperception (i.e., a measurement problem vs. a perceptual problem) are not mutually exclusive (see Harvey, 2005, for further explanation).

Notably, an experimental study showed that the misperception of sleep does not appear to be due to insomnia patients exhibiting a general deficit in time estimation abilities (Harvey & Tang, 2012; Tang & Harvey, 2005). Another study replicated this finding by demonstrating that there were no differences between good and poor sleepers in estimating time in nonsleep settings (Fichten, Creti, Amsel, Bailes, & Libman, 2005). Consistent with this evidence, Rioux, Tremblay, and Bastien (2006) compared insomnia patients and good sleepers on a finger-tapping time estimation task. They also reported no group differences and no relationship between insomnia severity and time estimation.

It is notable that several of the cognitive processes discussed in this chapter are interrelated. For example, two experimental studies illustrate the contribution of monitoring to misperception. In the first study, participants were randomly assigned to a clock monitoring group or a digital display monitoring group as they were trying to get to sleep. The clock monitoring group exhibited a greater discrepancy between their subjective estimate of sleep-onset latency and the objective estimate; that is, participants overestimated their sleep-onset latency when they monitored the clock (Tang et al., 2007). In the second study (Semler & Harvey, 2006), three groups of individuals with insomnia were randomly assigned to a self-focus group, a monitoring group, or a no-instruction group. Participants in the self-focus group were instructed to "pay attention to your image on the TV monitor" and in the monitoring group, to "pay attention to your thoughts, body, mood, and ability to perform" while completing a battery of challenging mental tasks. Self-focus was defined as focusing on internal thoughts and feelings—both present and past—while monitoring was explained as focusing on cues presenting a current threat. The results indicated that the self-focus group perceived their performance as worse on the test, compared to the no instruction group, though their performance did not in fact differ. Together, these results demonstrate that monitoring is one mechanism that likely contributes to misperception. Moreover, misperception among individuals with insomnia adversely affects daytime functioning.

Unhelpful Beliefs

Unhelpful beliefs play an important role in the maintenance of insomnia (Morin, 1993). These unhelpful beliefs may exacerbate intrusive and worrisome thoughts throughout the day and night, which contributes to the development and maintenance of sleep disturbance (Harvey, 2002). As we describe elsewhere (Kaplan et al., 2009), an example of an unhelpful belief in insomnia is an individual believing he or she needs to sleep continuously through the night with no awakenings to feel refreshed. Such a belief is unhelpful because awakenings are a natural part of nocturnal sleep (e.g., Åkerstedt et al., 2002). The subsequent worry related to this belief might take the form of an individual who, once awakened during the night, believes that this fragmented sleep will result in poorer work performance the following day.

Most research on unhelpful beliefs in insomnia has utilized the Dysfunctional Beliefs and Attitudes about Sleep Scale (DBAS; Espie, Inglis, Harvey, & Tessier, 2000; Morin, Vallières, & Ivers, 2007). When used in studies evaluating the effects of cognitive-behavioral therapy for insomnia, a decreased DBAS score predicts improved treatment outcome (Morin, Blais, & Savard, 2002). Also, a recent study reported that DBAS scores mediated treatment outcome following CBT-I including functional impairment, supporting the hypothesis that unhelpful beliefs contribute to the maintenance of insomnia (Sunnhed & Jansson-Fröjmark, 2015).

Researchers have also examined DBAS scores across insomnia subtypes and among healthy populations. Pooling data from five sleep clinics, researchers found that all insomnia subtypes exhibited higher DBAS scores opposed to good sleepers, indicating that patients with insomnia have more unhelpful beliefs about sleep than healthy sleepers (Carney, Edinger, et al., 2010). In addition, combining data from four insomnia-focused studies, researchers found that individuals can be clustered based on different subscales of the DBAS, and these different clusters based on unhelpful beliefs are related to insomnia severity (Sánchez-Ortuño & Edinger, 2010). In sum, strong evidence has accrued indicating a relationship between unhelpful beliefs about sleep and chronic insomnia.

Counterproductive Safety Behaviors

Safety behaviors are actions taken to avoid feared outcomes. They are maladaptive in two ways: (1) they prevent disconfirmation of the unhelpful beliefs, and (2) they increase the likelihood that the feared outcomes will occur (Salkovskis, Clark, Hackmann, Wells, & Gelder, 1999). Individuals with insomnia often employ safety behaviors in an attempt to cope with anxiety related to unhelpful beliefs about sleep (Ree & Harvey, 2004a). We previously described an individual who endorsed the unhelpful belief that only solid, uninterrupted sleep would allow unimpaired work performance the next day. To prevent nocturnal awakenings, this individual developed a routine of safety behaviors, including never going out in the evening, wearing earplugs, and using a sound machine as he or she slept. Engaging in these behaviors, though understandable, will prevent the individual from clearly learning that he or she can get adequate sleep even if the routine is broken. Paradoxically, the safety behaviors also may make the feared outcome more likely to occur. Not going out in the evening increases the chance that the person will become preoccupied with his or her sleep and may contribute to rumination/worry and sad mood. Earplugs can be effective in certain circumstances, but they can also contribute to sleep problems if they are uncomfortable or if they cause the person to strain to try to hear things in the environment. A sound machine might contribute to awakenings in the night (Kaplan et al., 2009).

In a direct examination of the relationship between beliefs about sleep and use of safety behaviors (Woodley & Smith, 2006), forty participants completed standard measures of insomnia severity, depression and anxiety, and also the DBAS. Following this, individuals kept a sleep diary for fourteen consecutive days and recorded the sleep safety behaviors used each day. Holding more unhelpful beliefs about sleep (i.e., higher DBAS scores) predicted the use of daily safety behaviors, though depression explained more of the variance in safety behavior use. Such research provides evidence for a relationship between sleep beliefs and safety behaviors and suggests depression as a third construct of importance in understanding chronic insomnia.

In order to better elucidate the role of safety behaviors in maintaining insomnia, a study examined the frequency of use and the perceived need for use of safety behaviors (Hood, Carney, & Harris, 2011). Using self-report measures with a large undergraduate sample, this study found that the frequency of safety behavior use was not associated with increased insomnia severity, whereas safety behavior use was associated with increased insomnia severity. Of note, this study also found that the perceived utility of safety behaviors was associated with increased perceived daytime disturbance. As the study's authors highlight, these findings indicate the importance of targeting safety behaviors during treatment: not just the frequency of their use, but also the perceived need of their use.

TREATMENT

The aim of cognitive therapy for insomnia (CT-I) is to reverse the five maintaining cognitive processes just reviewed (worry and rumination, selective attention and monitoring, misperception, unhelpful beliefs, and counterproductive safety behaviors). CT-I seeks to reverse these processes during both the night and the day. Essential to the delivery of CT-I are the cognitive therapy skills of Socratic questioning, guided discovery, and behavioral experiments. As we describe in more detail elsewhere (Harvey, Sharpley, Ree, Stinson, & Clark, 2007), the process of CT-I first involves case conceptualization in order to develop individualized cognitive models for the client; next it involves reversing the five maintaining processes using behavioral experiments; and then last it involves relapse prevention. Behavioral experiments that are carefully formulated to test negative beliefs and promote the development and testing of more adaptive views (Ree & Harvey, 2004b) are of particular importance to reversing the different maintaining processes. Examples of behavioral experiments for CT-I include demonstrating the discrepancies between objective and subjective measures of sleep using sleep diaries and actigraphy in order to reduce misperception; training in actively directing attention away from sleep-related stimuli in order to reduce monitoring; intentionally having a client experience one poor night of sleep (e.g., only six hours of sleep) in order for him or her to see that he or she can cope with an occasional poor night of sleep and thus addressing an unhelpful belief; comparing nights of sleep while drinking alcohol before bed versus not drinking alcohol before bed (although alcohol may help individuals fall asleep, it leads to more disrupted sleep throughout the night); and an experiment demonstrating how thought suppression in an attempt to stop worrying before bed may actually increase the number of thoughts in order to promote the adoption of new skills to combat worry and rumination (Soehner, Kaplan, Kanady, & Harvey, 2013).

In terms of evidence for CT-I, the detailed review of treatments for insomnia conducted by the American Academy of Sleep Medicine concluded that cognitive therapy had "received insufficient evaluation" (Morin et al., 2006). Since that publication, one open trial of CT-I and one randomized controlled trial of CT-I have been published. The open trial (*N* = 19) (Harvey et al., 2007) aimed to reverse the cognitive-maintaining processes reviewed in this chapter during both the night and the day. Assessments were completed pretreatment, posttreatment and at three-, six-, and twelve-month follow-up. The significant improvement in both nighttime and daytime impairment evident at the posttreatment assessment was retained up to the twelve-month follow-up. These preliminary results suggest that cognitive therapy is (1) acceptable to patients with insomnia, (2) helpful in improving sleep, and (3) effective in enhancing daytime functioning. The results were strongest for measures of daytime functioning and moderate for measures derived from the sleep diary. Replication of these findings within a sufficiently powered randomized controlled trial was a recommended next step.

More recently, researchers have conducted a randomized controlled trial of CT-I, including 188 adult patients with chronic insomnia who were recruited and treated at the University of California, Berkeley, or at the Université Laval (Harvey et al., 2014). The main goal was to examine the unique contribution of behavioral therapy (BT) and cognitive therapy (CT) relative to the full cognitive-behavioral therapy (full CBT). These treatments were individually delivered across eight weekly sessions. The results showed significant improvements across all three conditions on measures of insomnia symptom severity, nighttime sleep disturbances, and daytime functioning, and these improvements were generally sustained at six-month follow-up. The full CBT was associated with greatest improvements, the improvements associated with BT were faster but not as sustained, and the improvements associated with CT were slower and sustained. The latter result seems particularly interesting because the different trajectories of change may well provide unique insights into the process of behavior change via behavioral versus cognitive routes. They point to a need for future research to identify why an intervention targeting behavioral change generates faster improvement but is not as well sustained, while an intervention targeting cognitive processes generates slower but more sustained change. One methodological issue to keep in mind is that the CBT sessions were fifteen minutes longer than the CT and BT sessions so we cannot rule out the possibility that participants in the CBT group did better overall because they received more treatment. Together these findings raise several questions for future research. Is this pattern of findings specific to insomnia, or do these findings replicate in BT versus CT for other conditions? Are the behavioral adjustments that are core to BT easier for a patient to implement when a therapist is available for "coaching?" Do we need more emphasis on establishing the behavioral recommendations as habits that the patient automatically reinitiates if/when insomnia recurs? Are some features of the procedures used in CT more conducive to habit formation? Does change to cognitive processes take longer, but, once the skills are learned, are they more easily sustained?

CONCLUSIONS

The cognitive theory described in this chapter specifies five processes that function to maintain insomnia, namely, worry and rumination, selective attention and monitoring, misperception of sleep and daytime deficits, unhelpful beliefs, and counterproductive safety behaviors. The aim of CT-I is to reverse all five maintaining processes during both the night and the day. While progress has been made in testing the theoretical model and in developing a treatment to reverse the maintaining processes specified by the model, much further research remains to be done. For example, Ree and Harvey (2006) have examined biased interpretations, but these results have yet to be translated into treatment. Finally, expectations specific to the imminent sleep period also seem likely to also play a role (Born, Hansen, Marshall, Mölle, & Fehm, 1999).

ACKNOWLEDGMENTS

We would like to acknowledge Drs. David M. Clark and Melissa Ree who were key to developing this approach.

REFERENCES

Åkerstedt, T., Billiard, M., Bonnet, M., Ficca, G., Garma, L., Mariotti, M., . . . Schulz, H. (2002). Awakening from sleep. *Sleep Medicine Reviews, 6*(4), 267–286.

American Psychiatric Association. (2013). *Diagnostic and statistical manual of mental disorders* (5th ed.). Washington, DC: American Psychiatric Association.

Ancoli-Israel, S., & Roth, T. (1999). Characteristics of insomnia in the United States: Results of the 1991 National Sleep Foundation Survey: I. *Sleep, 22*(Suppl. 2), S347–S353.

Ansfield, M. E., Wegner, D. M., & Bowser, R. (1996). Ironic effects of sleep urgency. *Behaviour Research and Therapy, 34*(7), 523–531.

Baglioni, C., Battagliese, G., Feige, B., Spiegelhalder, K., Nissen, C., Voderholzer, U., . . . Riemann, D. (2011). Insomnia as a predictor of depression: A meta-analytic evaluation of longitudinal epidemiological studies. *Journal of Affective Disorders, 135*(1–3), 10–19.

Barclay, N. L., & Ellis, J. G. (2013). Sleep-related attentional bias in poor versus good sleepers is independent of affective valence. *Journal of Sleep Research, 22*(4), 414–421.

Beck, A. T. (1976). *Cognitive therapy and the emotional disorders.* New York: International Universities Press.

Borkovec, T. D. (1982). Insomnia. *Journal of Consulting and Clinical Psychology, 50,* 880–895.

Born, J., Hansen, K., Marshall, L., Mölle, M., & Fehm, H. L. (1999). Timing the end of nocturnal sleep. *Nature, 397*(6714), 29–30.

Broomfield, N. M., Gumley, A. I., & Espie, C. A. (2005). Candidate cognitive processes in psychophysiologic insomnia. *Journal of Cognitive Psychotherapy, 19*(1), 5–17.

Carney, C. E., Edinger, J. D., Morin, C. M., Manber, R., Rybarczyk, B., Stepanski, E. J., . . . Lack, L. (2010). Examining maladaptive beliefs about sleep across insomnia patient groups. *Journal of Psychosomatic Research, 68*(1), 57–65.

Carney, C. E., Harris, A. L., Falco, A., & Edinger, J. D. (2013). The relation between insomnia symptoms, mood, and rumination about insomnia symptoms. *Journal of Clinical Sleep Medicine, 9*(6), 567–575.

Carney, C. E., Harris, A. L., Moss, T. G., & Edinger, J. D. (2010). Distinguishing rumination from worry in clinical insomnia. *Behaviour Research and Therapy, 48*(6), 540–546.

Chambers, M. (1993). Alert insomniacs: Are they really sleep deprived? *Clinical Psychology Review, 13*(7), 649–666.

Clark, D. M. (1997). Panic disorder and social phobia. In D. M. Clark & C. G. Fairburn (Eds.), *Science and practice of cognitive behaviour therapy* (pp. 121–153). Oxford, UK: Oxford University Press.

Dalgleish, T., & Watts, F. N. (1990). Biases of attention and memory in disorders of anxiety and depression. *Clinical Psychology Review, 10*(5), 589–604.

Drake, C. L., Pillai, V., & Roth, T. (2014). Stress and sleep reactivity: A prospective investigation of the stress-diathesis model of insomnia. *Sleep, 37,* 1295–1304.

Easterbrook, J. A. (1959). The effect of emotion on cue utilization and the organization of behavior. *Psychological Review,* 66(3), 183–201.

Espie, C. A. (2002). Insomnia: Conceptual issues in the development, persistence, and treatment of sleep disorder in adults. *Annual Review of Psychology, 53,* 215–243.

Espie, C. A., Inglis, S. J., Harvey, L., & Tessier, S. (2000). Insomniacs' attributions. *Journal of Psychosomatic Research, 48*(2), 141–148.

Fichten, C. S., Creti, L., Amsel, R., Bailes, S., & Libman, E. (2005). Time estimation in good and poor sleepers. *Journal of Behavioral Medicine, 28*(6), 537–553.

Gross, R. T., & Borkovec, T. D. (1982). Effects of a cognitive intrusion manipulation on the sleep-onset latency of good sleepers. *Behavior Therapy, 13*(1), 112–116.

Guastella, A. J., & Moulds, M. L. (2007). The impact of rumination on sleep quality following a stressful life event. *Personality and Individual Differences, 42*(6), 1151–1162.

Harris, K., Spiegelhalder, K., Espie, C. A., MacMahon, K. M. A., Woods, H. C., & Kyle, S. D. (2015). Sleep-related attentional bias in insomnia: A state-of-the-science review. *Clinical Psychology Review, 42,* 16–27.

Harvey, A. G. (2001). Insomnia: Symptom or diagnosis? *Clinical Psychology Review, 21*(7), 1037–1059.

Harvey, A. G. (2002). A cognitive model of insomnia. *Behaviour Research and Therapy, 40*(8), 869–893.

Harvey, A. G. (2005). A cognitive theory and therapy for chronic insomnia. *Journal of Cognitive Psychotherapy, 19*(1), 41–59.

Harvey, A. G., Bélanger, L., Talbot, L., Eidelman, P., Beaulieu-Bonneau, S., Fortier-Brochu, E., . . . Morin, C. M. (2014). Comparative efficacy of behavior therapy, cognitive therapy, and cognitive behavior therapy for chronic insomnia: A randomized controlled trial. *Journal of Consulting and Clinical Psychology, 82*(4), 670–683.

Harvey, A. G., Sharpley, A. L., Ree, M. J., Stinson, K., & Clark, D. M. (2007). An open trial of cognitive therapy for chronic insomnia. *Behaviour Research and Therapy, 45*(10), 2491–2501.

Harvey, A. G., & Tang, N. K. Y. (2012). (Mis)perception of sleep in insomnia: A puzzle and a resolution. *Psychological Bulletin, 138*(1), 77–101.

Haynes, S. N., Adams, A., & Franzen, M. (1981). The effects of presleep stress on sleep-onset insomnia. *Journal of Abnormal Psychology, 90*, 601–606.

Hood, H. K., Carney, C. E., & Harris, A. L. (2011). Rethinking safety behaviors in insomnia: Examining the perceived utility of sleep-related safety behaviors. *Behavior Therapy, 42*(4), 644–654.

Jansson-Fröjmark, M., Bermås, M., & Kjellén, A. (2012). Attentional bias in insomnia: The dot-probe task with pictorial stimuli depicting daytime fatigue/malaise. *Cognitive Therapy and Research, 37*(3), 534–546.

Jones, B. T., Macphee, L. M., Broomfield, N. M., Jones, B. C., & Espie, C. A. (2005). Sleep-related attentional bias in good, moderate, and poor (primary insomnia) sleepers. *Journal of Abnormal Psychology, 114*(2), 249–258.

Kaplan, K. A., Talbot, L. S., & Harvey, A. G. (2009). Cognitive mechanisms in chronic insomnia: Processes and prospects. *Sleep Medicine Clinics, 4*(4), 541–548.

Levey, A. B., Aldaz, J. A., Watts, F. N., & Coyle, K. (1991). Articulatory suppression and the treatment of insomnia. *Behaviour Research and Therapy, 29*(1), 85–89.

Lundh, L.-G. G., Froding, A., Gyllenhammar, L., Broman, J.-E. E., & Hetta, J. (1997). Cognitive bias and memory performance in patients with persistent insomnia. *Cognitive Behaviour Therapy, 26*(1), 27–35.

MacLeod, C., Mathews, A., & Tata, P. (1986). Attentional bias in emotional disorders. *Journal of Abnormal Psychology, 95*, 15–20.

MacMahon, K. M. A., Broomfield, N. M., & Espie, C. A. (2006). Attention bias for sleep-related stimuli in primary insomnia and delayed sleep phase syndrome using the dot-probe task. *Sleep, 29*(11), 1420–1427.

Marchetti, L. M., Biello, S. M., Broomfield, N. M., Macmahon, K. M. A., & Espie, C. A. (2006). Who is pre-occupied with sleep?: A comparison of attention bias in people with psychophysiological insomnia, delayed sleep phase syndrome and good sleepers using the induced change blindness paradigm. *Journal of Sleep Research, 15*(2), 212–221.

Mercer, J. D., Bootzin, R. R., & Lack, L. C. (2002). Insomniacs' perception of wake instead of sleep. *Sleep, 25*, 564–571.

Meyer, T. J., Miller, M. L., Metzger, R. L., & Borkovec, T. D. (1990). Development and validation of the Penn State Worry Questionnaire. *Behaviour Research and Therapy, 28*(6), 487–495.

Morin, C. M. (1993). *Insomnia: Psychological assessment and management.* New York: Guilford Press.

Morin, C. M., Blais, F., & Savard, J. (2002). Are changes in beliefs and attitudes about sleep related to sleep improvements in the treatment of insomnia? *Behaviour Research and Therapy, 40*(7), 741–752.

Morin, C. M., Bootzin, R. R., Buysse, D. J., Edinger, J. D., Espie, C. A., & Lichstein, K. L. (2006). Psychological and behavioral treatment of insomnia: Update of the recent evidence (1998–2004). *Sleep, 29*(11), 1398–1414.

Morin, C. M., Vallières, A., & Ivers, H. (2007). Dysfunctional beliefs and attitudes about sleep (DBAS): Validation of a brief version (DBAS-16). *Sleep, 30*(11), 1547–1554.

Nolen-Hoeksema, S. (1991). Responses to depression and their effects on the duration of depressive episodes. *Journal of Abnormal Psychology, 100*(4), 569–582.

Perlis, M. L., Giles, D. E., Mendelson, W. B., Bootzin, R. R., & Wyatt, J. K. (1997). Psychophysiological insomnia: The behavioural model and a neurocognitive perspective. *Journal of Sleep Research, 6*(3), 179–188.

Pillai, V., Roth, T., & Drake, C. L. (2015). The nature of stable insomnia phenotypes. *Sleep, 38*(1), 127–138.

Posner, M. I., & Petersen, S. E. (1990). The attention system of the human brain. *Annual Review of Neuroscience, 13,* 25–42.

Rasskazova, E., Zavalko, I., Tkhostov, A., & Dorohov, V. (2014). High intention to fall asleep causes sleep fragmentation. *Journal of Sleep Research, 23*(3), 295–301.

Ree, M. J., & Harvey, A. G. (2004a). Investigating safety behaviours in insomnia: The development of the Sleep-Related Behaviours Questionnaire (SRBQ). *Behaviour Change, 21*(1), 26–36.

Ree, M. J., & Harvey, A. G. (2004b). Insomnia. In J. Bennett-Levy, G. Butler, M. Fennell, A. Hackman, M. Mueller, & D. Wesbrook (Eds.), *The Oxford guide to behavioural experiments in cognitive therapy* (pp. 287–308). New York: Oxford University Press.

Ree, M. J., & Harvey, A. G. (2006). Interpretive biases in chronic insomnia: An investigation using a priming paradigm. *Behavior Therapy, 37*(3), 248–258.

Rensink, R. A. (2002). Change detection. *Annual Review of Psychology, 53,* 245–277.

Rensink, R. A., O'Regan, J. K., & Clark, J. J. (1996). To see or not to see: The need for attention to perceive changes in scenes. *Investigative Ophthalmology and Visual Science, 37*(3), 1–6.

Rioux, I., Tremblay, S., & Bastien, C. H. (2006). Time estimation in chronic insomnia sufferers. *Sleep, 29*(4), 486–493.

Roth, T., Jaeger, S., Jin, R., Kalsekar, A., Stang, P. E., & Kessler, R. C. (2006). Sleep problems, comorbid mental disorders, and role functioning in the national comorbidity survey replication. *Biological Psychiatry, 60*(12), 1364–1371.

Sagaspe, P., Sanchez-Ortuno, M., Charles, A., Taillard, J., Valtat, C., Bioulac, B.,

. . . Philip, P. (2006). Effects of sleep deprivation on Color-Word, Emotional, and Specific Stroop interference and on self-reported anxiety. *Brain and Cognition, 60*(1), 76–87.

Salkovskis, P. M. (1996). *Frontiers of cognitive therapy*. New York: Guilford Press.

Salkovskis, P. M., Clark, D. M., Hackmann, A., Wells, A., & Gelder, M. G. (1999). An experimental investigation of the role of safety-seeking behaviours in the maintenance of panic disorder with agoraphobia. *Behaviour Research and Therapy, 37*(6), 559–574.

Sánchez-Ortuño, M. M., & Edinger, J. D. (2010). A penny for your thoughts: Patterns of sleep-related beliefs, insomnia symptoms and treatment outcome. *Behaviour Research and Therapy, 48*(2), 125–133.

Sarsour, K., Morin, C. M., Foley, K., Kalsekar, A., & Walsh, J. K. (2010). Association of insomnia severity and comorbid medical and psychiatric disorders in a health plan-based sample: Insomnia severity and comorbidities. *Sleep Medicine, 11*(1), 69–74.

Semler, C. N., & Harvey, A. G. (2004). An investigation of monitoring for sleep-related threat in primary insomnia. *Behaviour Research and Therapy, 42*(12), 1403–1420.

Semler, C. N., & Harvey, A. G. (2006). Daytime functioning in primary insomnia: Does attentional focus contribute to real or perceived impairment? *Behavioral Sleep Medicine, 4*(2), 85–103.

Semler, C. N., & Harvey, A. G. (2007). An experimental investigation of daytime monitoring for sleep-related threat in primary insomnia. *Cognition and Emotion, 21*(1), 146–161.

Soehner, A., Kaplan, K., Kanady, J., & Harvey, A. G. (2013). Cognitive therapy for insomnia. In C. Kushida (Ed.), *The encyclopedia of sleep* (Vol. 2, pp. 290–295). Waltham, MA: Academic Press.

Spiegelhalder, K., Espie, C., Nissen, C., & Riemann, D. (2008). Sleep-related attentional bias in patients with primary insomnia compared with sleep experts and healthy controls. *Journal of Sleep Research, 17*(2), 191–196.

Spiegelhalder, K., Kyle, S. D., Feige, B., Prem, M., Nissen, C., Espie, C. A., . . . Riemann, D. (2010). The impact of sleep-related attentional bias on polysomnographically measured sleep in primary insomnia. *Sleep, 33*(1), 107–112.

Sunnhed, R., & Jansson-Fröjmark, M. (2015). Cognitive arousal, unhelpful beliefs and maladaptive sleep behaviors as mediators in cognitive behavior therapy for insomnia: A quasi-experimental study. *Cognitive Therapy and Research, 39*(6), 841–852.

Takano, K., Iijima, Y., & Tanno, Y. (2012). Repetitive thought and self-reported sleep disturbance. *Behavior Therapy, 43*(4), 779–789.

Tang, N. K. Y., & Harvey, A. G. (2004). Correcting distorted perception of sleep in insomnia: A novel behavioural experiment? *Behaviour Research and Therapy, 42*(1), 27–39.

Tang, N. K. Y., & Harvey, A. G. (2005). Time estimation ability and distorted perception of sleep in insomnia. *Behavioral Sleep Medicine, 3*(3), 134–150.

Tang, N. K. Y., Schmidt, D. A., & Harvey, A. G. (2007). Sleeping with the enemy: Clock monitoring in the maintenance of insomnia. *Journal of Behavior Therapy and Experimental Psychiatry, 38*(1), 40–55.

Taylor, L. M., Espie, C. A., & White, C. A. (2003). Attentional bias in people with acute versus persistent insomnia secondary to cancer. *Behavioral Sleep Medicine, 1*(4), 200–212.

Voss, U., Kolling, T., & Heidenreich, T. (2006). Role of monitoring and blunting coping styles in primary insomnia. *Psychosomatic Medicine, 68*, 110–115.

Wicklow, A., & Espie, C. A. (2000). Intrusive thoughts and their relationship to actigraphic measurement of sleep: Towards a cognitive model of insomnia. *Behaviour Research and Therapy, 38*(7), 679–693.

Woodley, J., & Smith, S. (2006). Safety behaviors and dysfunctional beliefs about sleep: Testing a cognitive model of the maintenance of insomnia. *Journal of Psychosomatic Research, 60*(6), 551–557.

Woods, H., Marchetti, L. M., Biello, S. M., & Espie, C. A. (2009). The clock as a focus of selective attention in those with primary insomnia: An experimental study using a modified Posner paradigm. *Behaviour Research and Therapy, 47*(3), 231–236.

Woods, H., Scheepers, C., Ross, K. A., Espie, C. A., & Biello, S. M. (2013). What are you looking at?: Moving toward an attentional timeline in insomnia: A novel semantic eye tracking study. *Sleep, 36*(10), 1491–1499.

Zoccola, P. M., Dickerson, S. S., & Lam, S. (2009). Rumination predicts longer sleep onset latency after an acute psychosocial stressor. *Psychosomatic Medicine, 71*(7), 771–775.

CHAPTER 12

Cognitive-Behavioral Couple Therapy

Norman B. Epstein

Although cognitive therapy (CT) initially was developed as a treatment for problems in individuals' personal functioning such as depression and anxiety disorders (A. T. Beck, 1976; A. T. Beck, Rush, Shaw, & Emery, 1979), one of its basic goals was to produce a more realistic and appropriate alignment between events in people's lives and the individuals' subjective cognitive interpretations of them. Many of those life events involved interpersonal relationships, especially with significant others such as parents and romantic partners. Individuals in CT commonly told their therapists about distressing close relationships in the same manner that they would relate upsetting experiences with job stresses, failure to meet personal performance standards regarding life goals, and so on. Cognitive therapists could help these individuals in understanding the importance of identifying one's negative automatic thoughts about an intimate relationship and evaluating their validity through logical analysis and systematic examination of available evidence (e.g., "You get upset when you think your partner does not care about you. In what ways, even small ones, has your partner behaved toward you recently that might reflect caring?"). Behavioral experiments offered another avenue for testing negative expectancies (e.g., if a man predicted that his partner would not remember a discussion they had a few days ago, the therapist could encourage him to ask her about it and find out how much she recalled).

Thus, from its early days, the CT framework went far beyond internal logical analysis of negative cognitions to take people's interactions with their environments into account, as sources of data and as means of initiating change. However, a traditional individual therapy approach to relationship problems had a limitation shared by other individual therapy models; namely, that an individual's reports about events in an intimate relationship were solely that person's subjective perceptions. On occasions when a therapist invited a significant other to join a session for the purposes of corroborating the client's reports and engaging the partner as a source of support for the individual's treatment, it was not unusual for the therapist to discover that the partner was not quite as had been portrayed. In addition, it was clear that the members of the couple were locked in negative behavioral interaction patterns and distressed emotions that were both fueled by negative cognitions about each other. The issue was how to address the reciprocal influences among the cognitions, emotional responses, and behaviors of the two partners simultaneously. This could not simply involve two parallel individual cognitive therapies, as the partners were continuously influencing each other.

Initially, Epstein (1982), A. T. Beck (1988), and Dattilio and Padesky (1990) applied CT principles to distressed couple relationships, and Ellis and Harper's (1961) focus on irrational beliefs was extended by Ellis et al. (1989) to treating members of unhappy couples. These expansions of individually focused cognitive models took into account the fact both members of a couple could be contributing to negative interactions, and they used established cognitive assessment and intervention methods from individual therapy to identify and modify partners' distorted or inappropriate perceptions, inferences, and beliefs about each other. However, they still emphasized negative cognitions more than problematic dyadic behavioral patterns.

Fortunately, at the same time that Beck and colleagues were developing CT and other cognitively focused models were emerging, including Ellis's rational-emotive therapy and Meichenbaum's (1985) stress inoculation approach, the field of behavioral marital and family therapy based on social learning principles was gaining momentum. Major contributions by Liberman (1970), Patterson (1971), Weiss, Hops, and Patterson (1973), Jacobson and Margolin (1979), and Stuart (1980) focused on conjoint treatment to reduce significant others' exchanges of negative behavior and increase mutually pleasing actions. Those primarily behavioral approaches were based on an assumption that individuals' positive thoughts and emotions about significant others would follow from more positive behavioral interactions.

The primary focus of cognitive therapies on individuals' subjective internal experiences of their significant others and the primary focus of behavioral marital and family therapy on overt interactions offered complementary components for an integrative cognitive-behavioral model of therapy. Regarding cognitive-behavioral couple therapy (CBCT), Baucom and Epstein's (1990) text *Cognitive-Behavioral Marital Therapy* and Rathus and Sanderson's (1999) volume *Marital Distress: Cognitive Behavioral Interventions for Couples* focused on the interplay among cognitions, affect, and behavior, with major attention paid to assessment and intervention within each domain. They applied traditional CT concepts and methods for addressing partners' cognitions, as well as behavioral marital therapy procedures for improving couple communication, problem solving, and constructive expression of emotions such as anger. CBCT became more systemic by tracking interaction cycles in which partners continuously influence each other (e.g., partner B interprets partner A's behavior as disrespectful, becomes angry, and behaves vindictively toward partner A, who perceives B's behavior as unjustified and reciprocates the negative behavior, and so on), thus perpetuating a cycle of self-fulfilling prophecies.

Subsequently, Epstein and Baucom (2002) presented an enhanced CBCT model that added a broader ecological, contextual perspective in which a couple's functioning is influenced by multiple system levels, ranging from each partner's needs and traits to conflicts within the couple, to interactions with children and other family members, to extended family and friends, to job demands, to environmental stresses such as community violence and economic problems. The enhanced model includes a stress and coping component in which the success of a couple's relationship depends on their ability as individuals and as a dyad to cope with life demands in any of the contextual levels they experience (e.g., one partner's depression, a child's chronic illness, a partner's job stresses). Furthermore, the enhanced CBCT model gives partners' emotional responses a more prominent place in assessment and treatment, consistent with growing recognition of the importance of emotional experience in intimate relationships (Greenberg & Goldman, 2008; Johnson, 1996). Finally, the model differentiates between microlevel responses (e.g., an argument about who was responsible for leaving dirty dishes in the kitchen sink) and macrolevel patterns (e.g., a broad power struggle).

Initially, CBCT was designed to improve the overall quality of a couple's relationship by reducing aversive behavioral interactions, increasing pleasing behavior between partners, reducing distorted, unhelpful or inappropriate cognitions (e.g., unrealistic standards for how a partner should demonstrate "caring") that elicit conflict and emotional distress, and improving partners' regulation of emotions such as anger. The "bottom-line" goal was improved relationship satisfaction. However, in the past two decades the empirically supported applications of CBCT have expanded substantially in two major directions: (1) couple interventions for problems in individual functioning (e.g., depression, anxiety disorders, substance abuse, stress of coping with a serious physical illness) that previously were addressed primarily through individual treatments, and (2) interventions for specific types of challenging relational problems (e.g., infidelity, partner aggression) (Baucom, Epstein, Kirby, & LaTaillade, 2015; Epstein, Dattilio, & Baucom, 2016). Thus, cognitive-behavioral couple therapists increasingly have become valuable members of mental health treatment teams and have implemented effective strategies for assisting couples with relational patterns seriously affecting the members' well-being.

COGNITIVE-BEHAVIORAL MODEL

CBCT is truly an integration of concepts and methods from behaviorally oriented couple therapy, cognitive therapy, and a family systems model. The following sections present brief summaries of components of those three major theoretical models that together comprise this flexible therapeutic approach.

Behaviors Influencing the Quality of Couple Relationships

The concepts of *functional analysis* within the behavioral therapy field (that the occurrence of a behavior is influenced by eliciting stimuli and increased or decreased by its consequences) played a significant role in development of the microlevel assessment of couple interactions in behavioral couple therapy (Weiss et al., 1973). Even though individuals commonly think in linear causal terms when blaming their partners for relationship problems, behavioral couple therapists identified how each person elicits the other's actions and provides consequences for them. When one's goal is to reduce negative behaviors and increase positive behaviors between partners, it is crucial to observe samples of couple interaction directly and to track the sequences that occur. For example, a member of a couple may complain about a partner's nagging but may reinforce it by ignoring the partner's requests until the partner shifts to nagging.

Researchers who studied interactions of distressed couples developed microlevel behavioral coding systems to track the frequencies and sequences of actions associated with subjective relationship satisfaction (Gottman, 1994; Hahlweg et al., 1984; Weiss et al., 1973; Weiss & Summers, 1983). Dyadic patterns that have been found to be especially destructive include one partner pursuing/demanding and the other withdrawing or "stonewalling," partners locked in an escalating exchange of aversive behavior, and the couple engaged in mutual avoidance. Clinicians need not apply coding systems in assessing couple behavior, but it is valuable to observe interactions systematically with an eye toward identifying patterns that exacerbate conflict and unhappiness.

A limitation of pure behavioral observation is that it overlooks cognitive factors; namely, the subjective meanings that partners attach to each other's actions that make those acts pleasing or displeasing. As cognitive therapists know well, different people commonly interpret the same behavior differently, and a person's intent to express caring through a particular action may be perceived negatively by the recipient. For example, a man whose wife told him about upsetting interactions she had with a co-worker intended to be helpful to her by making suggestions about strategies she could use in dealing with the co-worker. However, she became angry, responding to him, "You clearly don't think I'm smart enough to figure out on my own what to do!" Therefore, in behavioral assessment with distressed couples, it is important to identify specific acts that partners experience negatively *and* to inquire what those behaviors mean to them.

Although individuals' interpretations of their partners' actions can be idiosyncratic, there also are some core dimensions of meanings that people commonly attach to types of behavior. Epstein and Baucom (2002) reviewed theoretical and research literature on basic human needs and motives, noting consistent evidence of themes regarding *communal needs* (e.g., affiliation, intimacy, nurturance) involving connections to others and *agentic needs* (e.g., autonomy, achievement, control) involving one's individual impact on the world. Therapists commonly encounter couples in which an individual has a strong negative emotional response to a partner's behavior that on the surface appears benign, but with more in-depth inquiry (using the CT "downward arrow" technique), it becomes clear that the upset recipient interpreted the behavior as highly relevant to a core personal need (e.g., "She took over my work on the checkbook because she has no confidence that I can do it competently by myself."). Thus, in CBCT, behavioral assessment is very important for isolating specific actions and couple patterns that are counterproductive, but full understanding of the effects of behavior on the members of the couple requires cognitive assessment as well.

Behavioral Skills

In addition to forms of positive and negative behavior that influence recipients' satisfaction by meeting emotional or instrumental needs, there are other types of dyadic behavior that comprise skills that couples require to exchange information accurately and solve life problems together. CBCT has incorporated standard behavioral therapy components of training couples in communication and problem-solving skills (Baucom & Epstein, 1990; Baucom et al., 2015; Epstein & Baucom, 2002; Rathus & Sanderson, 1999). Constructive communication involves one person expressing thoughts and emotions clearly and concisely, while the other engages in empathic listening, trying to understand the expresser's subjective experiences and reflecting back what she or he heard. Even if happy couples do not naturally communicate in that manner, when partners intentionally use the suggested skills, they reduce misunderstanding and convey that they care about each other's experiences.

Problem-solving skills include sequential steps designed to help a couple decide on a mutually acceptable solution to a stressful issue. The problem-solving steps are (1) defining the problem in observable behavioral terms (e.g., "We have trouble getting our children to go to bed at a reasonable time"); (2) brainstorming a variety of possible solutions, without evaluating them at this point, and specifying the role each partner would have in carrying it out; (3) listing the advantages and disadvantages of each potential solution; (4) collaborating on deleting solutions that have unfavorable disadvantages and selecting a solution to try; (5) trying the solution in daily life for a trial period between therapy sessions and gathering data on the outcome; and (6) discussing the outcome with the therapist and choosing to continue the solution if it worked well, revising it if it was moderately successful, or returning to the brainstormed list to pick another solution to try.

In CBCT, the initial assessment commonly includes the therapist asking the couple to discuss an issue in their relationship and observing their communication and problem-solving skill behavior, identifying targets for treatment. Using social learning principles, the therapist gives the couple instructions about the skills, models the skills live or shows the couple video examples, and coaches the partners as they practice during sessions.

Cognition in Close Relationships

CBCT has drawn heavily from CT concepts regarding automatic thoughts, underlying schemas, maladaptive assumptions, and cognitive distortions (A. T. Beck et al., 1979; J. S. Beck, 2011). Baucom, Epstein, Sayers, and Sher's (1989) typology of cognitions involved in relationship distress includes three forms that tend to occur as automatic thoughts in stream-of-consciousness thinking. *Selective attention* involves one's tendency to notice particular aspects of events occurring in one's relationship while overlooking others, *attributions* are inferences one makes about factors that have influenced one's own and a partner's actions (e.g., inferring that a partner failed to respond to a question because she did not care enough to listen), and *expectancies* involve predictions about the likelihood that particular events will occur in one's relationship (e.g., that telling a partner one feels sad will lead the partner to withdraw). Each type of automatic thought is a normal form of human cognition but is susceptible to distortions such as arbitrary inferences, dichotomous thinking, and overgeneralization.

Baucom et al.'s (1989) typology of relational cognitions also includes two forms that tend to comprise relatively stable schemas: *assumptions* that are beliefs about the natural characteristics of people and relationships (e.g., a husband's generalized assumption that women like to control men) and *standards* that involve beliefs about characteristics people and relationships "should" have (e.g., that a partner who cares about you should be willing to place your needs before his or her own in most situations).

Consistent with a basic premise of CT, members of couples typically fail to examine and evaluate the validity and appropriateness of their cognitions about their partner and relationship; these thoughts function as the individual's view of reality. When members of a couple are interacting, their automatic thoughts about each other occur at lightning speed, influencing their emotional and behavioral responses to each other (Epstein & Baucom, 2002). Consequently, CBCT clinicians must monitor the rapid process of couple interactions during sessions, guiding the partners in identifying and evaluating their cognitions and their consequences. Behavioral couple therapists illuminated the importance of "tracking" rapidly unfolding behavioral sequences, providing evidence that particular patterns are destructive to relationship satisfaction and stability (Gottman, 1994), but in CBCT the assessment process is even more complex, as the clinician also must probe for partners' cognitions about each other's behavior. Once a distorted or extreme cognition has been identified, the therapist can use a variety of cognitive therapy procedures to modify it. For example, when an individual makes a negative attribution about the intent underlying a partner's upsetting behavior, the therapist can coach the person in considering alternative causes of the partner's actions. A number of texts (Baucom & Epstein, 1990; Dattilio, 2010; Epstein & Baucom, 2002; Rathus & Sanderson, 1999) provide detailed descriptions of interventions for assessing and modifying counterproductive cognitions in couple therapy.

Systems Theory Components of CBCT

Bandura's (1977) social learning model, which forms a key component of the theoretical base of CBCT, emphasizes circular processes in *reciprocal determinism,* in which individuals are both influenced by and influence their interpersonal environments. Early texts on behavioral couple therapy (e.g., Jacobson & Margolin, 1979) described negative *circular processes* that occur between members of distressed couples, and researchers who applied microlevel behavioral coding to couple discussions documented destructive circular patterns such as escalation of reciprocal negative behavior exchanges (Gurman, 1994; Hahlweg & Jacobson, 1984). Similarly, CBCT models take into account processes through which partners influence each other's cognitions, emotions, and behaviors (Baucom & Epstein, 1990; Epstein & Baucom, 2002).

The early behavioral couple therapy texts made few explicit references to systems theory (Gurman, 2013), but more recent CBCT models have integrated systemic concepts into CBCT. For example, the systems concept of "punctuating" an ongoing interaction between members of a couple involves arbitrary points at which an observer begins to track the cause–effect sequence. Thus, a husband may propose that an argument began when his wife's critical statement led him to feel angry, which then led to his criticizing her in return. However, his wife may focus on how her critical remark was a response to his looking at a text message on his phone while they were discussing finances. Each person's seemingly biased perception ("selective abstraction" in CT terms) influences their definition of the problem. An astute couple therapist draws their attention to the complexities of their process, in which each person contributes to the negative pattern and thus has some responsibility for changing it. It is important to note that systemic thinking does not involve holding victims of intimate partner violence responsible for their partner's aggression; each individual must take personal responsibility for perpetration of harmful acts (Epstein, Werlinich, & LaTaillade, 2015).

CLINICAL APPLICATION

As previously mentioned, CBCT initially focused mainly on reducing overall unhappiness in couple relationships by reducing negative behavioral interactions, increasing mutually pleasing behavior, modifying forms of cognition (e.g., unrealistic standards regarding desirable qualities of a close relationship) that contributed to partners' dissatisfaction, and improving partners' awareness and expression of emotions (Baucom & Epstein, 1990; Rathus & Sanderson, 1999). In the past decade and a half, the CBCT model has been enhanced, and its applications have expanded dramatically.

CBCT for Problems in Individual Psychological Functioning

Initially, behavioral couple therapy was tested as an intervention for individuals' depression, based on evidence of an association between marital distress and depression, and indications that the causal influence between the two can go in both directions (Whisman, 2013). The couple interventions were designed to decrease negative behavioral interactions and enhance partners' mutual emotional support (Beach, Dreifuss, Franklin, Kamen, & Gabriel, 2008; Whisman & Beach, 2012). Studies (Beach & O'Leary, 1992; Jacobson, Fruzzetti, Dobson, Whisman, & Hops, 1993) indicated that when individuals experienced both problems, couple therapy reduced both, whereas individual cognitive therapy did not lessen relationship distress.

O'Farrell and colleagues (Birchler, Fals-Stewart, & O'Farrell, 2008; O'Farrell, 1993) developed and found empirical support for a treatment program that integrates behavioral couple therapy and interventions focused on a partner's substance use. The couple therapy focuses on increasing exchanges of pleasing and caring behavior, increasing shared rewarding activities, improving partners' communication and problem-solving skills, avoiding threats of separation, attending to the present rather than past problems, and avoiding physical aggression. Those dyadic interventions occur simultaneously with others for the individual's substance use (e.g., attending self-help meetings, using medication to inhibit drinking).

CBCT also has been applied with anxiety disorders, typically as an adjunctive intervention with standard individual or group CBT anxiety treatments. For example, Chambless (2012) uses couple therapy that includes psychoeducation about characteristics of an individual's anxiety disorder, as well as how anxiety symptoms affect and are commonly affected by couple interactions. The couple also receives communication and problem-solving skill training, preparation for coping jointly with symptoms, and planning of strategies for reducing patterns in which the couple accommodated their daily interactions to the individual's symptoms (e.g., a partner facilitates an agoraphobic individual's avoidance of public places by taking over activities that would require the person to leave the house). Similarly, Abramowitz et al. (2013) developed a couple-based approach to exposure and response prevention procedures for treating obsessive–compulsive disorder (OCD). It includes psychoeducation about how OCD is maintained, the strategies of exposure and response prevention exercises to confront feared situations, and coaching the couple in engaging in exposure together, with the partner playing the role of coach by encouraging the symptomatic person to stay in the anxiety-provoking situation of response prevention until the anxiety subsides.

Monson and Fredman's (2012) cognitive-behavioral conjoint therapy for posttraumatic stress disorder (PTSD) also includes psychoeducation regarding the causes and symptoms of PTSD, as well as mutual influences between an individual's symptoms and the couple's behavioral patterns (including avoidance), use of strategies for increasing positive couple interactions, interventions to improve emotion regulation, practice with communication skills to reduce the individual's emotional numbing and avoidance, and improvement of the couple's problem-solving skills. In addition, cognitive restructuring is used to reduce partners' beliefs that maintain PTSD symptoms and relationship problems (e.g., a "just world" belief that bad things happen to bad people).

Bulik, Baucom, Kirby, and Pisetsky (2011) applied CBCT in their program for anorexia nervosa (AN). Similar to the other applications of couple therapy for individual disorders, this therapy combines interventions specific to the eating disorder (e.g., psychoeducation about the disorder and the recovery process; reduction of secrecy surrounding the AN; fostering of couple collaboration to support the patient's goals for recovery such as normalized eating, weight gain, refraining from purging, and managing anxiety more effectively; strategies to avoid arguments about food) with traditional CBCT procedures of problem solving and communication skill training that reduce conflict and distress.

In all of these applications of CBCT for individual partners' problems, there are three modes of couple intervention (Baucom et al., 2015; Epstein & Baucom, 2002). In the first mode, *partner-assisted intervention,* the partner of a patient also receives psychoeducation about the disorder during joint sessions and serves in a supportive, collaborative role as the patient receives treatment. For example, in cases of panic disorder both members of the couple receive psychoeducation about causes, symptoms, and effective treatments, as well as effects that the disorder commonly has on a couple's relationship. They then both receive interoceptive exposure to conditions that simulate panic symptoms (e.g., breathing through a narrow straw to create sensations of suffocation; slowly spinning in a rotating desk chair to simulate disorientation), both to desensitize the patient to the distressing subjective feelings and increase the partner's empathy for the individual's anxiety experiences. In the second mode, *disorder-specific intervention,* the therapist guides the couple in being aware of interaction patterns that have been shaped by the disorder and may maintain the individual problem. For example, an individual's panic disorder that is associated with agoraphobia may have led the nonsymptomatic partner to take over the individual's tasks involving trips outside the home as a way of sparing the individual emotional distress. Couple interventions would involve showing them how their coping pattern backfires and maintains the individual's avoidance, and instituting changes in that pattern to encourage autonomous functioning. The third mode of couple intervention is *couple therapy,* which addresses the couple's overall functioning beyond a member's specific disorder. Because general stress in a relationship can exacerbate individual members' disorder symptoms (Whisman, 2013), improving behavioral patterns, cognitions about the relationship, and emotional expression can contribute to symptom reduction. For example, a depressed individual's sense of hopelessness about life can decrease as he or she experiences more pleasant shared activities and explicit verbal expressions of affection with a partner.

Finally, CBCT has been applied to help couples deal with severe physical illness. Baucom et al. (2009) developed a CBT-based program for women being treated for breast cancer and their male partners. Couples are taught expressive and listening skills and apply them to topics associated with the cancer (e.g., fear of mortality, stressful medical decisions). They also are taught problem-solving skills for making treatment decisions. A psychoeducation aspect of the program focuses on psychological and physical effects that cancer treatments commonly have on partners' sexual functioning. The program is intended to help the patients and partners reduce the negative impacts of cancer diagnosis and treatment by finding meaning and growth in their experiences, benefiting from mutual emotional support and effective decision making.

CBCT for Severe Relationship Problems

Many couples seek assistance for erosion in closeness and satisfaction that can be addressed through generic CBCT methods such as communication and problem-solving training, identification of behavior exchanges that will make partners feel important to each other, cognitive interventions to help partners have reasonable standards for their relationship and challenge negative attributions about each other's behavior, and skills for regulating emotions such as anger. However, a substantial number of couples present with major disruptions to their well-being as individuals and as a dyad, including partner aggression, infidelity, and sexual dysfunction. Just as CBCT clinicians need to apply specialized approaches with individual disorders such as depression and substance abuse, they need to tailor assessment and intervention for these severe relationship problems.

Partner Aggression

Clinicians commonly avoid conducting conjoint interventions with couples in which physical violence or battering (most often perpetrated by a male against a female partner) has occurred, to preclude therapy from increasing the risk of further violence and injury. The treatment of choice has been referring perpetrators to anger management groups and referring victims to shelters and clinicians who work to empower them to leave abusive relationships (O'Leary, 2008). Outcome research on anger management groups has indicated limited effectiveness. There also is substantial evidence that many couples engage in mutual exchanges of psychological and mild to moderate physical aggression when they are in conflict and do not intend to end their relationships (Epstein et al., 2015). These couples often do not label the aggressive behavior as abusive but view it as disrespectful and damaging to personal psychological well-being as well as relationship quality.

To meet the needs of couples who experience partner aggression but no battering and physical injury requiring medical attention, increasing attention has been paid to designing and evaluating couple therapy protocols that address risk factors for partner aggression: (1) "overlearned" or automatic aggressive behaviors used to express upset and influence one's partner, (2) deficits in communication and problem-solving skills, (3) negative cognitions that fuel anger and justify aggression, (4) poor regulation of anger, and (5) partners' difficulties in coping with life stresses (Epstein et al., 2015). These programs have been predominantly based on CBCT and solution-focused therapy models, which are structured and relatively time limited (Epstein et al., 2015; Stith, McCollum, & Rosen, 2011).

Regarding CBCT approaches, Heyman and Neidig's (1997) multi-couple group Physical Aggression Couples Treatment (PACT) program and Epstein and colleagues' CBCT protocol for individual couples within their Couples Abuse Prevention Program (CAPP; Epstein et al., 2015; LaTaillade, Epstein, & Werlinich, 2006) include components of psychoeducation about risk factors for partner aggression and effective treatments, anger management training, training in communication and problem-solving skills, use of CT techniques for challenging one's own anger-eliciting thoughts, and building of mutual emotional support and intimacy. Couples are screened carefully with questionnaires and separate individual interviews to select out cases at risk for injurious physical violence, and therapists regularly monitor each couple's level of aggression.

Infidelity

It is virtually inevitable that therapists who work with couples will be presented with cases involving affairs. Based on empirical evidence that individuals who have been betrayed by a partner commonly experience trauma symptoms, Baucom, Snyder, and Gordon (2009) developed a predominantly CBCT-based program that helps both partners cope with the impact of such a major stressor, gain insight into factors (e.g., the perpetrator's low self-esteem, long-term erosion in the couple's emotional connection) that placed the perpetrator at risk of engaging in the affair, make decisions about the future of their relationship, and develop strategies for reducing risk factors for further relationship problems and infidelity if they choose to stay together. The emphasis on partners developing a conceptualization of how conditions contributed to the affair (focusing on taking responsibility rather than blame) and identifying specific behaviors that they can engage in (e.g., improving their communication skills, increasing shared activities to enhance intimacy) draw heavily on CBCT.

Sexual Dysfunction

Although some couples directly describe sexual issues during their initial assessment interviews, many do not mention such concerns initially (or sometimes ever) unless the therapist asks about them. The common lack of disclosure can be due to a variety of reasons, such as feeling embarrassment, viewing sexual problems as less important than other distressing issues, being resigned to what they perceive as an untreatable problem, or assuming that a couple therapist lacks expertise in treating sexual dysfunction (which often actually is the case). Furthermore, the fairly recent development and extensive marketing of medications for men with erectile dysfunction has contributed to a common belief that sexual problems are purely physiological and that individual and couple psychotherapy are irrelevant. However, research indicates that psychological and relationship factors have major influences on sexual desire, arousal, and orgasm (Binik & Hall, 2014), and pro-sexual medications such as Viagra and Cialis have limited effects when those other characteristics are interfering with relaxation, intimacy, and pleasure. Given that cognitions such as perfectionistic standards for sexual performance and partners' tendencies to engage in "spectatoring" (hyper-focusing on how one's body is responding) have been implicated in sexual dysfunctions (Metz & McCarthy, 2011), as has negative communication regarding relationship conflicts (Metz & Epstein, 2002), modern sex therapy tends to be heavily cognitive-behavioral. It commonly involves psychoeducation regarding physiological processes in women's and men's sexual responses (with an emphasis on normalizing imperfect and inconsistent responses), as well as regarding physical, psychological, and relational factors influencing positive response or dysfunction. Couples are introduced to a CT model and are taught to identify and challenge negative thoughts related to sex (e.g., "I should automatically get physically aroused, no matter how tired or distracted I may be." "Sex without intercourse is second-rate."). They also are taught communication and problem-solving skills, and are engaged in a variety of exercises (most done jointly) for enhancing sensual and erotic experiences, increasing physical and emotional relaxation, reducing spectatoring, and decreasing performance anxiety through a desensitization process involving graduated nondemand sensual/sexual couple behaviors (e.g., Metz & McCarthy, 2004, 2011).

RESEARCH

Behavioral and cognitive-behavioral approaches to couple therapy are the most extensively researched couple therapies, with considerable evidence that they improve partners' overall relationship satisfaction as well as couple communication assessed with self-report questionnaires and behavioral observation (Baucom, Shoham, Mueser, Daiuto, & Stickle, 1998; Gurman, 2013). In addition, outcome studies on CBCT for specific individual disorders and couple relationship problems have produced evidence of effectiveness. As described earlier, studies indicate that behavioral couple therapy for co-occurring depression and relationship distress reduces both problems (Whisman & Beach, 2012).

Research on CBCT for Individual Disorders

Regarding couple interventions for anxiety disorders, Chambless (2012) reported improvements in anxiety symptoms in two couple-based treatment case studies, one involving a partner with OCD and the other with generalized anxiety disorder (GAD). Abramowitz et al. (2013) conducted a pilot study with eighteen couples to test their couple-based CBT intervention to enhance individual exposure and response prevention for moderate to severe OCD symptoms, assessing individual symptoms and couple functioning at pretherapy, immediately posttherapy, and at six- and twelve-month follow-ups. The results indicated a large improvement in OCD symptoms at posttherapy and at the follow-ups, as well as a significant decrease in depression at posttherapy, which was maintained on follow-up self-reports but not on clinician ratings. Impressively, the effect size for the decrease in OCD symptoms was larger than effects reported from individual CBT intervention studies. The couple-based intervention also led to significantly improved self-reported relationship satisfaction and constructive couple communication at posttherapy but not at the twelve-month follow-up.

Initial empirical support for Monson and Fredman's (2012) cognitive-behavioral conjoint therapy for PTSD was found in two pilot studies. Monson, Schnurr, Stevens, and Guthrie (2004) tested the approach with seven male Vietnam War veterans with PTSD and their wives. There were large statistically significant improvements in PTSD symptoms on ratings by clinicians and the veterans' partners, as well as a moderate effect size for changes in PTSD symptoms reported by the veterans. The veterans also showed significant large effect sizes for improved depression and anxiety symptoms. There was a trend toward an increase in wives' relationship satisfaction but no improvement in veterans' relationship satisfaction. In Monson et al.'s (2011) uncontrolled pilot study with couples in which a member had a PTSD diagnosis, five of the six patients who completed the treatment no longer met PTSD diagnostic criteria, and effect sizes for decreases in PTSD symptoms rated by the patients, partners, and clinicians were large. Again, there were no notable improvements in relationship satisfaction. Thus, the CBCT approach was helpful for the target PTSD symptoms, but more research is needed to understand its effects on couple functioning.

Bulik et al. (2011) compared changes resulting from their CBCT-based Uniting Couples in the Treatment of Anorexia Nervosa (UCAN) protocol with those from McIntosh et al.'s (2005) randomized controlled trial for adult anorexia nervosa that included individual treatment with CBT, interpersonal psychotherapy, or social support/case management. On average, the UCAN patients gained two to four times as much weight (statistically significant) as those in the McIntosh et al. treatments. Another advantage of the UCAN treatment was that only 5% of the patients dropped out, compared to an average 37% dropout across treatments in the McIntosh et al. (2005) study.

Regarding O'Farrell and colleagues' behavioral couple therapy for substance abuse, Powers, Vedel, and Emmelkamp (2008) conducted a meta-analysis of twelve randomized controlled outcome studies for couples, with one member diagnosed with substance use disorder. The analysis indicated that behavioral couple therapy was more effective than individual therapy in reducing substance use and relationship distress.

Research on CBCT for Specific Relationship Problems

Outcome research on CBCT for partner aggression has indicated positive effects, without increased risk of conjoint therapy provoking violence. O'Leary, Heyman, and Neidig (1999) compared their PACT program to gender-specific anger management group treatment in a longitudinal investigation. Husbands and wives had significantly higher marital adjustment scores at posttreatment than at pretreatment. Husbands scored lower on measures of psychological and physical aggression at posttreatment, as well as higher on taking responsibility for their violence and lower in blaming their wives for the husbands' violence, while wives reported decreases in self-blame and taking responsibility for their husbands' aggression. Results at a one-year follow-up also indicated decreases in husbands' psychological and physical aggression, and both husbands and wives reported higher marital satisfaction. However, PACT and gender-specific treatment were equally effective.

In a clinical trial evaluating the CAPP project, clinic couples who were identified as experiencing psychological aggression and mild to moderate physical aggression were assigned randomly to the CBCT intervention or TAU at the family therapy clinic involving major systems-based therapy models. In both conditions, no-violence contracts are written, and treatment is focused on reducing couple patterns that contribute to partner aggression. Findings indicated that both treatment conditions increased relationship satisfaction, decreased psychological partner aggression, decreased venting of anger, reduced negative attributions about one's partner, decreased aggressive thoughts during conflict, increased overall trust in the partner, decreased anxiety, and increased positive moods prior to engaging in a conflict-resolution discussion with one's partner (Epstein, Ott, & Werlinich, 2015; Hrapczynski, Epstein, Werlinich, & LaTaillade, 2011; Kahn, Epstein, & Kivlighan, 2015; LaTaillade et al., 2006). CBCT, but not TAU, led to increased anger control and increased perceived opportunities for autonomy provided by one's partner (Epstein et al., 2015). CBCT also produced significant decreases in behaviorally coded negative communication by both males and females, whereas TAU produced no change. Couple therapies produced a significant decrease in males' use of physical aggression (physical assault and injury) and a trend toward such a decrease in females' physical aggression.

There have been no randomized clinical trials evaluating the effects of Baucom et al.'s (2009) CBCT-based treatment for couples experiencing affairs, but Baucom et al. (2006) examined preliminary evidence from two samples. One sample was from a pilot study of nine case studies of couples who had experienced affairs during the past year but had ended the affair. The second sample was nineteen affair couples from a large clinical trial comparing two types of behavioral couple therapy for distressed couples (Atkins, Eldridge, Baucom, & Christensen, 2005). Results indicated that for improvements in relationship distress, effect sizes for partners who had been betrayed were substantial for the two samples (0.70 and 0.79, respectively) but were mixed (0.08 and 1.02) for the unfaithful partners. Baucom et al. (2006) suggest that the lack of improvement among unfaithful partners in the pilot sample may be due to their being recruited on the basis of the injured partners' distress regarding the affair, whereas couples in the Atkins et al. (2005) sample were selected based solely on partners' overall marital distress. Further follow-up research is needed to see whether such interventions decrease the probability of future infidelity.

Finally, there have been no controlled trials of CBCT for sexual dysfunctions as yet. This may continue to be the case, as funding for such expensive studies on the topic of psychosexual treatments for sexual dysfunction is not readily available.

CONCLUSIONS

CBCT has developed substantially in the past three decades from its roots in a relatively narrow framework that was focused on shifting the balance between negative and positive behaviors exchanged by members of a couple through use of behavioral contracts and skills training. The first major development was integration of concepts and methods regarding couple behavioral interactions with principles and clinical methods of cognitive therapy, as well as systems theory. CBCT captured the complex interactions between two individuals as they respond to each other behaviorally and continuously process each other's actions cognitively and emotionally. The model then was enhanced by viewing the couple's interactions within an ecological framework of multiple influences, distinguishing between microlevel relationship events and macrolevel patterns, and noting the importance of the couple's ability to cope individually and as a dyad with a range of life stressors both normative and unexpected. CBCT has become a flexible therapeutic model that has been applicable to treating relational factors in a variety of individual disorders, as well as specific relationship problems such as partner aggression, infidelity, and sexual dysfunction. The multifaceted nature of modern CBCT gives it great potential as a clinical intervention model and also requires that practitioners develop their understanding and clinical skills regarding individual psychological functioning, relationship dynamics, and complex systemic influences on couples' lives.

REFERENCES

Abramowitz, J. S., Baucom, D. H., Wheaton, M. G., Boeding, S., Fabricant, L. E., Paprocki, C., & Fischer, M. S. (2013). Enhancing exposure and response prevention for OCD: A couple-based approach. *Behavior Modification, 37,* 189–210.

Atkins, D. C., Eldridge, K. A., Baucom, D. H., & Christensen, A. (2005). Infidelity and behavioral couple therapy: Optimism in the face of betrayal. *Journal of Consulting and Clinical Psychology, 73,* 144–150.

Baucom, D. H., & Epstein N. (1990). *Cognitive-behavioral marital therapy.* New York: Brunner/Mazel.

Baucom, D. H., Epstein, N. B., Kirby, J. S., & LaTaillade, J. J. (2015). Cognitive-behavioral couple therapy. In A. S. Gurman, J. L. Lebow, & D. K. Snyder (Eds.), *Clinical handbook of couple therapy* (5th ed., pp. 23–60). New York: Guilford Press.

Baucom, D. H., Epstein, N., Sayers, S., & Sher, T. G. (1989). The role of cognitions in marital relationships: Definitional, methodological, and conceptual issues. *Journal of Consulting and Clinical Psychology, 57,* 31–38.

Baucom, D. H., Gordon, K. C., Snyder, D. K., Atkins, D. C., & Christensen, A. (2006). Treating affair couples: Clinical considerations and initial findings. *Journal of Cognitive Psychotherapy: An International Quarterly, 20,* 375–392.

Baucom, D. H., Porter, L. S., Kirby, J. S., Gremore, T. M., Wiesenthal, N., Aldridge, W., . . . Keefe, F. J. (2009). A couple-based intervention for female breast cancer. *Psycho-Oncology, 8,* 276–283.

Baucom, D. H., Shoham, V., Mueser, K. T., Daiuto, A. D., & Stickle, T. R. (1998). Empirically supported couple and family interventions for marital distress and adult mental health problems. *Journal of Consulting and Clinical Psychology, 66,* 53–88.

Baucom, D. H., Snyder, D. K., & Gordon, K. (2009). *Helping couples get past the affair: A clinician's guide.* New York: Guilford Press.

Beach, S. R. H., Dreifuss, J. A., Franklin, K. J., Kamen, C., & Gabriel, B. (2008). Couple therapy and the treatment of depression. In A. S. Gurman (Ed.), *Clinical handbook of couple therapy* (4th ed., pp. 545–566). New York: Guilford Press.

Beach, S. R. H., & O'Leary, K. D. (1992). Treating depression in the context of marital discord: Outcome and predictors of response for marital therapy vs. cognitive therapy. *Behavior Therapy, 23,* 507–528.

Beck, A. T. (1976). *Cognitive therapy and the emotional disorders.* New York: International Universities Press.

Beck, A. T. (1988). *Love is never enough.* New York: Harper & Row.

Beck, A. T., Rush, A. J., Shaw, B. F, & Emery, G. (1979). *Cognitive therapy of depression.* New York: Guilford Press.

Beck, J. S. (2011). *Cognitive therapy: Basics and beyond* (2nd ed.). New York: Guilford Press.

Binik, Y. M., & Hall, K. S. K. (Eds.). (2014). *Principles and practice of sex therapy* (5th ed.). New York: Guilford Press.

Birchler, G. R., Fals-Stewart, W., & O'Farrell, T. J. (2008). Couple therapy for alcoholism and drug abuse. In A. S. Gurman (Ed.), *Clinical handbook of couple therapy* (4th ed., pp. 523–544). New York: Guilford Press.

Bulik, C. M., Baucom, D. H., Kirby, J. S., & Pisetsky, E. (2011). Uniting couples (in the treatment of) anorexia nervosa (UCAN). *International Journal of Eating Disorders, 44,* 19–28.

Chambless, D. L. (2012). Adjunctive couple and family intervention for patients with anxiety disorders. *Journal of Clinical Psychology: In Session, 68,* 548–560.

Dattilio, F. M. (2010). *Cognitive-behavior therapy with couples and families: A comprehensive guide for clinicians.* New York: Guilford Press.

Dattilio, F. M., & Padesky, C. A. (1990). *Cognitive therapy with couples.* Sarasota, FL: Professional Resource Exchange.

Ellis, A., & Harper, R. A. (1961). *A guide to rational living.* Englewood Cliffs, NJ: Prentice-Hall.

Ellis, A., Sichel, J. L., Yeager, R. J., DiMattia, D. J., & DiGiuseppe, R. (1989). *Rational-emotive couples therapy.* New York: Pergamon Press.

Epstein, N. (1982). Cognitive therapy with couples. *American Journal of Family Therapy, 10,* 5–16.

Epstein, N. B., & Baucom, D. H. (2002). *Enhanced cognitive-behavioral therapy for couples: A contextual approach.* Washington, DC: American Psychological Association.

Epstein, N. B., Dattilio, F. M., & Baucom, D. H. (2016). Cognitive-behavior couple therapy. In T. L. Sexton & J. Lebow (Eds.), *Handbook of family therapy* (4th ed., pp. 361–386). New York: Routledge.

Epstein, N. B., Ott, E. M., & Werlinich, C. A. (2015, November). *Couple therapy for partner violence: Effects on cognitions, anger, and autonomy.* Paper presented at the annual meeting of the National Council on Family Relations, Vancouver, Canada.

Epstein, N. B., Werlinich, C. A., & LaTaillade, J. J., (2015). Couple therapy for partner aggression. In A. S. Gurman, J. L. Lebow, & D. K. Snyder (Eds.), *Clinical handbook of couple therapy* (5th ed., pp. 389–411). New York: Guilford Press.

Gottman, J. M. (1994). *What predicts divorce?: The relationship between marital processes and marital outcomes.* Hillsdale, NJ: Erlbaum.

Greenberg, L. S., & Goldman, R. N. (2008). *Emotion-focused couples therapy: The dynamics of emotion, love, and power.* Washington, DC: American Psychological Association.

Gurman, A. S. (2013). Behavioral couple therapy: Building a secure base for therapeutic integration. *Family Process, 52,* 115–138.

Hahlweg, K., & Jacobson, N. S. (Eds.). (1984). *Marital interaction: Analysis and modification.* New York: Guilford Press.

Hahlweg, K., Reisner, L., Kohli, G., Vollmer, M., Schindler, L., & Revenstorf, D. (1984). Development and validity of a new system to analyze interpersonal communication (KPI: Kategoriensystem für Partnerschaftliche Interaktion). In K. Hahlweg & N. S. Jacobson (Eds.), *Marital interaction: Analysis and modification* (pp. 182–198). New York: Guilford Press.

Heyman, R. E., & Neidig, P. H. (1997). Physical aggression couples treatment. In W. K. Halford & H. J. Markman (Eds.), *Clinical handbook of marriage and couples intervention* (pp. 589–617). Chichester, UK: Wiley.

Hrapczynski, K. M., Epstein, N. B., Werlinich, C. A., & LaTaillade, J. J. (2011). Changes in negative attributions during couple therapy for abusive behavior: Relations to changes in satisfaction and behavior. *Journal of Marital and Family Therapy, 38,* 117–132.

Jacobson, N. S., Fruzzetti, A. E., Dobson, K., Whisman, M., & Hops, H. (1993). Couple therapy as a treatment for depression: II. The effects of relationship quality and therapy on depressive relapse. *Journal of Consulting and Clinical Psychology, 61,* 516–519.

Jacobson, N. S., & Margolin, G. (1979). *Marital therapy: Strategies based on social learning and behavior exchange principles.* New York: Brunner/Mazel.

Johnson, S. M. (1996). *The practice of emotionally focused marital therapy.* New York: Brunner/Mazel.

Kahn, S. Y., Epstein, N. B., & Kivlighan, D. M. (2015). Couple therapy for partner aggression: Effects on individual and relational well-being. *Journal of Couple and Relationship Therapy, 14,* 95–115.

LaTaillade, J. J., Epstein, N. B., & Werlinich, C. A. (2006). Conjoint treatment of intimate partner violence: A cognitive behavioral approach. *Journal of Cognitive Psychotherapy, 20,* 393–410.

Liberman, R. P. (1970). Behavioral approaches to couple and family therapy. *American Journal of Orthopsychiatry, 40,* 106–118.

McIntosh, V., Jordan, J., Carter, F., Luty, S., Mckenzie, J., Bulik, C., . . . Joyce, P. (2005). Three psychotherapies for anorexia nervosa: A randomized controlled trial. *American Journal of Psychiatry, 162,* 741–747.

Meichenbaum, D. (1985). *Stress inoculation training.* New York: Pergamon Press.

Metz, M. E., & Epstein, N. (2002). The role of relationship conflict in sexual dysfunction. *Journal of Sex and Marital Therapy, 28,* 139–164.

Metz, M. E., & McCarthy, B. W. (2004). *Coping with erectile dysfunction.* Oakland, CA: New Harbinger.

Metz, M. E., & McCarthy, B. W. (2011). *Enduring desire.* New York: Routledge.

Monson, C. M., & Fredman, S. J. (2012). *Cognitive-behavioral conjoint therapy for PTSD.* New York: Guilford Press.

Monson, C. M., Fredman, S. J., Adair, K. C., Stevens, S. P., Resick, P. A., Schnurr, P. P., et al. (2011). Cognitive-behavioral conjoint therapy for PTSD: Pilot results from a community sample. *Journal of Traumatic Stress, 24,* 97–101.

O'Farrell, T. J. (1993). *A behavioral marital therapy couples group program for alcoholics and their spouses.* New York: Guilford Press.

O'Leary, K. D. (2008). Couple therapy and physical aggression. In A. S. Gurman (Ed.), *Clinical handbook of couple therapy* (4th ed., pp. 478–498). New York: Guilford Press.

O'Leary, K. D., Heyman, R. E., & Neidig, P. H. (1999). Treatment of wife abuse: A comparison of gender-specific and couples approaches. *Behavior Therapy, 30,* 475–505.

Patterson, G. R. (1971). *Families: Applications of social learning to family life.* Champaign, IL: Research Press.

Powers, M. B., Vedel, E., & Emmelkamp, P. M. G. (2008). Behavioral couples therapy (BCT) for alcohol and drug use disorders: A meta-analysis. *Clinical Psychology Review, 28,* 952–962.

Rathus, J. H., & Sanderson, W. C. (1999). *Marital distress: Cognitive behavioral interventions for couples*. Northvale, NJ: Jason Aronson.

Stith, S. M., McCollum, E. E., & Rosen, K. H. (2011). *Couples therapy for domestic violence: Finding safe solutions*. Washington, DC: American Psychological Association.

Stuart, R. B. (1980). *Helping couples change: A social learning approach to marital therapy*. New York: Guilford Press.

Weiss, R. L., Hops, H., & Patterson, G. R. (1973). A framework for conceptualizing marital conflict, a technology for altering it, some data for evaluating it. In L. A. Hamerlynck, L. C. Handy, & E. J. Mash, (Eds.), *Behavior change: Methodology, concepts, and practice* (pp. 309–342). Champaign, IL: Research Press.

Weiss, R. L., & Summers, K. J. (1983). Marital Interaction Coding System—III. In E. E. Filsinger (Ed.), *Marriage and family assessment: A sourcebook for family therapy* (pp. 85–115). Beverly Hills, CA: SAGE.

Whisman, M. A. (2013). Relationship discord and the prevalence, incidence, and treatment of psychopathology. *Journal of Social and Personal Relationships, 30*, 163–170.

Whisman, M. A., & Beach, S. R. H. (2012). Couple therapy for depression. *Journal of Clinical Psychology: In Session, 68*, 526–535.

CHAPTER 13

Cognitive-Behavioral Family Therapy

Frank M. Dattilio
Michelle Hanna Collins

Cognitive-behavioral family therapy (CBFT) has its roots in the 1960s and 1970s (see Dattilio, 2010, 2014, for a more detailed discussion of the history).

It was not until the end of the 1980s that the late Ian Falloon (1988) encouraged behavioral family therapists to adopt an open-systems approach that involved the complex dynamics existing within the family constellation. Falloon emphasized the need to focus on the physiological status of the individual, as well as his or her cognitive, behavioral, and emotional responses. This was in addition to considering the interpersonal transactions that occur within the family, workplace, and social and cultural-political networks (Dattilio, 2014). Falloon encouraged clinicians to use a more contextual approach, whereby each potentially causative factor was considered in relation to other factors.

Later in the 1980s, cognitive processes were introduced as a component of treatment within the specific behavioral paradigm of couples and family therapy (Dattilio, 1983, 1989; Ellis, 1982; Epstein, Schlesinger, & Dryden, 1988). While the thought processes of various family members during therapy has always been considered important in a variety of theoretical orientations (e.g., reframing and the strategic approach, "problem-talk" in solution-focused therapy, and life stories in narrative therapy), it was not until the cognitive-behavioral therapies came into vogue that they gained additional emphasis (Dattilio, 2001a). In the 1990s, theorists established cognitive assessment and intervention methods that were derived from individual therapy and adapted by cognitive-behavioral therapists for use with family interventions. These interventions were used to identify and modify distorted cognitions that family members have about each other (Alexander & Parsons, 1982; Bedrosian, 1983). As with individual psychotherapy, cognitive-behavioral interventions with families were designed to enhance the family members' skills for evaluating and modifying their own problematic cognitions, as well as skills for communicating and solving problems constructively. Bedrosian (1983) specifically applied Beck's model of cognitive therapy to understanding and treating dysfunctional relationship dynamics, as did Barton and Alexander (1981). This effort spawned the approach that later became known as "functional family therapy" (Alexander & Parsons, 1982). Furthermore, during the same decade, the implementation of cognitive-behavioral techniques witnessed a rapid expansion into what constitutes contemporary CBFT (Dattilio, 1993; Epstein & Schlesinger, 1996; Epstein et al., 1988; Falloon et al., 1984; Schwebel & Fine, 1994).

Contemporary CBFT approaches maintain an ardent bond to the systemic approaches and emphasize the role of family schemas (Dattilio, 2005a). These schemas are jointly held beliefs among the family members that have developed as a result of years of integrated interaction within the family unit. For example, a family schema may be that family problems should remain within the family unit and never be discussed with anyone outside of the immediate household. Consequently, treatment may focus on what occurs if a family member feels the legitimate need to violate this schema and share information with an outside source in an attempt to derive external support.

In addition to family schemas, some CBFT approaches place specific emphasis on a particular clinical problem. This has involved treatment for abdominal pain in children (Sanders, Shepherd, Cleghorn, & Woolford, 1994), family intervention with cases of psychosis (Bird et al., 2010), family-focused therapy for anxiety disorders (Chambless, 2012), and structured family CBT for children with obsessive–compulsive disorder (Piacentini et al., 2011).

A more recent addition involves the triple p-positive parenting program that has become widely recognized as a family support strategy. This is a five-level program that aims to prevent severe behavioral, emotional, and developmental problems in children by enhancing parents' knowledge, skills, and confidence. These interventions include a universal population-level media information campaign targeting all parents, two levels of brief primary care consultations targeting mild behavior problems, and two more intensive parent training and family intervention programs for children at risk for more severe behavioral problems. Thus far, randomized outcome trials have yielded favorable results with this approach (Sanders, 2012). For a more comprehensive review of the literature on the research and clinical applications of CBFT, the reader is referred to Dattilio and Epstein (2016) and Dattilio (2010, 2014).

CLINICAL APPLICATION

Clinical Assessment

Much of CBFT's success rests on the accuracy of careful investigation through extensive interviewing and assessment procedures (Schwebel & Fine, 1994; Dattilio, 2005b). The more specific goals of assessment are to identify strength and problematic characteristics of the family and the environment, as well as to place current family functioning in the context of its developmental stages. Identifying cognitive, affective, and behavioral aspects of family interactions is also essential, particularly in determining targets of intervention. While the description of assessment in this chapter is limited, the reader is directed to a more extensive review of procedures in Dattilio (2010, 2014).

Unlike working with couples, family therapists typically do not separate family members unless there are specific reasons. For example, sometimes families enter into treatment circuitously, in which parents will arrive at a therapist's office because they are experiencing difficulty with their teenage son or daughter who refuses to pursue treatment. Therefore, in such cases, exceptions must be made. Most of the time, however, it is advantageous for therapists to see all family members together. It should be noted that CBT therapists deviate from traditional family therapists who insist that everyone attend therapy in order for treatment to begin. Sometimes this is just not realistic, and therefore modifications have to be considered. The therapist can focus on engaging with those members who are motivated to attend and later potentially draw in absent members. CBTs maintain the assumption that the difficulties that a family presents in ensuring the attendance of all members may be a sample of broader problematic dynamics. Thus, from the initial contact, a therapist is observing the family process and formulating a hypothesis about patterns that may be contributing to the family's overall dysfunction.

During the initial family interview, therapists may begin to probe family members' cognitions regarding the reasons for seeking therapy at this particular time and whether or not a crisis or a disturbance may have brought them into therapy. The therapist should probe each family member about their individual perspective on the stated concerns and about any changes that each member believes should be made to make family functioning more salubrious.

An important question to ask family members is "What works well in their family functioning, and what might account for times when the family functions in a productive, cohesive fashion?" Learning about what works in the family often provides the therapist with vital information about what is dysfunctional. An example might be that the family does not handle crisis episodes well and that a major breakdown of communication and physical altercations ensues. The assessment phase actually continues throughout the course of treatment and is not limited to the initial set of visits.

The Use of Inventories and Questionnaires

One aspect of CBFT that sets it aside from other modalities of family therapy is the use of standardized questionnaires in gathering information on family functioning. These measures can often be helpful to a therapist who may be limited in time. More importantly, they are useful in many ways since they provide structured questions about aspects of the family's functions that the therapist may not think to ask. These questionnaires and inventories are usually distributed during the initial meeting, and family members may be asked to complete them without collaborating. A variety of measures have been developed specifically to provide an overview of key aspects of family functioning, particularly in the areas of overall satisfaction, family cohesion, quality of communication, decision-making values, and level of conflict. Some examples include the Family of Origin Inventory (Stuart, 1995), which is a comprehensive inventory that allows parents to describe how the experiences of their respective families of origin influenced their lives, marriages, and immediate family. Other measures include the Family Environment Scale (Moos & Moos, 1986), the Family Assessment Device (Epstein, Baldwin, & Bishop, 1983), and the Self-Report Family Inventory (Beavers, Hampson, & Hulgus, 1985). These inventories may serve as a guideline for gathering more accurate information. They can also help to identify areas of strength as well as concerns and to provide insight into types of positive and negative interactions that affect the family's functioning. Some family members may be more likely to report concerns on questionnaires as opposed to doing so verbally during the family interviews.

Behavioral Observations and Change

Because of the limitations of self-report inventories, it is extremely important for family therapists to directly observe samples of family members' interactions. "Joining" the family is a very important aspect for therapists in that they become intrinsically involved with the family process, even during the course of treatment. In this respect, the therapist becomes an acting and reacting member of the therapeutic system. The therapist joins the family by emphasizing the aspects of his or her personality and experience that are syntonic with the family's. At the same time, he or she also retains the freedom to be spontaneous with experimental probes and recommendations for testing certain hypotheses with the family. Part of the goal of behavioral observation is to identify specific behavioral patterns by each individual family member and the sequence of acts among the family as a whole that are either constructive and pleasing or destructive and aversive. Identifying family members who tend to be more spontaneous, as opposed to others who fade into the background, offers important information with regard to family dynamics. One benefit of imposing very little structure in family therapy is the ability to sample the family's communication in natural ways within the treatment setting.

A valuable way to observe what happens within families is to instruct the members to engage in genuine problem-solving discussions during the actual course of a session and use behavioral rating scales to track how family members interact. During these discussions, the therapist can actually observe the difficulties in communication as well as problem solving. Depending on the posture that the therapist chooses, he or she may become more directive in the process and focus on certain interventions or remain more passive with his or her observation. A good example is when parents complain that their teenage child rarely expresses his or her feelings. Through observation, the clinician may notice that whenever the child does express his or her feelings, the parents either turn away or overtly cut him or her off and deny the child's feelings by making a disparaging comment (Dattilio, 2014). Such circular causal processes in family interactions are observed when a clinician notes how one family member's behavior affects the others and vice versa.

Assessing Cognitions

Family interviews also involve providing opportunities to elicit idiosyncratic cognitions and to track influential processes that cannot be assessed by standardized questionnaires. Socratic questioning is one method that involves a series of systematic questions that are employed to dismantle individual family members' defenses during both the exploration and/or assessment phase and at the beginning of treatment. An example of such defenses would be family members who cover for father's alcoholism by engaging in denial that he has an addiction in order to maintain homeostasis in the family unit. This technique aids the family therapist in piecing together a chain of thoughts that mediate between events and relationships and each individual's emotional and behavioral responses. One approach that uses Socratic questioning involves a technique known as the "downward arrow," developed by Beck, Rush, Shaw, and Emery (1979). This technique was developed to uncover the underlying assumption of a family member that generates dysfunction or distorted thoughts. Helping family members to identify automatic thoughts and associated emotions and behavior is a crucial requisite for modifying distortions and extreme cognitions about themselves and their family.

After a period of psychoeducation, in which the therapist educates families about the model of treatment, the concept of automatic thoughts is addressed, along with coaching family members in observing their own patterns of thought during sessions that are associated with negative emotional and behavioral responses to one another. To achieve this goal, family members are typically asked to keep small notebooks handy between sessions and jot down brief descriptions of circumstances in which they feel distressed about their family relationship or conflict. Some family members may prefer to rely on their smartphones or MP3 players in order to keep this log, along with descriptions of automatic thoughts as well as the resulting emotional and behavioral responses toward other family members. A modified version of the Daily Record of Dysfunctional Thoughts (Beck et al., 1979) is utilized for this purpose. This can also be uploaded into their smartphones or MP3 players.

Identifying Cognitive Distortions and Documenting Them

Family members are eventually trained to become adept at identifying the types of cognitive distortions involved in their automatic thoughts that create difficulties for them. An example of such thoughts is the children who state, "Our parents don't consider our feelings. They only think of themselves." A primary exercise is to have each family member refer to the list of cognitive distortions and labeling, along with any automatic thoughts that they experienced during the past week. The therapist can discuss with family members any aspects of the thoughts that were inappropriate or extreme, and whether the distortion contributed to negative emotions and behaviors at the time.

In the event that the family therapist believes that the family members' cognitive distortions are associated with any form of specific psychopathology, such as depression or a thought disorder, this can be addressed further, and a referral can be made for individual treatment.

Testing and Reinterpreting Automatic Thoughts

The process of restructuring automatic thoughts involves the individual considering alternative explanations. An example might be an adolescent male who believes that his older brother who refuses to share his cologne enjoys depriving him. Hence, his automatic thought might be, "He doesn't give a crap about my needs, yet he's always asking me for favors." The therapist may subsequently coach him in identifying that he might have been engaging in the "mind reading" distortion and that it might be important for him to gather more information from his brother by addressing the issue in a nonemotional way to see whether it is truly his brother's intention to "deprive" him or whether something else is occurring (i.e., he has very little cologne left). Gathering and weighing the evidence for one's thoughts is an integral part of the work conducted in family therapy. Family members are able to provide valuable feedback that will help each other evaluate the validity of their cognitions along with good communication skills, which are described later in this chapter. After a family member challenges his or her thoughts or beliefs, he or she is subsequently asked to rate his or her belief from 0 to 100 on the "Alternative Explanations" section of the Dysfunctional Thought Record. Often, revised thoughts may not be assimilated unless they are considered credible and implemented by family members.

Behavioral Experiments

The use of logical analysis to reduce family members' expectancies concerning certain events may not be forceful unless they have firsthand evidence to substantiate it. Consequently, CBFTs often guide family members in devising so-called behavioral experiments in which they test their predictions that a particular action will lead to certain responses from other family members. An example might be a youth who expects that his parents and siblings will think that his suggestion for a family vacation will be viewed as stupid and be rejected by other family members; he might bring this up during a family mealtime and see how it is received. When these plans are devised during joint family therapy sessions, the therapist can ask the other family members what they predict the responses might be during such an experiment. Family members can anticipate potential obstacles to the success of the experiment, and appropriate adjustments can be made. In addition, the therapist can examine what evidence the youth had for anticipating that his idea may be rejected.

Communications Training

Communications training and the improvement of family members' skills in expressing thoughts and emotions, as well as learning to listen effectively to each other, are very important aspects of family therapy. This intervention can have an indelible impact on problematic behavioral interactions, reduce family members' distorted cognitions about one another, and contribute to regulated experiences and expression of emotions. Presentation of specific instructions to family members about the specific behaviors in each type of expressive and reflective skill is part of the didactic aspect of therapy. Guidelines for speakers and listeners are provided and may involve specific training during family sessions. The use of strategies such as the

"Pad and Pencil Technique" may be very helpful in limiting the degree to which family members interrupt each other during heated exchanges (Dattilio, 2010).

The therapist may serve as a good role model for expressive and reflective skills. Coaching family members in using these guidelines, beginning with discussions or relatively benign topics, and working their way up to more substantive topics are all part of the process. It is important to start with more benign topics, so that negative emotions do not interfere with the constructive development of skills; as the family members improve their skills, more emotionally charged issues can be addressed and processed. Family members are also asked to practice these skills as homework assignments with increasingly conflictual topics. As these communication skills are practiced and more information surfaces about family members' motives and desires, important issues can be processed during the course of treatment. Following these guidelines also increases family members' perceptions that the others are more respectful and have better intentions than might have been expected.

Problem-Solving Training

The use of verbal and written instructions for problem-solving training, along with modeling and behavioral rehearsal and coaching, can help family members develop more effective coping skills. A number of steps can be followed in problem-solving training. The following is a set of steps adopted from Epstein and Schlesinger (1996) that may be used as a guideline.

- Define the problem in specified behavioral terms. Compare perceptions and arrive at an agreeable description of the problem.
- Generate a possible set of solutions.
- Evaluate the advantages and disadvantages of each solution.
- Select a feasible solution.
- Implement the chosen solution and evaluate its effectiveness.

These steps are outlined in more detail in Dattilio (2010). It is essential to agree on a trial period for implementing designated solutions and assessing their effectiveness. Once again, the use of homework practice for the development of problem-solving skills is very important (Kazantzis, Deane, Ronan, & L'Abate, 2005).

Behavioral Change Agreements

The occasional use of contracts is necessary to facilitate the exchange of desired behavior among family members. Every attempt is made to avoid making one family member's behavior change contingent on the others.

However, the more realistic goal may be for each person to identify and enact specific behaviors that would be likely to please other family members regardless of what actions the other members take. An example would involve a parent asking permission to enter a child's bedroom despite the fact that the child often enters their parents' bedroom at will. Sometimes, however, this cannot be avoided, and the mere agreement of exchange may be crucial in facilitating the modification of conflict. Every attempt should be made, however, to avoid encouraging family members to "stand on ceremony" and wait for others to behave positively before they engage in positive behaviors themselves. Such agreements may be helpful in reducing the propensities for family members to engage in standoffs with each other.

Homework Assignments

CBFTs have identified homework assignments as a cornerstone of treatment in family therapy (Dattilio, 1998, 2002; Schwebel & Fine, 1994). Research in family therapy has also indicated that homework assignments are crucial for change in this context (Dattilio, Kazantzis, Shinkfield, & Carr, 2011). Homework serves to keep the therapy session alive during the interim period and promotes a transfer from therapy sessions to day-to-day living. In essence, homework helps to galvanize what is learned during the therapy process.

Repeated practice only strengthens awareness of various issues that have unfolded during the course of treatment. These assignments can increase the expectations for family members to follow through with making changes rather than simply discussing change during the course of therapy and then not following through at home. Various types of homework assignments are used with families. Some of the more common ones involve activities scheduling, biblio- or video-therapy assignments, self-monitoring, behavioral task assignments, and/or cognitive restructuring of dysfunctional thoughts.

Interventions for Deficits and Excesses in Emotional Responses

CBT is sometimes characterized as neglecting or downplaying the emotional component of treatment, but this description is actually misleading. A variety of interventions can be used either to enhance the emotional experience of inhibited family members or to moderate extreme responses. Family members sometimes report experiencing little emotion. In these cases, the therapist may want to set clear guidelines for behavior within and outside of the therapy sessions for family members to express themselves in a way that will not lead to recrimination by other members.

Some of the techniques mentioned previously, such as downward arrow questioning, may be used to inquire about underlying emotions, as well as cognitions. Coaching family members in noticing internal cues to their emotional states is also helpful, along with repeating phrases that have an emotional impact on family members. Helping family members refocus their attention on emotional aspects is often extremely important during the course of treatment. Engaging family members in role play concerning important relationship issues in order to elicit emotional responses is sometimes crucial in encouraging emotions to flow appropriately in therapy.

Sometimes family members will experience intense emotions that affect them and significant others adversely. In this manner, the therapist can help them compartmentalize emotional responses by scheduling specific times to discuss distressing topics and coach them in self-soothing activities such as relaxation techniques. These activities help to improve the abilities of family members to monitor and challenge upsetting automatic thoughts. They also help to encourage family members to seek social support from family and others and develop their ability to tolerate distressing feelings. Enhancing a family member's skills in expressing emotions constructively so that others will notice is also an important aspect of treatment. Training techniques and emotional regulation, as well as tolerance building, are also significantly helpful when working with particularly volatile families.

RESEARCH

Unfortunately, the existing empirical literature in CBFT is quite lean. Faulkner, Klock, and Gale (2002) conducted a content analysis on articles published in the marital/couple and family therapy literature from 1980 to 1999. The *American Journal of Family Therapy, Contemporary Family Therapy, Family Process,* and the *Journal of Marital and Family Therapy* were among the top journals from which 131 articles that used quantitative research methodology were examined. Of these 131 articles, fewer than half involved outcome studies. Disappointingly, none of the studies that were reviewed included CBFT.

This is likely because research in family therapy is not easy to conduct as opposed to individual or couple therapy. Because multiple dynamics exist with families, this renders a more arduous course of study. However, many of the components of CBFT draw from cognitive-behavioral couple therapy, for which there are a number of substantial controlled outcome studies (see Dattilio, 2014 and Dattilio & Epstein, 2016, for an extensive review). These studies indicate the effectiveness of CBT for relationships, although the majority of the studies have primarily focused on the behavioral interventions utilizing communications training, problem-solving training, and behavioral contracts. A small number of studies focus on the impact of cognitive restructuring procedures. Additional studies are undoubtedly necessary in order for us to draw conclusions about the relative efficacies of the empirically supported treatments with families using a cognitive-behavioral approach. However, there is encouraging support for CBFT as a treatment mode that can be helpful to many distressed families (Dattilio, 2010, 2014; Dattilio & Epstein, 2016).

The research supports the effectiveness of behaviorally oriented family interventions, namely, psychoeducation and training in communications and problem-solving skills. Additional research has also been conducted on the straight behavioral approach for cases of aggressive behavior (Patterson, 1982) and the application of operant principles to parent–child interactive therapies for conduct problems (Sanders & Dadds, 1993; Webster-Stratton & Hancock, 1998), as well as for child anxiety and aggression (Dadds, Barrett, Rapee, & Ryan, 1996), depression (Birmaher, Brent, & Kolko, 2000; Brent, Holder, & Kolko, 1997), eating disorders (Wardle et al., 2003), as well as other psychiatric disorders (Mueser & Glynn, 1995).

The application of behavioral family therapy has also been studied in the treatment of schizophrenia (Falloon et al., 1984). Reducing relapse rates and improving patient social functioning have helped lessen hardships to families (Hahlweg & Wiedemann, 1999). Effective parenting strategies have also been used in the treatment of attention-deficit/hyperactivity disorder (Barkley, 1997; Chronis, Chacko, Fabiano, Wymbs, & Pelham, 2004). CBT with couples and families has gained popularity and respect among clinicians, including family therapists of various modalities, especially as a result of its inclusion as an empirically validated mode of treatment (Davis & Piercy, 2007; Dattilio, Piercy, & Davis, 2014; Dattilio & Epstein, 2016).

Recently, attention has been given to case-based reports within the family therapy literature. Traditionally, case-based research has not been considered as scientific by many in the field, owing to the lack of controlled conditions and objectivity. However, case study material can provide the basis for drawing casual inferences in properly designed clinical cases (Dattilio, 2006a) and is often preferred among students and trainees (Dattilio, Edwards, & Fishman, 2010; Edwards, Dattilio, & Bromley, 2004).

THE COGNITIVE-BEHAVIORAL MODEL

Consistent and compatible with systems theory, the cognitive-behavioral model of working with families is based on the premise that members of the family simultaneously influence and are influenced by each other's thoughts, emotions, and behaviors (Dattilio, 2001; Leslie, 1988). To become familiar with the family system as a whole is to know the individual parts and the manner in which they interact. As each family member observes his or her own cognitions, behaviors and emotions regarding family interactions, as well as cues regarding the responses of other family members, these perceptions lead to the formation of assumptions about family dynamics. This subsequently develops into schemas, or what are referred to as "cognitive structures." These cognitions, emotions, and behaviors may elicit responses from some members who typically constitute much of the moment-to-moment interaction with other family members. This interplay stems from the more stable schemas that serve as the foundation for the family's functioning (Dattilio, 2010). When this cycle involves negative content that affects cognitive, emotional, and behavioral responses, the volatility of the family's dynamics tends to escalate, rendering family members vulnerable to a negative spiral of conflict. Family schemas are a subset of a broad range of schemas that individuals develop about many aspects of life experiences (Dattilio, 2014).

Family Schema Development

The development and operation of schemas in family systems are similar to those with individuals and couples and are predicated on previous and current life experiences as perceived by each family member. For example, a couple sharing the belief that "parents should keep secrets from children about marital conflicts" may contribute to a child's belief that he or she should not know about his or her parents' marital problems. Parents' beliefs certainly have an effect on how their children interpret various life events. The term "family schema" is highlighted more clearly in the recent literature by Dattilio (2010, 2014). The concept entails stable, entrenched, long-standing beliefs that family members jointly hold about family life. Shared schemas evolve within the marital relationship and eventually contribute to what Dattilio (1993) refers to as "joint family schema." These schemas serve as a template for family members in their functioning within the family unit. Schemas can be a helpful guide for family members in navigating complex aspects of family life, but when they are extreme or distorted, they can contribute to family conflict.

To the extent that the family schema involves cognitive distortions, it may result in dysfunctional interactions. Schemas further influence how family members subsequently process information in new situations. For example, they may influence what the individual selectively perceives, the inferences he or she makes about the causes of another's behavior, and whether he or she is pleased or displeased with the family relationship. Existing schemas may often be difficult to modify and require a great deal of effort in restructuring. Schemas usually change only when there is enough new convincing information that serves to modify a family member's beliefs.

Family-of-Origin Schemas

While individual family members maintain their own basic beliefs about themselves, the world, and their future, they also develop schemas about characteristics of their family of origin, which are commonly generalized to some degree to conceptions about other close relationships. It was suggested in the past that greater emphasis should be placed on examining not only cognitions of individual family members, but also the family schema (Bedrosian & Bozicas, 1994; Dattilio, 1993, 2005a). Although family schemas typically constitute jointly held beliefs about most family phenomena, such as day-to-day dilemmas and interactions, they can also pertain to nonfamily phenomena, as well as other issues, such as cultural and spiritual matters. The vast majority of family schemas are shared, but individual family members may sometimes deviate from the joint schema. The beliefs developed in each parent's family of origin may be either conscious or beyond a conscious awareness, and whether or not they are explicitly expressed suggests how they may contribute to the joint family schema (see Dattilio, 2010, 2014, for a more expansive discussion).

Schemas are often at the heart of family conflicts (Dattilio, 2005a). For this reason, they should be addressed during the early phase of treatment while the assessment phase is still ongoing. One of the guidelines used for assessing schemas from family of origin is Richard Stuart's Family of Origin Inventory (1995). This subject is discussed in more detail under the section heading of "The Use of Inventories and Questionnaires." These schemas may be ingrained because they are deeply rooted in experiences from one's family of origin. They are also likely to be culturally based and imposed early in one's formative years, rendering them more resistant to modification and change (Dattilio & Bahadur, 2005).

Belief systems that hail from one's family of origin have usually been strong and consistently reinforced and have been internalized during key formative periods of life (Dattilio, 2006b). A classic example is a father whose schema from his family of origin is that fighting and arguing among parents lead to separation and divorce and therefore arguing must be avoided at all costs (Dattilio, 2010). Consequently, he may go out of his way to appease his wife and child to avoid intrafamilial conflict, with the anticipation that this may break up the family. This has a trickle-down effect to the offspring who view the father's role as passive and may respond in one of two ways. On the one hand, the child may respond to overcompensate for father's passivity by being more aggressive and arguing with his mother. On the other hand, the child may choose a different stance and remain passive, much like his own father, but then resent it and engage in passive-aggressive behaviors, or even develop depression, which may cause other problems in the family. Therefore, addressing such schemas and modifying behaviors within the family dynamics are essential to incur change.

COGNITIVE DISTORTIONS

Just as in the case of individuals, families are prone to engage in cognitive distortion. These distortions typically emanate from belief systems held not only by family members, but families as a whole and involve all of the traditional cognitive distortions first introduced in the basic model of cognitive therapy of depression (Beck et al., 1979).

Schema Restructuring

Schema restructuring involves the reworking of misperceptions and distorted thinking that occur among family members. It also explores and makes use of family of origin and the early-life experiences of parents and how schemas trickle down to affect the family members in the immediate family (Dattilio, 2006a). This includes addressing issues of attachment and emotional regulation. Exploring maladaptive schemas regarding issues of attachment and bonding, boundaries, fairness, power, and control are all essential in working with families in conflict. Many of these maladaptive schemas develop early within the nuclear family and tend to strengthen and become more resistant to change.

Emphasis is placed on the core themes that pertain to the family relationship dynamics. By addressing these themes in an analytic and structured fashion, family therapists may help families make sense of conflict, marital gridlock, and dysfunctional interaction patterns. Using education and direct confrontation also helps family members to become aware of their thinking and behavior and to take action toward changing them. The therapist also works as an agent to identify enabling factors in the spouse, parents, or other family members who may be serving to keep these behavioral patterns ongoing.

Identifying Automatic Thoughts and Cognitive Distortions

Automatic thoughts are cognitions that occur spontaneously and seem plausible to the individual. They consist of assessments or interpretations of events. Identifying automatic thoughts with families involves superficial or moment-to-moment thoughts that family members present during the course of assessment and treatment. These conscious automatic thoughts provide a pathway to uncover underlying beliefs and schemas that carry more significant weight with regard to family conflicts. A good example is a teenager who voiced the following frustration:

> "The rules in our family are all screwed up. Half the time, my parents say one thing and then do another and it's confusing. Then, I get yelled at for not following the rules. It's not fair and it makes me believe that they just do what they feel like at the time. I wish they'd get their acts together." The son's automatic thought, "My parents say one thing and do another" leads him to the underlying belief, "They just do what they feel like at the time."

Another example is a parent who may experience difficulty tolerating expressions of a desire for sexual activity by his or her adolescent children and might experience the automatic thought, "These kids just don't have any morals." This viewpoint may stem from an underlying belief or schema that the youth of today have less respect for traditional values and as a result maintain a carefree attitude about relationships in general.

Sometimes cognitions can also occur beyond an individual's level of conscious awareness. The more expansive underlying schemas are typically uncovered through a family member's automatic thoughts. However, not all automatic thoughts are expressions of schemas. Some automatic thoughts may express a family member's attributions about causes of an event that he or she has observed (e.g., "My son didn't call home and inform me that he had to work overtime. His job is more important than our family").

Undoubtedly, schemas are crucial in the application of CBFT. They constitute stable cognitive structures as opposed to fleeting inferences or perceptions. Consequently, they are typically more difficult to modify. While dealing with individual family members' thoughts is central to cognitive-behavioral therapy, dealing with joint family schemas is essential as well. It should be noted that the cognitive-behavioral theory does not suggest that cognitions cause all family members' behavior; however, it does stress that cognitive appraisal significantly influences family members' behaviors, interactions, and emotional responses to one another (Epstein et al., 1988; Wright & Beck, 1993).

CONCLUSIONS

CBFT has grown exponentially within the past several decades among family therapists who use it as either a straightforward approach within a system perspective or integrated into other approaches with couples and family therapy. While in the past the CBFT approach has focused mostly on the treatment of specific disorders with individual family members rather than on alleviating general conflicts and distress in family constellations, it has more recently been used as a general approach to treating families. Forms of CBFT have chosen to highlight some of the demonstrated efficacy of the behavioral aspect, which involves training parents in behavioral interventions for their children's anxiety or conduct disorders, or addressing issues of attention-deficit/hyperactivity disorder, as well as other behavioral problems. These problems may involve addressing core symptoms of inattention, impulsivity, hyperactivity, and even psychiatric conditions. As noted earlier, methods of CBFT have been used in conjunction with other interventions, particularly in addressing the issue of schemas and restructuring thought processes among family members who are in conflict. The results of various studies that have been conducted indicate that CBFT interventions are very effective in improving family functioning.

The CBFT approach has gained widespread adoption among family therapists throughout the globe who have found the basic approach to be easily integrated with other modalities, and also to provide an effective mechanism for restructuring maladaptive thinking patterns and dysfunctional behaviors. The unique aspect of CBFT is that it clearly embraces issues of attachment and emotional regulation, as well as maintaining an overall respect for the neurobiological functioning of human beings. CBFT is featured in all of the primary family therapy textbooks used within university graduate school training programs, as well as in medical school residence curriculums.

In some of the more recent surveys conducted among couples and family therapists, clinicians have designated their primary treatment modality as being CBFT, while respondents who use other approaches have stated that they use cognitive-behavioral techniques in combination with other methods of treatment (*Psychotherapy Networker*, 2007; Northey, 2002). As a result, the cognitive-behavioral approach, in one form or the other, will likely continue to be one of the more espoused treatment modalities among couples and family therapy.

REFERENCES

Alexander, J. F., & Parsons, B. V. (1982). *Functional family therapy*. Monterey, CA: Brooks/Cole.

Barkley, R. A. (1997). *ADHD and the nature of self-control*. New York: Guilford Press.

Barton, C., & Alexander, J. F. (1981). Functional family therapy. In A. S. Gurman & D. P. Kniskern (Eds.), *Handbook of family therapy* (pp. 403–443). New York: Brunner/Mazel.

Beavers, W. R., Hampson, R. B., & Hulgus, Y. F. (1985). The Beavers systems approach to family assessment. *Family Process, 24*, 398–405.

Beck, A. T., Rush, A. J., Shaw, B. F., & Emery, G. (1979). *Cognitive therapy of depression*. New York: Guilford Press.

Bedrosian, R. C. (1983). Cognitive therapy in the family system. In A. Freeman (Ed.), *Cognitive therapy with couples and groups* (pp. 95–106). New York: Plenum Press.

Bedrosian, R. C., & Bozicas, G. D. (1994). *Treating family of origin problems: A cognitive approach*. New York: Guilford Press.

Bird, V., Premkumar, P., Kendall, T., Whittington, C., Mitchell, J., & Kuipers, E. (2010). Early intervention services, cognitive-behavioral therapy and family intervention in early psychosis: Systematic review. *British Journal of Psychiatry, 197*(5), 350–356.

Birmaher, B., Brent, D. A., & Kolko, D. (2000). Clinical outcome after short-term psychotherapy for adolescents with major depressive disorder. *Archives of General Psychiatry, 57,* 29–36.

Brent, D. A., Holder, D., & Kolko, D. (1997). A clinical psychotherapy trial for adolescent depression comparing cognitive, family and supportive therapy. *Archives of General Psychiatry, 54,* 77–88.

Chambless, D. L. (2012). Adjunctive couple and family intervention for patients with anxiety disorders. *Journal of Clinical Psychology, 68*(5), 548–560.

Chronis, A. M., Chacko, A., Fabiano, G. A., Wymbs, B. T., & Pelham, W. E., Jr. (2004). Enhancements to the behavioral parent training paradigm for families of children with ADHD: Review of future directions. *Clinical Child and Family Psychology Review, 7,* 1–27.

Dadds, M. R., Barrett, P. M., Rapee, R. M., & Ryan, S. (1996). Family process and child anxiety and aggression: An observational analysis. *Journal of Abnormal Child Psychology, 24*(6), 715–734.

Dattilio, F. M. (1983, Winter). The use of operant techniques and parental control in the treatment of pediatric headache complaints: Case report. *Pennsylvania Journal of Counseling, 1*(2), 55–58.

Dattilio, F. M. (1989). A guide to cognitive marital therapy. In P. A. Keller & S. F. Heyman (Eds.), *Innovations in clinical practice: A source book* (Vol. 8, pp. 27–42). Sarasota, FL: Professional Resource Exchange.

Dattilio, F. M. (1993). Cognitive techniques with couples and families. *Family Journal, 1,* 51–56.

Dattilio, F. M. (1998). *Case studies in couples and family therapy: Systemic and cognitive perspectives.* New York: Guilford Press.

Dattilio, F. M. (2001). Cognitive-behavior family therapy: Contemporary myths and misconceptions. *Contemporary Family Therapy, 23,* 3–18.

Dattilio, F. M. (2002). Homework assignments in couple and family therapy. *Journal of Clinical Psychology, 58*(5), 570–583.

Dattilio, F. M. (2005a). Restructuring family schemas: A cognitive behavioral perspective. *Journal of Marital and Family Therapy, 32*(1), 15–30.

Dattilio, F. M. (2005b). Clinical perspectives on involving the family in treatment. In J. L. Hudson & R. M. Rapee (Eds.), *Psychopathology and the family* (pp. 301–321). London: Elsevier.

Dattilio, F. M. (2006a). Case-based research in family therapy. *Australian and New Zealand Journal of Family Therapy, 27*(4), 208–213.

Dattilio, F. M. (2006b). Restructuring schemata from family-of-origin couple therapy. *Journal of Cognitive Psychotherapy, 20*(4), 359–373.

Dattilio, F. M. (2010). *Cognitive-behavioral therapy with couples and families: A comprehensive guide for clinicians.* New York: Guilford Press.

Dattilio, F. M. (2014). Family therapy. In S. Hofmann & W. Rief (Eds.), *Cognitive behavior therapy: A complete reference guide* (Vol. 1, pp. 311–330). Hoboken, NJ: Wiley.

Dattilio, F. M., & Bahadur, M. (2005). Cognitive-behavior therapy with an East Indian family. *Contemporary Family Therapy, 27*(2), 137–160.

Dattilio, F. M., Edwards, D. A., & Fishman, D. N. (2010). Case studies within a mixed methods paradigm: Towards the resolution of the alienation between researcher and practitioner in psychotherapy research. *Psychotherapy, 47*(4), 427–441.

Dattilio, F. M., & Epstein, N. B. (2016). Cognitive-behavioral couple and family therapy. In T. L. Sexton & J. L. Lebow (Eds.), *The family therapy handbook* (2nd ed., pp. 89–119). New York: Routledge.

Dattilio, F. M., Kazantzis, N., Shinkfield, G., & Carr, A.G. (2011). Survey of homework use and barriers impeding homework completion in couples and family therapy. *Journal of Marital and Family Therapy, 37*(2), 121–136.

Dattilio, F. M., Piercy, F. P., & Davis, S. D. (2014). The divide between "evidence based" approaches and practitioners of traditional theories of couple and family therapy. *Journal of Marital and Family Therapy, 40*(1), 1–7.

Davis, S. D., & Piercy, F. P. (2007). What clients of couple therapy model developers and their former students say about change, part 1: Model dependent common factors across three models. *Journal of Marital and Family Therapy, 33*(3), 318–343.

Edwards, D., Dattilio, F. M., & Bromley, D. B. (2004). Developing evidence-based practice: The role of case-based research. *Professional Psychology: Research and Practice, 35*(6), 589–597.

Ellis, A. (1982). Rational-emotive family therapy. In A. M. Home & M. M. Ohlsen (Eds.), *Family counseling and therapy* (pp. 302–328). Itasca, IL: Peacock.

Epstein, N. B., Baldwin, L. M., & Bishop, D. S. (1983). The MacMaster family assessment device. *Journal of Marital and Family Therapy, 9,* 171–180.

Epstein, N., & Schlesinger, S. E. (1996). Treatment of family problems. In M. A. Reinecke, F. M. Dattilio, & A. Freeman (Eds.), *Cognitive therapy with children and adolescents: A casebook for clinical practice* (pp. 299–326). New York: Guilford Press.

Epstein, N., Schlesinger, S. E., & Dryden, W. (1988). Concepts and methods of cognitive-behavior family treatment. In N. Epstein, S. E. Schlesinger, & W. Dryden (Eds.), *Cognitive-behavior therapy with families* (pp. 5–48). New York: Brunner/Mazel.

Falloon, I. R. H. (Ed.). (1988). *Handbook of behavioral family therapy.* New York: Guilford Press.

Falloon, I. R. H., Boyd, L., & McGill, C. W. (1984). *Family care of schizophrenia.* New York: Guilford Press.

Faulkner, R. A., Klock, K., & Gale, J. E. (2002). Qualitative research in family therapy: Publication trends from 1980 to 1999. *Journal of Marital and Family Therapy, 28*(1), 69–74.

Hahlweg, K., & Widemann, G. (1999). Principles and results of family therapy in schizophrenia. *European Archives of Psychiatry and Clinical Neuroscience, 249*(Suppl. 4), IV/108–IV/115.

Kazantzis, N., Deane, F. P., Ronan, K. R., & L'Abate, L. L. (Eds.). (2005). *Using homework assignments in cognitive-behavior therapy.* New York: Routledge.

Leslie, L. A. (1988). Cognitive-behavioral and systems models of family therapy: How compatible are they? In N. B. Epstein, S. E. Schlesinger, & W. Dryden (Eds.), *Cognitive-behavior therapy with families* (pp. 49–83). New York: Brunner/Mazel.

Moos, R. H., & Moos, B. H. (1986). *Family environment scale manual* (2nd ed.). Palo Alto, CA: Consulting Psychologists Press.

Mueser, K. T., & Glynn, S. M. (1995). *Behavioral family therapy for psychiatric disorders.* Boston: Allyn & Bacon.

Northey, W. F. (2002). Characteristics and clinical practices of marriage and family therapists: A national survey. *Journal of Marital and Family Therapy, 28*, 487–494.

Patterson, G. R. (1982). *Coercive family process.* Eugene, OR: Castalia Press.

Piacentini, J., Bergman, R. L., Chang, S., Langley, A., Peris, T., Wood, J. J., . . . McCracken, J. (2011). Controlled comparison of family cognitive behavioral therapy and psychoeducation/relaxation training for child obsessive–compulsive disorder. *Journal of the American Academy of Child and Adolescent Psychiatry, 50*(11), 1149–1161.

Psychotherapy Networker. (2007). The top 10: The most influential therapist of the past quarter century. *Psychotherapy Networker, 31*(2), 24–68.

Sanders, M. R. (2012). Development, evaluation, and multinational dissemination of the triple P-positive parenting program. *Annual Review of Clinical Psychology, 8*, 345–379.

Sanders, M. R., & Dadds, M. R. (1993). *Behavioral family intervention.* Boston: Allyn & Bacon.

Sanders, M. R., Shepherd, R. W., Cleghorn, G., & Woolford, H. (1994). The treatment of recurrent abdominal pain in children: A controlled comparison of cognitive-behavioral family intervention and standard pediatric care. *Journal of Consulting and Clinical Psychology, 62*, 306–314.

Schwebel, A. I., & Fine, M. A. (1994). *Understanding and helping families: A cognitive-behavior approach.* Hillsdale, NJ: Erlbaum.

Stuart, R. B. (1995). *Family of origin history.* New York: Guilford Press.

Wardle, J., Cooke, L. J., Gibson, E. L., Sapochnik, M., Sheiham, A., & Lawson, M. (2003). Increasing children's acceptance of vegetables: A randomized trial of parent-led exposure. *Appetite, 40*, 155–162.

Webster-Stratton, D., & Hancock, L. (1998). Parent training for young children with conduct problems: Content, methods and therapeutic processes. In C. E. Schaefer (Ed.), *Handbook of parent training* (pp. 98–152). New York: Wiley.

Wright, J. H., & Beck, A. T. (1993). Family cognitive therapy with inpatients. In J. H. Wright, M. E. These, A. T. Beck, & J. W. Ledged (Eds.), *Cognitive therapy with inpatients* (pp. 176–190). New York: Guilford Press.

CHAPTER 14

Cognitive-Behavioral Therapy for the Reduction of Suicide Risk

Cory F. Newman

Suicide is a public health problem of immense proportions, both at home in the United States and internationally. Here, there has been a disturbing upward trend in suicide rates, particularly among military personnel, with a total of approximately 41,000 deaths by suicide annually (Centers for Disease Control and Prevention, 2013). Worldwide, the number of suicides per year is estimated to be about one million (World Health Organization, 2013). As such, suicide is a target of major importance for mental health intervention. Fortunately, cognitive-behavioral interventions that specifically target suicidality are showing promise in significantly reducing potentially lethal self-directed violence in patients at high risk. This chapter will describe the core elements of recently developed cognitive-behavioral treatment packages to reduce suicide risk and will summarize the empirical support for these methods.

ASSESSMENT

The initial meeting with a new patient—whether in routine practice or in a crisis situation—customarily involves a thorough assessment of the patient's reasons for presenting for treatment, psychiatric symptoms, mental status, and level of risk to self and/or others (if any). The clinician also obtains a psychosocial history, as well as information regarding the patient's previous psychiatric and/or addiction treatments (including pharmacotherapy and hospitalizations).

In those instances when a new patient presents with suicidal ideation, intent, and/or recent self-harming behaviors, the clinician will need to conduct a more comprehensive suicide risk assessment per se (see Bryan, 2015; Wenzel, Brown, & Beck, 2009). This assessment involves several components, including directly interviewing the patients about their suicidal thoughts, asking them *why* they have a wish to die, observing their behavior directly, obtaining information from other pertinent sources (e.g., medical records, verbal reports from accompanying family members, family history), and using psychometrically sound assessment inventories, including self-report and interview-based questionnaires (a sample of which is summarized in Table 14.1).

If an ambulatory patient has already engaged in self-directed violence, the clinician assesses such variables as the patient's level of *intent* (e.g., impulsive versus planned; crying out for help versus wanting to die), degree of *lethality* of the method used (e.g., taking several pills or superficially cutting one's wrist, versus trying to hang or gas oneself), presence and extent of actual physical *injury,* whether or not the suicide attempt was *interrupted* (and by whom), and situational context and triggers. It is also important to determine if the current suicide attempt was the first time or the latest in a historical pattern, as patients who have a history of multiple suicide attempts are particularly at risk. Repeat attempters require less provocation to become suicidal, are less responsive to positive life events, and are especially prone to underutilizing therapy when compared to suicidal patients who do not have such a history (Joiner & Rudd, 2000). Similarly, it is very informative to ask whether the patient is glad to have survived the suicide attempt or regretful about still being alive. Regret about surviving the attempt is an indicator that a high level of risk persists (Henriques, Wenzel, Brown, & Beck, 2005).

It is good practice to inquire in depth about the patient's most recent suicidal crisis as part of the goal of constructing a chain analysis (similar to an explanatory flow chart) of the sequence of precipitating events. In addition, it is important to probe the patient's resultant suicidal thoughts, emotions, and behaviors, as well as the consequences (Brown, Wright, Thase, & Beck, 2012). Asking the patients specific questions to flesh out their narrative of the suicidal crisis will help elucidate their personal risk factors, both external (e.g., stressful life circumstances) and internal (e.g., beliefs that romanticize suicide). This process assists in formulating a preliminary case conceptualization and in providing patients with valuable psychoeducation about their vulnerabilities and related targets for intervention.

TABLE 14.1. Inventories to Assess Suicidality

Beck Scale for Suicide Ideation (BSSI; Beck, Kovacs, & Weissman, 1979)
The BSSI is an interview-based instrument that addresses multiple factors pertinent to a patient's potential suicidality. Notably, the BSSI includes a second section that inquires about the patient's *worst past episode* of suicidality. This adds important information, as there is evidence that future risk for suicide is significantly linked to past severity of suicidality, even if the patient's current risk level is low (Beck, Brown, Steer, Dahlsgaard, & Grisham, 1999; Joiner et al., 2003).

Beck Hopelessness Scale (BHS; Beck, Weissman, Lester, & Trexler, 1974)
The BHS is a 20-item "true–false" self-report inventory that assesses patients' views of their future, with such items as "I might as well give up because there is nothing I can do about making things better for myself." Hopelessness has been shown to be a mediator between depression and suicidality, and has predictive validity for deaths by suicide (Brown, Jeglic, Henriques, & Beck, 2006).

Beck Depression Inventory-II (BDI-II; Beck, Steer, & Brown, 1996)
This twenty-one-item self-report measure of the severity of depression contains items pertinent to hopelessness (#2) and suicidality (#9). When patients fill out the BDI-II at each session, therapists can eyeball these two scoring items for a quick, concise understanding of the patients' current level of suicide risk, and can ask the patients to discuss their inventory responses as part of the session agenda.

Columbia-Suicide Severity Rating Scale (C-SSRS; Posner et al., 2011)
The C-SSRS is an interview-based scale measuring patients' past and current suicidal ideation and behavior. It addresses the four constructs of severity, intensity, behavior, and lethality.

Suicide Cognitions Scale (SCS; Bryan et al., 2014)
The SCS is an eighteen-item self-report instrument. Patients rate their strength of belief in each item on a 0–5 Likert-type scale. The two main constructs underlying the items are the suicidal schemas of *unbearability* and *unlovability.*

Assessment of risk does not just occur at the first meeting; it is conducted at each session if there is ongoing care for an at-risk patient. Therapists can explain to their patients that they will ask about their suicidal ideation, intentions, and behaviors as a routine part of each session's agenda, never taking for granted that "everything is okay now" and realizing that they need to be vigilant for emergent recurrences of increased risk. Self-report measures such as the Beck Depression Inventory-II and the Beck Hopelessness Scale (BDI-II and BHS, respectively, see Table 14.1), completed by the patient at each session, are also convenient ways to keep track of the patient's problems with depressed mood, hopelessness, and suicidal ideation.

COGNITIVE-BEHAVIORAL MODEL OF SUICIDALITY

The Suicidal "Mode"

Unlike the more traditional *syndromal* model that viewed patients' suicidality as secondary to their psychiatric diagnoses, a cognitive-behavioral approach uses a model that examines the antecedent and consequent contextual influences as well as the patient's *belief systems* that interact to initiate and maintain suicidal feelings and behaviors (Clemans, 2015). A key concept is the *suicidal mode* (Rudd, Joiner, & Rajab, 2004), composed of four integrated systems:

1. *Cognition,* or the "suicidal belief system" (see "cognitive vulnerabilities," below).
2. *Emotion,* including negative affect states that may be poorly regulated and easily triggered.
3. *Physiology,* which pertains to the somatic experiences associated with the suicidal crisis, such as physical pain and sleep problems.
4. *Behavior,* which includes not only the suicidal actions themselves, but also the patient's maladaptive coping strategies (e.g., social withdrawal, misuse of alcohol and other drugs, avoidance of important activities, and nonsuicidal self-injury such as cutting oneself to distract from emotional pain).

Internal or external stimuli can activate the suicidal mode, with the threshold for activation and the severity of the episode being a function of the interaction between baseline predispositions (e.g., Does the patient typically feel hopeless or have a history of previous suicide attempts?) and the severity of acute risk factors (e.g., Did the patient just suffer a grievous loss?). The cognitive-behavioral model also pays close attention to the function or purpose of the suicidal behavior. For example, does the patient receive negative reinforcement for cutting himself (e.g., reduction of emotional pain), or perhaps positive reinforcement (e.g., a dramatic increase in others showing concern)? Does the patient's self-harming behavior feel "congruent" with her belief system ("I am a bad person who deserves to die," or "Only by dying can I escape my problems")? Conversely, does the patient respond with hope and increased desire to live in response to positive stimuli (e.g., responsivity to expressions of care from others and to therapy)? Exploring these aspects of the model contributes greatly to the formulation of a cognitive-behavioral case conceptualization (see Kuyken, Padesky, & Dudley, 2009) that can increase the practitioner's accurate empathy, and guide the construction of a treatment plan for the suicidal patient.

Cognitive Vulnerabilities Associated with Suicidality

A CBT approach to the assessment and treatment of suicidality pays close attention to the cognitive characteristics associated with suicide risk. For example, *hopelessness* has been found to be a significant factor in differentiating nonsuicidal persons from those who are potentially at elevated risk for suicide (Beck, Brown, Berchick, Stewart, & Steer, 1990; Beck, Steer, Beck, & Newman, 1993; Beck, Steer, Kovacs, & Garrison, 1985; Brown, Beck, Steer, & Grisham, 2000; Brown, Jeglic, Henriques, & Beck, 2006; Smith, Alloy, & Abramson, 2006). Hopelessness refers broadly to the belief that life's difficulties will not improve and that the future holds little or no promise. This general outlook seems to exacerbate clinical depression and confers an added risk for suicide.

In addition to general hopelessness, there are specific beliefs (especially in combination) that have been found to be related to suicide risk. In particular, suicidal patients have a tendency to believe that they are *unlovable,* that their problems are *unsolvable,* that their pain is *unbearable,* and/or that they are a *burden* to others (Ellis & Rufino, 2015; Joiner et al., 2009; Peak et al., 2015). Interventions need to focus on helping patients to value and appreciate themselves, to better recognize their importance to others (and to work on building and maintaining their relationships), to improve their distress tolerance, and to become better problem solvers. Regarding this last-named point, it has been found that suicidal patients perceive more problems but generate fewer solutions than nonsuicidal patients (Weishaar, 1996) and are slow to appreciate the practical and self-efficacy-enhancing benefits of actively keeping up with important tasks in everyday life. To counter this, treatment planning with suicidal patients can include teaching the skills of systematic problem solving (Nezu, Nezu, & D'Zurilla, 2013), bearing in mind the patients' struggles with lethargy, hopelessness, low motivation, and low self-efficacy.

Cognitive *rigidity* or *inflexibility* has also been identified as a common characteristic in suicidal thinking (Miranda, Valderrama, Tsypes, Gadol, & Gallagher, 2013). Suicidal persons are prone to evaluate themselves and their lives in all-or-none terms. Situational self-reproach becomes blanket self-condemnation. An adverse event seems inexorable and devastating. Competent CBT practitioners recognize that it does little good to combat this cognitive habit without first offering their patients sincere empathy for their emotional distress. Patients then become more receptive to learning to evaluate themselves and their lives on a continuum and are more likely to notice signs of hope that they might otherwise overlook.

Morbid perfectionism is also a cognitive risk factor for suicide (Flett, Hewitt, & Heisel, 2014). This level of perfectionism is more harmful than a mere stubborn desire to get things right. It entails a patient's internal demand to have things be "just so" and to be punitive toward oneself and angry at the world if things turn out differently. Within this mindset, the minor setbacks of everyday life become triggers for emotional crises, and larger disappointments become reasons to want to die (e.g., "If I don't pass the Bar Exam this time, I will kill myself").

THE THERAPEUTIC RELATIONSHIP WITH THE SUICIDAL PATIENT

Accurate empathy and trust are cornerstones of any therapeutic relationship, but these factors take on added significance when patients are suicidal. In order to be *accurately* empathic, the therapist needs to be able to grasp the patient's level of pain and despair that makes death seem a more attractive option than life and to be able to communicate this understanding sincerely. Likewise, the therapist must be able to articulate an understanding of the patient's reasons for wanting to die, thereby averting giving the patient the stigmatic message that his or her thoughts and feelings are "crazy," and instead giving the patient the impression that the therapist "gets it." At the same time, the therapist must be able to offer genuine messages of hope.

The issue of trust goes both ways in the therapeutic relationship with the suicidal patient. For example, the therapist wants to be able to trust that the patient will openly disclose suicidal thoughts and feelings, rather than conceal them. In turn, suicidal patients want to be able to trust that if they admit to harboring suicidal thoughts and feelings, the therapist will not secretly judge them as being hopeless and/or an unwanted clinical burden. To maximize trust, the therapist must be transparent about the decision-making process that goes into the consideration of an inpatient stay. One way to do this is to openly consider questions such as:

- To what degree is the patient willing and able to collaborate with an outpatient safety plan?
- Is it feasible to increase the frequency of outpatient sessions, intersession phone contacts, and therapeutic homework assignments?
- Are there people in the patient's everyday life who can be called upon (with the patient's consent) to spend extra time with and keep a caring eye on the patient between sessions?
- What are the patient's personal obligations that would be interrupted by a hospital stay? For example, would missing work, missing school, or not being available to take care of loved ones at home add significantly *more* stress to the patient's life, and perhaps make an inpatient stay counterproductive in the long run?
- If the patient attempts suicide during the course of therapy, what are the parameters for resuming outpatient CBT once the patient is discharged from the hospital?

Regarding this last point, one may argue that it is best if therapists do *not* issue the patient the ultimatum that "if you try suicide I will no longer be your therapist." While no therapist wants to be permissive about suicidal behavior, it does little good to have a "zero tolerance policy" for suicidal behavior when treating patients whose central problem is suicidality. Rather than denying care, the CBT practitioner can engage the patient in *revising the treatment plan* so that it will now take into account the evidence for heightened risk (Ramsay & Newman, 2005).

INTERVENTIONS

It is somewhat misleading to categorize "interventions" as being distinct from the therapeutic relationship or the case conceptualization, as these important factors interact (see Newman, 2015). Similarly, the term "interventions" does not refer solely to what transpires in the therapist's office. It also refers to the patients' homework assignments, in which they practice in everyday life what they learned in their CBT sessions. Homework assignments can also include self-help readings that supplement and are congruent with the treatment (e.g., *Choosing to Live: How to Defeat Suicide Through Cognitive Therapy,* Ellis & Newman, 1996). Such readings can be discussed during sessions so as to be certain that the patient is comprehending the most hopeful and constructive contents, as well as the exercises.

Safety Planning

In the past, it was common practice to institute "antisuicide contracts" with suicidal patients. The intention was to encourage such patients to commit to treatment, to collaborate constructively with the therapist, and to emphasize that both parties were taking the threat of suicide seriously. Combined with a positive therapeutic relationship, and in the context of a broad, well-articulated treatment plan, such antisuicide contracts made sense as an important part of the therapeutic process. However, when used in a cursory fashion, antisuicide contracts could counteract a sense of collaboration between therapist and patient, and could be construed as being more about protecting the therapist than about understanding and treating the patient. Indeed, evidence for the efficacy of such contracts is lacking (Kleepsies & Dettmer, 2000; Rudd, Mandrusiak, & Joiner, 2006; Stanford, Goetz, & Bloom, 1994).

Instead, the field has come around to the idea that "safety planning" is a more useful way to introduce formal methods for keeping suicidal patients safe between therapy sessions when they are not under direct clinical supervision and may be vulnerable to exacerbations in mood and related suicidality (Stanley & Brown, 2012; Wenzel et al., 2009). Safety planning entails the implementation of good, standard risk management methods, including identifying, promoting, and utilizing the patients' interpersonal and intrapersonal resources.

The typical components of outpatient risk management include scheduling between-session phone contacts, increasing the frequency of sessions, making arrangements for the patient to spend time in public places around other people and activities (e.g., cafes, bookstores, parks, sporting or community events, malls) and/or with selected others who can provide some measure of oversight (e.g., friends, family, support group cohorts, 12-step sponsor), and doing advance problem-solving to reduce the likelihood of the patient's being in situations that might increase risk. These risk management methods clearly involve a strong *interpersonal* component, in which the patient is prepared to reach out to (and spend time with) others. Patients should have ready access to important contact information, including phone numbers for their practitioners and suicide hot lines. The interpersonal part of the safety plan can also be utilized to enact a *lethal means restriction*—that is to say that important people in the patient's life are enlisted to help remove whatever poses a potential danger to the patient. For example, a trusted family member can take possession of the patient's firearm(s) for safe storage (see Simon, 2007), or a person in the patient's household can take charge of doling out the patient's medications in small increments to lower the risk of deliberate overdose.

The *intrapersonal* piece in safety planning has to do with the patient learning to spot early warning signs of increasing suicidality and being ready and agreeable to use the full array of self-help coping skills he or she has learned in CBT. The key, central self-help skills are described in some detail in this chapter, but it is worth briefly noting here that they can also include mindfulness techniques, physical exercise, and healthy self-soothing.

An additional "tool" to be included in the safety plan is called the *hope kit* (Wenzel et al., 2009). This is a compilation of memorabilia and contact information that patients can easily access (e.g., from a shoebox, a phone app, a computer file) when they are in need of positive reminders about themselves and their lives. A hope kit is typically composed of photos that represent positive times and events, birthday and greeting cards that the patient has received over the years, artifacts that represent success experiences (e.g., award or honor certificates, congratulatory messages), mementos from favored activities (e.g., trips, clubs), emotionally significant and meaningful writings the patient has composed, including the best examples of previous therapy homework assignments, a list of important people in the patient's life (along with their contact information), and any other items that favorably represent the patient's life and times. The general purposes of the hope kit are to assemble and highlight evidence that suicidal patients do indeed have important attachments to life, and to remind them why their existence is worth preserving and nurturing. Sometimes the therapist will ask their suicidal patients to bring their hope kits to session, so that they may discuss their contents and add to them.

Building Psychological Self-Help Skills

Safety planning represents the short-term part of the CBT package for treating suicidality. Longer-term treatment methods entail helping patients develop and practice psychological skills, including modifying harmful beliefs. Some of these interventions include (1) developing hopefulness and reasons for living, (2) rationally responding to suicidogenic beliefs, (3) constructing a compassionate narrative of one's own life, (4) improving problem solving, and (5) engaging in activities that bring a sense of accomplishment and enjoyment, among others (see Ellis & Newman, 1996; Wenzel et al., 2009).

Developing Hopefulness and Reasons for Living

Compassionate, collaborative CBT therapists validate their patients' experiences of subjective emotional pain, but also invite them to consider ways in which this pain may be eased within the scope of an improved life, with a more hopeful future. A simple, straightforward, but often powerful technique is a thorough discussion (and writing) about the pros and cons of committing suicide versus committing to life (Ellis & Newman, 1996; Jobes, 2006; Brown et al., 2012). This method gives patients overt permission to identify the "advantages" of suicide that they have already been harboring and to talk about the topic openly with the therapist (see Figure 14.1). Often, obvious cognitive biases are identified in the course of fleshing out the "pros of dying" (e.g., "My parents will be better off if I kill myself"), and these can be subjected to rational responding (see below). Meanwhile, the therapist engages the patient in a process of considering the advantages of committing to life, something that the patient may have been discounting or neglecting. A further utilization of this technique is to discuss the pros and cons of the patient's life and death in relation to their effects on the patient's loved ones. This often motivates patients to think about the well-being of their family as a deterrent to suicide.

Rationally Responding to Suicidogenic Beliefs

Suicidal patients are taught to identify their beliefs that potentially support their suicidal feelings and intentions, and to use cognitive restructuring techniques (see Newman, 2015) in an attempt to modify these dangerous beliefs. Many suicidal patients evince rigid, maladaptive beliefs that are not easy to relinquish. However, it is therapeutic to try to create "reasonable doubt" in the minds of such patients about their notions (for example) that

[Sample responses]

	PRO	CON
TRYING SUICIDE	1. My parents will be better off if I kill myself. 2. I won't be overwhelmed by my problems anymore. 3. People will really understand that I was serious about wanting to die.	1. I would never have a chance to turn my life around. 2. I might wind up in a coma and become an even bigger burden to my family. 3. I would always be remembered for killing myself, rather than something good. 4. My mother would probably get suicidal too.
COMMITTING TO LIVING	1. This could be a turning point in my life. 2. My family won't be stigmatized. 3. I can live and try to help others who might feel suicidal.	1. I might have to go through more misery and disappointment in my life. 2. I might be fooling myself to think things can get better, and then I will just suffer for a longer time. 3. People will stop taking me seriously when I tell them I want to die.

FIGURE 14.1. Advantages/disadvantages analysis.

death is the only "solution" to their problems, or that they are so bad that they "deserve" to die. Suicidal patients do not necessarily have to disavow their negative beliefs completely in order to benefit from learning to generate alternative beliefs that support their lives. Similarly, it is not essential that patients buy into their newly generated adaptive beliefs 100% in order for them to benefit from learning how to *generate* rational responses such as "If I continue to live, I will have a chance to leave a better legacy than if I were to kill myself now." Rational responding is not the same thing as "thought replacement." The more apt description is that rational responding plants seeds of hope that can sprout over time with the help of a strong therapeutic relationship and a comprehensive treatment plan.

Constructing a Compassionate Narrative of One's Own Life

In order to gain a broader perspective on their lives, to escape the time trap of being unduly focused on the pain of the moment, to improve specific autobiographical recall, and to imagine a better future, suicidal patients are encouraged to write a compassionate narrative of their lives. It is best if this technique is done in stages, across sessions, so that it can grow into a detailed, thorough story, and so that it can become a useful, ongoing homework assignment. This method dovetails nicely with the *hope kit,* which itself tells a positive story of the patient's life from the past to the present. An additional narrative can be added that describes positive possibilities for the future. For example, the patients can be asked to list three positive and/or interesting things they might experience each year going forward—things that they would miss if they were to commit suicide (see Ellis & Newman, 1996). If the patient professes to have no ideas, therapists can help, such as by suggesting important future family events and landmarks (e.g., a sibling's wedding), positive experiences (e.g., vacation trips the patient may make), and personal goals (e.g., learning to play the guitar, moving to a new apartment, getting a dog). Along the same lines, the future narrative can also include attending to unfinished business, such as making amends with an old friend or finishing an educational degree. In the process, the patient invests more in life, and creates new attachments to goals and people. The written aspects of the compassionate narrative—as the technique would suggest—must be composed in a congenial tone, and the therapist (who is witness to the narrative) gives the patient feedback to shape the tenor of the story.

Improving Problem Solving

Suicidal patients sometimes feel overwhelmed by life's problems (and/or by their *perceptions* of life's problems) and see no way out other than escaping from life itself. This is where therapists need to teach their patients basic problem-solving skills, including describing problems objectively, brainstorming solutions, weighing pros and cons, implementing chosen methods, evaluating the outcomes, and beginning the process with another problem (Nezu et al., 2013). Even when patients have bona fide crises and hardships, therapists offer empathy along with a lesson in the benefits of doing "damage control" to begin to turn things around for the better.

Activities for Accomplishment and Enjoyment

Deeply depressed individuals often experience anhedonia, lethargy, and low motivation that lead to their abandoning (or not considering) activities that could boost their mood and sense of self-efficacy. In CBT, the therapists empathically acknowledge that it is difficult to do things when one is inclined to be inert. Nonetheless, the therapists help patients brainstorm a list of activities in which to engage, particularly those that have the potential to be enjoyable and/or to provide a sense of accomplishment. Sometimes an excellent source of ideas for this list comes from a review of the things that the patient *used to do* and/or has been *meaning to do*. Deeply depressed patients are prone to minimizing the meaning or importance of such activities, and often assume that taking part in the activities will fail to make them feel better anyway. Effective therapists encourage the patients to increase their level of activity step by step as a therapeutic experiment to test hypotheses about the potential impact. When patients begin to do positive, constructive things, it often improves their morale, provides some hope, and helps in the process of connecting with others and/or solving problems. All of this serves as a counterweight to suicidality.

Relapse Prevention

After the patients have practiced and solidified their use of the above skills to the point where they have reduced their suicidal thinking and connected better with their lives, it is time to work on relapse prevention. This involves such methods as reviewing and documenting the patient's self-help strategies (e.g., including samples from their homework assignments), updating the safety plan to incorporate new ideas (e.g., new activities, additional people and professionals to contact), and organizing and assembling coping cards that contain the best of the patients' rational responses to the re-emergence of old stress reactions. It should be noted that "coping cards" used to mean hard copies of writings, perhaps on index cards. Nowadays, the therapeutic content can just as easily be kept on a patient's phone or other digital device, a strategy that may elicit greater compliance in younger patients. An additional relapse prevention method—a guided imagery exercise—is described by Green and Brown (2015). Here, the therapist guides the patients to imagine anticipated situations in the future that could have the potential to trigger a suicidal crisis. Patients then have to provide a detailed account of the coping methods they would use in such situations. The patients' facility in performing this task provides an assessment of their readiness for the completion of regularly scheduled sessions.

EMPIRICAL SUPPORT FOR CBT WITH SUICIDAL PATIENTS

There is a growing body of research suggesting that CBT-related approaches that specifically target suicidality lead to a reduction in suicidal behavior, at least during the critical period of time following a suicide attempt when the risk for further attempts is high, and up to two years of assessed follow-up.

Commonalities among the CBT-based treatment approaches reviewed here are more prominent than their relatively minor procedural and terminology differences. What they have in common is an assessment process that uses empathic interviewing, psychometrically supported measures, and a combination of functional analyses and cognitive conceptualizations in order to understand the chain reaction of external events (precipitants and consequences) and internal reactions (thoughts, feelings, physiological responses, and behaviors) that comprise the suicidal crises. Further, these approaches are alike in that they emphasize the teaching of psychological skills. Suicidal patients are taught to self-monitor, to reflect on their intended actions rather than respond reflexively, to engage in constructive actions and rational responding to combat a sense of helplessness and hopelessness, to reach out to their social supports so as to counteract a sense of isolation, and to contact mental health professionals (including those by whom they are being treated, and others who are "on call," such as those in hospitals and on crisis hotlines). These methods can be used as part of a larger, general package of CBT for the full range of problems that patients bring to treatment, or they can be stand-alone treatments. When they are used as single-session interventions in emergency departments (Stanley & Brown, 2012) or as brief treatments in inpatient facilities (e.g., Ellis & Ruffino, 2015), they can be learned and applied by well-trained mental health professionals regardless of their self-identified theoretical orientation.

A landmark randomized controlled trial showing the efficacy of a brief Beckian cognitive therapy protocol in reducing suicide attempts in a high-risk population was conducted by Brown et al. (2005). The 120 patients in this study had presented with a suicide attempt in the emergency department (ED) and were recruited within forty-eight hours for random assignment either to a treatment-as-usual condition or a ten-session cognitive therapy package (identified as cognitive therapy for suicide prevention, or *CT-SP*) in addition to treatment as usual (all of which was conducted postdischarge). The primary outcome variable was repeat suicide attempt(s) during a follow-up period of eighteen months. Participants in the cognitive therapy group were 50% less likely to reattempt suicide during follow-up, and they showed significantly lower depression and hopelessness. A very similar version of brief CBT was successfully tested in a military sample of active-duty Army soldiers who had made a suicide attempt within the past month or who had suicidal ideation with intent to die in the past week (Rudd et al., 2015). Half of the cohort (n = 76) was randomly assigned to the treatment-as-usual condition, and the other half (n = 76) was randomly assigned to brief CBT (twelve sessions) plus treatment as usual. Similar to the Brown et al. treatment study (2005), the Rudd et al. (2015) program utilized a CBT approach that specifically focused on the symptoms of suicidality (including the patients' belief systems pertinent to their thoughts about life and death), as well as on safety planning and relapse prevention.

During the two-year follow-up period, those receiving CBT were 60% less likely to make a suicide attempt.

The Collaborative Assessment and Management of Suicidality (CAMS; Jobes, 2006, 2012) is a therapeutic approach that self-identifies as being applicable in conjunction with treatments across the theoretical spectrum but nonetheless borrows heavily from CBT methods. In a nonrandomized control comparison study, CAMS was associated with reductions in suicidal ideation in comparison to treatment as usual and was significantly linked to decreases in emergency department utilization during the six-month follow-up period (Jobes et al., 2005). In a randomized trial, a brief course of outpatient CAMS was shown to reduce suicidal thinking and general symptom distress significantly, and to increase hopefulness and reasons for living at twelve-month follow-up more so than an enhanced care-as-usual approach (Comtois et al., 2011). When provided to hospitalized patients in an individual therapy format, CAMS led to significantly greater improvements on measures specific to suicidal ideation and suicidal cognitions compared to inpatients who did not receive the CAMS interventions (Ellis, Rufino, Allen, Fowler, & Jobes, 2015). Two caveats are that the Ellis et al. (2015) study used a nonrandomized design, and the six-week stay at the Menninger Clinic (where the study was conducted) provided a longer period of treatment than is customary in most inpatient facilities (thus calling into question the generalizability of results across institutions).

There is evidence, however, that even a one-time suicide-specific intervention in the ED may be sufficient to help acutely suicidal patients remain safe when they leave. *Safety Planning Intervention* (SPI; Stanley & Brown, 2012) consists of the same steps as described earlier, but in a condensed, written format that serves as a guide to aftercare and follow-up when suicidal patients exit the ED. The basic elements of the written SPI are: (1) identifying early warning signs of heightened suicide risk, (2) employing prepared, internal coping strategies, (3) utilizing social settings and contacts to distract from suicidal preoccupation, (4) contacting friends and family members for support in times of crisis; (5) contacting mental health practitioners or agencies, and (6) restricting access to lethal means. Stanley and Brown report that SPI has been used as part of other evidence-based psychotherapy interventions in clinical trial research. The authors are in the process of testing its efficacy as a stand-alone intervention in an urban ED and in a Department of Veterans Affairs project.

Another CBT approach that has been applied to suicidal individuals in inpatient settings is post-admission cognitive therapy (PACT, not to be confused with physical aggression couples treatment, used in another chapter; Ghahramanlou-Holloway, Cox, & Green, 2012). PACT emphasizes helping patients face the stressors that are often encountered following discharge from hospital; stressors that if not managed properly can easily trigger a relapse of suicidal thoughts, feelings, urges, and behaviors. Indeed, the period of time when patients are re-acclimating to life outside of the hospital is a period of high risk for another suicide attempt (Ghahramanlou-Holloway, Neely, & Tucker, 2015). PACT has the same treatment objectives as outpatient CBT (e.g., identifying and modifying the cognitive, emotional, and behavioral factors that comprise the patient's "suicidal mode"), but also helps patients develop the problem-solving skills they will need on the outside. The goals include improving the patient's self-efficacy in dealing with the demands of their life situation and increasing their compliance with adjunctive medical, social, psychiatric, and substance abuse interventions both during and after hospitalization. PACT is currently under evaluation in a multisite randomized controlled trial.

It is also important to acknowledge the contribution of dialectical behavior therapy (DBT) to the treatment literature on suicide risk reduction. Although DBT is a distinct treatment that involves components of care that are not routinely included in standard CBT packages (e.g., a skills group to go along with individual treatment; regular between-sessions phone contacts), DBT and the CBT approaches mentioned in this review have the same common theoretical roots. Brown et al. (2012) note that their *CT-SP* treatment and DBT both focus on preventing suicidal behavior by teaching high-risk patients specific coping skills. Thus, it is appropriate to note the empirical support for DBT with suicidal patients, such as the Linehan et al. (2006) randomized controlled trial with two-year follow-up. Similarly, it is important to mention that CBT can be applied to suicidal children and adolescents (a full description of which goes beyond the scope of this chapter). One representative randomized controlled trial was conducted by Esposito-Smythers and Spirito (2004) on hospitalized adolescents with a substance use disorder and at least one suicide attempt in the previous three weeks. Their data showed the superiority of CBT over enhanced treatment as usual on outcomes related to substance use, suicide attempts, ED visits, and arrests. The adolescents who received CBT also showed better treatment adherence. Another CBT approach currently being applied to the treatment of suicidal adolescents is the aptly named Treatment of Adolescent Suicide Attempters (TASA; Brent et al., 2009). The authors emphasize the importance of safety planning and increased frequency of therapeutic contact early in treatment.

CONCLUSIONS

Helping a patient to relinquish suicidal intentions and behaviors is a *process*. It is rarely a sudden epiphany for the patient to choose to live as a committed stance. More often, the therapist makes gradual inroads by establishing a genuinely caring therapeutic relationship, constructing a clear and comprehensive framework for the work of therapy, collaborating with the patient on an agreed-upon treatment plan, and offering a steady flow of words of empathy, support, encouragement, and hope. In other words, no single intervention in any given session is likely to put a definitive end to the patient's risk for suicide. However, each intervention contributes to a lowering of risk, especially if the therapist succeeds in motivating the patient to practice a range of self-help methods between therapy sessions. In sum, the therapist offers the suicidal patient *hope* and a *plan,* made formidable by the therapist's ability to present interventions in ways that fit the case conceptualization, thus demonstrating *accurate* empathy for the patient's unique experiences.

Although we have seen that brief CBT interventions for suicidality can be efficacious, a longitudinal approach to the treatment of suicidality may be best, as there is evidence that even when patients respond well to treatment they are prone to residual symptoms—including sub-optimally modified dysfunctional beliefs about suicide—that may keep the patients at elevated risk in the face of future triggers. Likewise, when a patient survives a suicide attempt, the crisis is *not* necessarily over. Patients who have recently tried suicide often are at continued heightened risk for further suicidal behavior in the aftermath (Monti, Cedereke, & Ojehagen, 2003).

In outpatient work with suicidal individuals, spotty attendance and early dropout from treatment take on added significance. There is evidence that those patients who are most at risk (e.g., having a history of multiple suicide attempts) are the same patients who tend to be least likely to avail themselves of regular therapy sessions (see Berk, Henriques, Warman, Brown, & Beck, 2004; Joiner & Rudd, 2000). Similarly, suicidal patients who opt to discontinue therapy without having a formal concluding session to summarize their gains and formulate a maintenance plan, and/or while still demonstrating hopelessness (e.g., as assessed via their last-completed BHS) are at higher ongoing risk for suicide than those who complete treatment with a better sense of hope and direction (Dahlsgaard, Beck, & Brown, 1998). The upshot of these findings is that therapists cannot remain passive when their suicidal patients are absent from treatment in an unanticipated way. Instead, it is important to reconnect with the patients, such as by calling and leaving caring messages that invite them to come in for an appointment as soon as possible (Brown et al., 2012).

Even when therapy with a suicidal patient has formally ended, it is a good idea for therapists occasionally to contact the former patient, perhaps mailing a card (e.g., holiday, birthday) or a note to say "Hello" and "How are you?" A randomized controlled trial by Motto and Bostrom (2001) demonstrated that such posttherapy communications, initiated by former therapists of patients who had received treatment for suicidality, made a significant difference in lowering risk during follow-up compared to those patients who had not been on the receiving end of such posttherapy greetings. The message is clear; therapists ought to strive to help their suicidal patients successfully complete a course of therapy. Later, the therapist may consider putting forth occasional gestures of outreach in a way that is professionally appropriate. This is all in the spirit of making the most of the therapeutic relationship and helping the patients to maintain their therapeutic gains.

REFERENCES

Beck, A. T., Brown, G. K., Berchick, R. J., Stewart, B. L., & Steer, R. A. (1990). Relationship between hopelessness and ultimate suicide: A replication with psychiatric outpatients. *American Journal of Psychiatry, 147,* 190–195.

Beck, A. T., Brown, G. K., Steer, R. A., Dahlsgaard, K. K., & Grisham, J. R. (1999). Suicide ideation at its worst point: A predictor of eventual suicide in psychiatric outpatients. *Suicide and Life-Threatening Behavior, 29,* 1–9.

Beck, A. T., Kovacs, M., & Weissman, A. (1979). Assessment of suicidal intention: The Scale for Suicide Ideation. *Journal of Consulting and Clinical Psychology, 47,* 343–352.

Beck, A. T., Steer, R. A., Beck, J. S., & Newman, C. F. (1993). Hopelessness, depression, suicidal ideation, and clinical diagnosis of depression. *Suicide and Life-Threatening Behavior, 23,* 139–145.

Beck, A. T., Steer, R. A., & Brown, G. K. (1996). *Manual for the Beck Depression Inventory-II.* San Antonio, TX: Psychological Corporation.

Beck, A. T., Steer, R. A., Kovacs, M., & Garrison, B. (1985). Hopelessness and eventual suicide: A 10-year prospective study of patients hospitalized with suicidal ideation. *American Journal of Psychiatry, 142,* 559–563.

Beck, A. T., Weissman, A., Lester, D., & Trexler, L. (1974). The measurement of pessimism: The Hopelessness Scale. *Journal of Consulting and Clinical Psychology, 42,* 499–505.

Berk, M. S., Henriques, G. R., Warman, D. M., Brown, G. K., & Beck, A. T. (2004). A cognitive therapy intervention for suicide attempters: An overview of the treatment and case examples. *Cognitive and Behavioral Practice, 11,* 265–277.

Brent, D. A., Greenhill, L. L., Compton, S., Emslie, G., Wells, K., Walkup, J., . . . Blake, T. J. (2009). The Treatment of Adolescent Suicide Attempters (TASA) study: Predictors of suicidal events in an open treatment trial. *Journal of the American Academy of Child and Adolescent Psychiatry, 48,* 987–996.

Brown, G. K., Beck, A. T., Steer, R. A., & Grisham, J. R. (2000). Risk factors for suicide in psychiatric outpatients: A 20-year prospective study. *Journal of Consulting and Clinical Psychology, 68,* 371–377.

Brown, G. K., Jeglic, E., Henriques, G. R., & Beck, A. T. (2006). Cognitive therapy, cognition, and suicidal behavior. In T. E. Ellis (Ed.), *Cognition and suicide: Theory, research, and therapy* (pp. 53–74). Washington, DC: American Psychological Association.

Brown, G. K., Ten Have, T., Henriques, G. R., Xie, S. X., Hollander, J. D., & Beck, A. T. (2005). Cognitive therapy for the prevention of suicide attempts: A randomized controlled trial. *Journal of the American Medical Association, 294,* 563–570.

Brown, G. K., Wright, J. H., Thase, M. E., & Beck, A. T. (2012). Cognitive therapy for suicide prevention. In R. I. Simon & R. E. Hales (Eds.), *Textbook of suicide assessment and management* (pp. 233–249). Washington, DC: American Psychiatric Publishing.

Bryan, C. J. (Ed.). (2015). *Cognitive behavioral therapy for preventing suicide attempts: A guide to brief treatments across clinical settings.* New York: Routledge.

Bryan, C. J., Rudd, M. D., Wertenberger, E., Etienne, N., Ray-Sannerud, B. N., Peterson, A. L., . . . Young-McCaughom, S. (2014). Improving the detection and prediction of suicidal behavior among military personnel by measuring suicidal beliefs: An evaluation of the Suicide Cognitions Scale. *Journal of Affective Disorders, 159,* 15–22.

Centers for Disease Control and Prevention. (2013). *Web-based Injury Statistics Query and Reporting System* (WISQARS) [Online]. Atlanta: National Center for Injury Prevention and Control. Available from *www.cdc.gov/injury/wisqars/index.html.*

Clemans, T. A. (2015). A cognitive behavioral model of suicide risk. In C. J. Bryan (Ed.), *Cognitive behavioral therapy for preventing suicide attempts: A guide to brief treatments across clinical settings* (pp. 51–64). New York: Routledge.

Comtois, K. A., Jobes, D. A., O'Connor, S. S., Atkins, D. A., Janus, K. I., Chessen, C. E., . . . Yuodelis-Flores, C. (2011). Collaborative Assessment and Management of Suicidality (CAMS): Feasibility trial for next day appointment services. *Depression and Anxiety, 28,* 963–972.

Dahlsgaard, K. K., Beck, A. T., & Brown, G. K. (1998). Inadequate response to therapy as a predictor of suicide. *Suicide and Life-Threatening Behavior, 28,* 197–204.

Ellis, T. E., & Newman, C. F. (1996). *Choosing to live: How to defeat suicide through cognitive therapy.* Oakland, CA: New Harbinger.

Ellis, T. E., & Rufino, K. A. (2015). A psychometric study of the Suicide Cognitions Scale with psychiatric inpatients. *Psychological Assessment, 27,* 82–89.

Ellis, T. E., Rufino, K. A., Allen, J. G., Fowler, J. C., & Jobes, D. A. (2015). Impact of a suicide-specific intervention within inpatient psychiatric care: The Collaborative Assessment and Management of Suicidality (CAMS). *Suicide and Life-Threatening Behavior, 45,* 556–566.

Esposito-Smythers, C., & Spirito, A. (2004). Adolescent substance use and suicidal behavior: A review with implications for treatment research. *Alcoholism: Clinical and Experimental Research, 28,* 77S–88S.

Flett, G. L., Hewitt, P. L., & Heisel, M. J. (2014). The destructiveness of perfectionism revisited: Implications for the assessment of suicide risk and the prevention of suicide. *Review of General Psychology, 18,* 156–172.

Ghahramanlou-Holloway, M., Cox, D., & Greene, F. (2012). Post-admission cognitive therapy: A brief intervention for psychiatric inpatients admitted after a suicide attempt. *Cognitive and Behavioral Practice, 19,* 116–125.

Ghahramanlou-Holloway, M., Neely, L. L., & Tucker, J. (2015). Treating risk for self-directed violence in inpatient settings. In C. J. Bryan (Ed.), *Cognitive behavioral therapy for preventing suicide attempts: A guide to brief treatments across clinical settings* (pp. 91–109). New York: Routledge.

Green, K. L., & Brown, G. K. (2015). Cognitive therapy for suicide prevention: An illustrated case example. In C. J. Bryan (Ed.), *Cognitive behavioral therapy for preventing suicide attempts: A guide to brief treatments across clinical settings* (pp. 65–88). New York: Routledge.

Henriques, G., Wenzel, A., Brown, G. K., & Beck, A. T. (2005). Suicide attempters' reaction to survival as a risk factor for eventual suicide. *American Journal of Psychiatry, 162,* 2180–2182.

Jobes, D. A. (2006). *Managing suicidal risk: A collaborative approach.* New York: Guilford Press.

Jobes, D. A. (2012). The Collaborative Assessment and Management of Suicidality (CAMS): An evolving evidence-based clinical approach to suicidal risk. *Suicide and Life-Threatening Behavior, 42,* 640–653.

Jobes, D. A., Wong, S. A., Kiernan, A., Conrad, A. K., Drozd, J. F., & Neal-Walden, T. (2005). The collaborative assessment and management of suicidality vs. treatment as usual: A retrospective study with suicidal outpatients. *Suicide and Life-Threatening Behavior, 35,* 483–497.

Joiner, T. E., & Rudd, M. D. (2000). Intensity and duration of suicidal crises vary as a function of previous suicide attempts and negative life events. *Journal of Consulting and Clinical Psychology, 68,* 909–916.

Joiner, T. E., Steer, R. A., Brown, G., Beck, A. T., Petit, J. W., & Rudd, M. D. (2003). Worst-point suicidal plans: A dimension of suicidality predictive of past suicide attempts and eventual death by suicide. *Behaviour Research and Therapy, 41,* 1469–1480.

Joiner, T. E., Van Orden, K. A., Witte, T. K., Selby, E. A., Ribeiro, J. D., Lewis, R., . . . Rudd, M. D. (2009). Main predictors of the interpersonal-psychological theory of suicidal behavior: Empirical tests in two samples of young adults. *Journal of Abnormal Psychology, 188,* 634–646.

Kleepsies, P. M., & Dettmer, E. L. (2000). An evidence-based approach to evaluating and managing suicidal emergencies. *Journal of Clinical Psychology, 56,* 1109–1130.

Kuyken W., Padesky, C. A., & Dudley, R. (2009). *Collaborative case conceptualization: Working effectively with clients in cognitive-behavioral therapy.* New York: Guilford Press.

Linehan, M. M., Comtois, K. A., Murray, A. M., Brown, M. Z., Gallop, R. J., Hedard, H. L., . . . Lindenboim, N. (2006). Two-year randomized controlled trial and follow-up of dialectical behavior therapy vs. therapy by experts for suicidal behavior and borderline personality disorder. *Archives of General Psychiatry, 63,* 757–766.

Miranda, R., Valderrama, J., Tsypes, A., Gadol, E., & Gallagher, M. (2013). Cognitive inflexibility and suicidal ideation: Mediating role of brooding and hopelessness. *Psychiatry Research, 210,* 174–181.

Monti, K. M., Cedereke, M., & Ojehagen, A. (2003). Treatment attendance and suicidal behavior 1 month and 3 months after a suicide attempt: A comparison between two samples. *Archives of Suicide Research, 7,* 167–174.

Motto, J. A., & Bostrom, A. G. (2001). A randomized controlled trial of post-crisis suicide intervention. *Psychiatric Services, 52,* 828–833.

Newman, C. F. (2015). Cognitive restructuring/cognitive therapy. In A. M. Nezu & C. M. Nezu (Eds.), *Oxford handbook of cognitive and behavioral therapies* (pp. 118–141). New York: Oxford University Press.

Nezu, A. M., Nezu, C. M., & D'Zurilla, T. (2013). *Problem-solving therapy: A treatment manual.* New York: Springer.

Peak, N. J., Overholser, J. C., Ridley, J., Braden, A., Fisher, L., Bixler, J., & Chandler, M. (2015). Too much to bear: Psychometric evidence supporting the Perceived Burdensomeness Scale. *Psychiatry Research, 228,* 554–550.

Posner, K., Brown, G. K., Stanley, B., Brent, D. A., Yershova, K. V., Oquendo, M. A., . . . Mann, J. J. (2011). The Columbia-Suicide Severity Rating Scale: Initial validity and internal consistency findings from three multisite studies with adolescents and adults. *American Journal of Psychiatry, 168,* 1266–1277.

Ramsay, J. R., & Newman, C. F. (2005). After the attempt: Repairing the therapeutic alliance following a serious suicide attempt by a patient. *Suicide and Life-Threatening Behavior, 35,* 413–424.

Rudd, M. D., Bryan, C. J., Wertenberger, E. G., Peterson, A. L., Young-McCaughan, S., Mintz, J., . . . Bruce, T. O. (2015). Brief cognitive-behavioral therapy effects on post-treatment suicide attempts in a military sample: Results of a randomized clinical trial with 2-year follow-up. *American Journal of Psychiatry, 172,* 441–449.

Rudd, M. D., Joiner, T. E., & Rajab, M. H. (2004). *Treating suicidal behavior: An effective, time-limited approach.* New York: Guilford Press.

Rudd, M. D., Mandrusiak, M., & Joiner, T. E. (2006). The case against no-suicide contracts: The commitment to treatment statement as a practice alternative. *Journal of Clinical Psychology, 62,* 243–251.

Simon, R. I. (2007). Gun safety management with patients at risk for suicide. *Suicide and Life Threatening Behavior, 37,* 518–526.

Smith, J. M., Alloy, L. B., & Abramson, L. Y. (2006). Cognitive vulnerability to depression, rumination, hopelessness, and suicidal ideation: Multiple pathways to self-injurious thinking. *Suicide and Life-Threatening Behavior, 36,* 443–454.

Stanford, E., Goetz, R., & Bloom, J. (1994). The no harm contract in the emergency assessment of suicidal risk. *Journal of Clinical Psychiatry, 55,* 344–348.

Stanley, B., & Brown, G. K. (2012). Safety planning intervention: A brief intervention to mitigate suicide risk. *Cognitive and Behavioral Practice, 19,* 256–264.

Weishaar, M. E. (1996). Cognitive risk factors in suicide. In P. M. Salkovskis (Ed.), *Frontiers of cognitive therapy* (pp. 226–249). New York: Guilford Press.

Wenzel, A., Brown, G. K., & Beck, A. T. (2009). *Cognitive therapy for suicidal clients: Scientific and clinical applications.* Washington, DC: American Psychological Association.

World Health Organization. (2013). Suicide prevention (SUPRE). Retrieved from *www.who.int/mental_health/prevention/suicide/suicideprevention.*

CHAPTER 15

Cognitive Therapy for Bipolar Disorder

Sheri L. Johnson
Andrew D. Peckham

DEFINING BIPOLAR DISORDER

Bipolar disorders are each defined by manic symptoms, and the various forms of bipolar disorders are differentiated from each other by the severity and duration of manic symptoms. The DSM-5 criteria for bipolar I disorder (BD I) specify the presence of at least one lifetime episode of mania. Mania, in turn, is defined by a period of at least one week (unless interrupted by hospitalization) of excessively expansive, euphoric, or irritable mood and of excessive activity accompanied by three or more of the following symptoms: overly high self-confidence or grandiosity, racing thoughts, distractibility, little need for sleep, pressured speech, increased goal-directed activity, and reckless behavior (American Psychiatric Association, 2013). Bipolar II disorder (BD II) is defined by at least one hypomania and at least one major depressive episode during the lifetime. Hypomanic episodes, in turn, are defined by a less intense period of mood elevation than mania; although symptom criteria are parallel, hypomanic episodes do not reach the duration or impairment of a full manic episode. Cyclothymic disorder is defined by chronic fluctuations between high and low moods that are not severe enough to qualify as episodes, yet persist for two years (or one year among children and adolescents). Most treatment literature focuses on BD I.

Major depressive episodes are not required for diagnosis of BD I, and 20–30% of people with a lifetime episode of mania will report no history of major depressive episodes (Judd et al., 2002; Kupka et al., 2007). Even for those who do experience depression, symptoms of depression and mania appear to fluctuate independently over time (Johnson, Morriss, et al., 2011) and are predicted by different risk factors (Cuellar, Johnson, & Winters, 2005). All in all, depression and mania do not appear to function as opposite ends of the same dimension,

In planning treatment, therapists are faced with the complexity of this disorder. Clients are more likely to seek treatment for depression than for mania, and depression is related to increased risk of suicidality. Recent evidence from a representative sample suggests that BD I is the psychiatric disorder with the highest rates of completed suicide (Nordentoft, Mortensen, & Pedersen, 2011), with rates of completed suicide that are twenty to thirty times those observed in the general population (Pompili et al., 2013; Schaffer et al., 2015). Family members, though, will often be at least as deeply concerned by manic episodes. Each episode of mania can damage occupational stability, interpersonal relationships, and financial resources. Perhaps because of these consequences of serious episodes for functioning, consumers report that restoring quality of life is more important than symptom reduction as a therapeutic goal (Michalak et al., 2012). Although many will struggle with functional outcome, the incredible heterogeneity of BD I deserves mention, as a growing body of work highlights the fact that milder forms of BD may be related to high levels of creative accomplishment in artistic and scientific domains (Johnson, Murray, et al., 2012). It is also important to note that comorbidity is extremely common and may influence treatment needs. Anxiety disorders are as common as are depression for those with BD I. Among those diagnosed with BD I, rates of lifetime comorbid anxiety disorders are about 75%, and rates of lifetime comorbid alcohol/substance use disorders are estimated to be about 40% (Merikangas et al., 2007).

With regard to treatment, all major national guidelines emphasize the importance of mood-stabilizing medications, such as lithium, anticonvulsant medication, or antipsychotic medications, for BD I. Recommendations are not as firm regarding medication for BD II, and in one novel treatment trial, psychotherapy achieved comparable outcomes to medication for BD II (Swartz, Frank, & Cheng, 2012).

Given that the median time to relapse even on mood-stabilizing medication is one year for those with BD I disorder (Keller, Lavori, Coryell, Endicott, & Mueller, 1993), major treatment guidelines recommend psychotherapy as an adjunct to medication treatment for BD I. The British NICE (National Institute for Health and Clinical Excellence) treatment guidelines recommend providing structured psychotherapy in addition to medication if moderate or severe depression is present, if depressive symptoms persist after medications are started, or if medications are not effective; family therapy is also recommended if the client is in close contact with family members (NICE, 2014).

THE COGNITIVE MODEL OF BD

Cognitive models of BD are rooted in Beck's theory that patterns of thinking about the self, personal world, and the future confer vulnerability for emotional disorders (Beck, 1976). Extended to BD, this theory predicts that depression is caused and maintained by negative attitudes, attributions, and biases favoring depression-congruent information; whereas mania is linked to overly optimistic and positive cognitive styles (Leahy & Beck, 1988). Although some models characterize manic cognition as the inverse of depressive cognition (e.g., overly positive instead of overly negative), elevated mood is only one of the cardinal symptoms of manic episodes and is not universally present during mania. Irritability and anger are also cardinal symptoms of mania, and one might not expect these to relate to overly positive cognition. Some models, then, focus on the idea that mania is related to excessive goal pursuit (Johnson, Edge, Holmes, & Carver, 2012). When goal pursuit goes well, elevated mood may occur; when goal pursuit is thwarted, frustration may be incurred (Wright, Lam, & Brown, 2008). More specifically, theory and evidence suggest that cognitions involving reward and heightened striving for ambitious goals are relevant to mania. During euthymic periods, models posit that cognitive vulnerabilities for both depression and mania are each present; these underlying vulnerabilities will be expressed after life events or mood shifts.

Although certain facets of cognition appear to be stably present even during remission, some cognitive processes, such as confidence and heightened self-esteem, appear tethered to mood state (Johnson, Edge et al., 2012). Clinically, increased confidence in one's own ideas and capabilities are a widely observed feature during mania and hypomania. The compelling nature of these shifts is perhaps best captured by Kay Jamison, who wrote: "When you're high it's tremendous. The ideas and feelings are fast and frequent like shooting stars, and you follow them until you find better and brighter ones. Shyness goes, the right words and gestures are suddenly there, the power to captivate others a felt certainty. There are interests found in uninteresting people. Sensuality is pervasive and the desire to seduce and be seduced irresistible. Feelings of ease, intensity, power, well-being, financial omnipotence, and euphoria pervade one's marrow" (Jamison, 1995, pp. 67–68). As confidence increases, risk-taking may occur (Leahy, 1999).

There are several challenges to empirically testing links of cognition with BD I. Given that the aftermath of episodes can be devastating for self-confidence, one might expect that many people with BD will struggle with negative cognitions about themselves and their future. The key question for this model is whether those types of thoughts then predict changes in mood symptoms over time. Only longitudinal designs can test this question. Beyond this, the considerable heterogeneity in symptoms associated with BD I should relate to cognitive profiles. For example, one might expect to see maladaptive negative cognition only among those people with a history of depressive episodes. Among those with comorbid anxiety disorders, anxiety-relevant cognition such as vigilance for threat and beliefs about personal safety may be important to consider.

Notwithstanding the complexities of theory and research design, considerable research is available on cognitive profiles in BD I. Researchers in this area have most commonly used measures of negative cognitive styles such as the Dysfunctional Attitudes Scale (DAS, Weissman & Beck, 1978), which assesses rigid negative thinking about dependency on others, self-control, and achievement, or the Attributional Style Questionnaire (ASQ; Peterson et al., 1982), which assesses negative attributional style (the tendency to attribute negative events as having global, stable, and internal qualities. Some researchers have also considered whether BD I relates to increased attention to negative stimuli or reduced attention to positive stimuli.

In general, this body of findings indicates that the cognitive profile of bipolar depression is highly similar to that of unipolar depression (for review, see Cuellar et al., 2005). That is, during periods of bipolar depression, people show dysfunctional assumptions and beliefs (Hollon, Kendall, & Lumry, 1986; Jabben et al., 2012; Reilly-Harrington et al., 2010; Scott & Pope, 2003), a negative attributional style (Lyon, Startup, & Bentall, 1999; Reilly-Harrington et al., 1999), and reduced attention to positive stimuli (Garcia-Blanco et al., 2014; Jabben et al., 2012) compared to healthy control participants. Moreover, the extent of negative cognition and related processes, like rumination, appears to be related to the severity of depressive symptoms within BD (Johnson & Fingerhut, 2004; Reilly-Harrington et al., 2010; Van der Gucht et al., 2009).

Not unlike findings in the unipolar depression literature (cf. Just, Abramson, & Alloy, 2001), it is less clear whether these negative cognitive styles can still be observed after bipolar depressive symptoms remit. On the one hand, people who are either manic (Goldberg et al., 2008) or hypomanic (Lex, Hautzinger, & Meyer, 2011) have been found to obtain higher DAS total scores than healthy controls. Nonetheless, evidence for the presence of negative cognitive style in remission is mixed (e.g., Lex et al., 2008; Scott et al., 2000; Tracy et al., 1992; Wright, Lam, & Newsom-Davis, 2005), though one might expect this variability, given that many people with BD will never experience a full-blown depressive episode.

In longitudinal research, there is evidence that negative cognitions in BD also help to predict increases in depression over time (Johnson &

Fingerhut, 2004) and that negative attributional style in response to stress as measured by the ASQ interacts with negative life events to predict increases in depression (Alloy et al., 1999). Thus, rigid and negative cognition are consistent predictors of depression in BD.

In contrast to depression, the evidence that mania is related to overly positive cognitive styles has been mixed. Not all facets of cognition appear to be overly positive. For example, research does not indicate that people with BD tend to pay greater attention to positive stimuli during remission (Peckham, Johnson, & Gotlib, 2016) or during mania (Garcia-Blanco et al., 2014) as compared to controls.

In contrast to globally positive cognition, goal striving may be a distinctive aspect of mania-relevant cognitive style (cf. Johnson, Edge, et al., 2012). This is supported by a modified factor structure for the DAS-24 items in a BD I sample, which consists of subscales of goal attainment (extreme and rigid attitudes about attaining high goals), interpersonal dependency, and achievement (beliefs about perfectionism and success) (Lam, Wright, & Smith, 2004). Dysfunctional beliefs about goal attainment differentiated remitted BD I from those with remitted unipolar depression, and goal attainment factor scores correlated significantly with the frequency of hospitalizations for mania (Lam et al., 2004). In another sample, people with BD I, but not BD II, endorsed significantly greater maladaptive beliefs on the goal attainment subscale than did control participants (Fletcher, Parker, & Manicavasagar, 2013). DAS goal attainment beliefs have also been found to correlate with a greater willingness to increase activity in response to hypothetical scenarios (Lee, Lam, Mansell, & Farmer, 2010). Across several studies, people with BD have been found to be more willing than those without the disorder to endorse a willingness to pursue highly ambitious goals (Johnson, Carver, & Gotlib, 2012; see Johnson, Edge, et al., 2012, for a review). Taken together, these findings indicate that people with BD may hold strong beliefs about goal attainment.

More importantly, dysfunctional beliefs about goal attainment may predict manic outcomes. Endorsement of extremely ambitious goals predicted increases in manic symptoms over time (Johnson, Edge, et al., 2012) and onset of bipolar spectrum disorder (Alloy, 2012). One potential mechanism could involve tendencies for those who are highly invested in goal pursuit to overvalue hypomanic qualities such as heightened productivity and energy. In two studies, the DAS-goal attainment factor strongly related to the Sense of Hyper-Positive Self Scale (SHPSS), a measure that captures the degree to which individuals identify with and aspire to have a high-arousal positive mood state (Lam et al., 2005; Lee et al., 2010). In turn, higher SHPSS scores predicted faster relapse during cognitive-behavioral treatment (CBT; Lam et al., 2005). In other studies, cognitive styles relevant to high goal striving have predicted mania symptoms. For example, the Achievement Striving subscale of the NEO Conscientiousness Scale predicted increases in manic symptoms among people with BD I (Lozano & Johnson, 2001). Also, people with BD have been found to endorse higher levels of Autonomy on the Sociotropy-Autonomy Scale (SAS; Beck, Epstein, Harrison, & Emery, 1983), which includes content relevant to goal striving; high scores on the Autonomy scale predicted a greater chance of manic episodes over time (Alloy et al., 2009). On the whole, findings indicate that goal attainment beliefs are important cognitive variables to consider in treatment.

Beyond goal striving, BD has been tied to dynamic shifts in self-confidence after a success or increase in positive mood, or relatedly, to risk-taking. On the self-rated Cognitive Checklist for Mania-Revised (Beck, Colis, Steer, Modrak, & Goldberg, 2006), subscales relevant to goal engagement, confidence, and self-worth in relationships were found to be more elevated among people with a current manic episode compared to people with mixed or depressive episodes (Beck et al., 2006), although in another study, items relevant to excitement and risk-taking (but not confidence specifically) were related to current manic symptoms (Fulford, Tuchman, & Johnson, 2009). Two of the widely used self-report mania cognition measures, the Hypomania Interpretations Questionnaire (HIQ; Jones, Mansell, & Waller, 2006) and the Hypomanic Attitudes and Positive Predictions Inventory (HAPPI; Mansell, 2006), capture confidence in response to hypomania and high mood (e.g., "If I was feeling 'sped up' inside, I would probably think it was because I am in good spirits and can take on challenges."). Elevations on both of these measures have been documented in BD (Jones et al., 2006; Dodd, Mansell, Morrison, & Tai, 2011). Overconfidence may be apparent even during subtly positive mood states. In one laboratory study, euthymic individuals with BD I were significantly less likely to follow advice after a positive mood induction (Mansell & Lam, 2006). In another study, positive mood in remitted BD was associated with ranking oneself as more superior to others (Gilbert, McEwan, Hay, Irons, & Cheung, 2007). Thus, at least in some studies, those with BD appear to experience increases in confidence and risk-taking during manic and hypomanic states, as well as positive mood states.

Beyond the focus on goal attainment and confidence, several extensions of cognitive models of BD have received support. First, Holmes and her group have conducted considerable research to document that imagery may be more powerful than semantic content in eliciting emotion states (Holmes & Mathews, 2010). Their work suggests that people with a broad range of mood and anxiety disorders endorse experiencing more imagery than others do (Holmes & Mathews, 2010). For those with BD, Holmes and colleagues propose that intense mental imagery may interact with interpretations of internal and external triggers to exacerbate symptoms (Holmes, Geddes, Colom, & Goodwin, 2008). They have shown that those with BD report experiencing more frequent and intense mental imagery, and that mental imagery is correlated with mood instability and suicidal thinking (Hales, Deeprose, Goodwin, & Holmes, 2011; Ng, Di Simplicio, & Holmes, 2016). This highlights the need to consider imagery in asking patients about their cognitive styles.

Others have emphasized cognitive interpretations of internal states as an important contributor to symptom expression. In one such model, Jones and colleagues proposed that cognitive responses to physiological symptoms might amplify symptoms of hypomania (Jones, 2001). In support of this idea, people at risk for and those diagnosed with BD were more likely than others to positively interpret small increases in energy and mood—for example, interpreting increases in restlessness as a sign of having enough energy to take on big challenges (Johnson & Jones, 2009; Jones et al., 2006; Jones & Day, 2008).

Mansell emphasizes that people with BD may hold both extremely positive and catastrophically negative interpretations of internal states and that such beliefs can spur maladaptive attempts to cope with these states by increasing or decreasing activation levels (Mansell, Morrison, Reid, Lowens, & Tai, 2007). The HAPPI was developed to assess these extreme beliefs about internal states (Mansell, 2006). Several studies have found that overall HAPPI scores and their subscales are significantly higher in those with BD compared to healthy controls (e.g., Mansell, 2006), and another found that the HAPPI subscale specifically related to interpreting internal states as uncontrollable predicted increases in depression (Dodd, Mansell, Morrison, & Tai, 2011). Questions remain, though, about the extent to which uncontrollability on the HAPPI reflects genuine difficulties regulating mood and symptoms, versus an overly negative response to symptoms. A trial of CBT based on this model is underway (Mansell et al., 2014), with a goal of helping people become more aware of their responses to symptoms and develop alternative strategies. Findings from this type of specific intervention will provide a strong test of the model.

In sum, findings support a cognitive model of BD. That is, during depressive episodes, people with BD I endorse negative cognitive styles, and when present after remission, these negative cognitive styles predict the course of bipolar depression. This provides an evidence base for addressing negative cognition as a way to reduce depression risk. Original cognitive theory suggested that mania might be tied to overly positive cognition. Over the past two decades, research has suggested that mania might be tied to a narrower band of cognitions related to stable goal striving and fluctuating confidence. In considering the nature of cognition, research suggests that clinicians would do well to consider imagery as well as semantic facets of cognition, and to carefully consider cognitive responses to symptomatic states.

CLINICAL APPLICATION

A diversity of cognitive techniques have been developed and described for addressing BD, leading to publication of a series of CBT manuals (Basco & Rush, 2005; Lam, Jones, & Hayward, 2010; Newman, Leahy, Beck, Reilly-Harrington, & Gyulai, 2002). CBT manuals universally provide suggestions for psychoeducation and for addressing both depression and mania. Many self-help books are now also available to support implementation of these strategies by the client (e.g., Basco, 2015; Caponigro, Lee, Johnson, & Kring, 2012; Jones, Hayward, & Lam, 2009; Otto et al., 2008). Although these techniques are frequently offered individually, they can be offered within a group context as well (e.g., Patelis-Siotis et al., 2001). Here we focus on four general clinical goals: providing psychoeducation, helping the client develop skills for early recognition of incipient symptoms, addressing overly negative cognitive styles relevant to depression, and preventing manic symptoms and their aftermath.

Psychoeducation

Most manuals suggest that treatment should begin with psychoeducation regarding the disorder. Information is generally provided about the biological basis of the disorder, the high rates of recurrence, and the medications used to treat BD. Many treatment manuals address medication adherence from a CBT framework, including addressing maladaptive beliefs and assumptions about medication, and integrating behavioral approaches to support adherence. Most interventions raise the topic of stigma, in hopes of fostering more positive attitudes about the illness. Good psychoeducation helps set the tone of optimism and helps clients understand that learning new techniques for identifying and reducing cognitive and behavioral triggers can reduce the risk of relapse.

Early Recognition of Symptoms

As one facet of psychoeducation, people with BD are taught to reliably identify prodromal signs of mood episodes. Building awareness and skills for recognizing prodromal signs of depression and mania provides a foundation for implementing early intervention and management (Lam, Wong, & Sham, 2001). By noting symptoms before they become pronounced, there is a greater chance that the person will be able to detect changes early enough to enact intervention strategies. Because manic symptoms can be ego-syntonic, fostering an awareness of early signs of mania can be more elaborate than what might be implemented for depression. Several strategies can help promote better symptom awareness, including charting previous symptoms and prospectively monitoring for symptoms over time.

To chart previous symptoms, the most commonly used technique is the Life Chart, which was initially developed by the National Institute of Mental Health (NIMH; Roy-Byrne, Post, Uhde, Poreu, & Davis, 1985). Web-based life-charting programs have been developed. Clinicians may choose to vary the detail of life charts by limiting the time period covered. Life charts provide a way for the clinician and the patient to graph manic and depressive episodes over the life course, the treatments that have (or have not) helped, and triggers that preceded episodes. These triggers may include sleep disruptions, medication changes, substance use, or life events. Considerable literature suggests that major negative life events can trigger depressive symptoms, whereas major goal attainments can trigger increases in manic symptoms (Johnson, Edge, et al., 2012). Identifying triggers may restore some sense of control and predictability, which is all too frequently missing for clients as they struggle with the major mood fluctuations.

For each episode, it is helpful to carefully outline the types of symptoms and behavioral changes that were present. Denoting the earliest changes is one way to emphasize early prodromes and warning signs. Changes in cognition can also be considered by asking individuals how their sense of self-esteem and their abilities may have shifted. Overconfident assertions like "I was invincible and could conquer anything" may be more recognizable as maladaptive when considered during a period of wellness.

Life charts can also help counteract tendencies toward "all or nothing" thinking and the catastrophic interpretation of minor manic symptoms that Mansell has described (Mansell et al., 2007). Although serious mood episodes can incur high costs, clients who develop one or two manic symptoms sometimes experience terror about relapse that overwhelms coping efforts. By plotting the severity of episodes, clients can more clearly see that episodes vary in their severity and that some episodes have been contained without the same degree of aftermath.

A final, albeit delicate, step in constructing a life chart is to consider the consequences that have emerged from various episodes. Clinicians can inquire about the changes in relationships, jobs, finances, and lifestyle that emerged as a consequence of different episodes. Many clients want the chance to grieve for these losses. For others, reviewing the losses consequent to episodes powerfully enhances motivation to learn skills to prevent relapse. The clinician who deeply understands the losses that have occurred is in a stronger position to help a person reengage in treatment strategies when the siren call of hypomania begins to emerge. When reviewing the consequences of mania, though, it is important to be sensitive to the degree of grief, shame, and distress that clients may feel and to provide encouragement that the goal of treatment is to reduce these consequences in the future.

Beyond charting history, a core goal is for a person to begin to implement a program for early detection of manic symptoms on an ongoing basis. The most common approach to this is to help the person learn self-monitoring skills. Because manic symptoms can be so ego-congruent, one consumer described having the sense that manic symptoms were like "a big black dirt mark on my forehead that I was the last to see." Overt training to detect these symptoms is a standard part of many psychological approaches. Tools involve reviewing diagnostic criteria symptoms to help clients put key symptoms into their own words, reviewing signals that family members tend to monitor, or drawing notes from a life chart. Regardless of the source, these symptoms can be turned into a personalized list of potential warning signs to monitor. Items should be phrased as objectively as possible—it is easier to monitor for "less than six hours of sleep" than for "less need for sleep." Having a list of symptoms provides another reminder that mania varies in severity, and so it provides another window into challenging "all or nothing" catastrophic thinking about mania.

As the self-monitoring list is developed, it is important for clients to test how well the form works. We ask participants to complete the list two to four times initially, to consider whether (1) the thresholds for concern are so well defined that they can be easily judged, (2) high scores are specific to emergent manic symptoms, and (3) the form appears sensitive to incipient symptoms. As the list develops, it is helpful to review it with family members or partners, who can provide advice about missing items, thresholds, and strategies. Doing so often helps others appreciate that the person with bipolar disorder is taking on a new level of responsibility for managing his or her symptoms. For all, it is helpful to remember that one symptom alone is not likely to mean that a relapse is impending, as this knowledge can reduce anxiety that patients and family members experience around small mood shifts. With practice, patients learn to internalize the checklist, so that completing a paper-and-pencil copy each day is not needed.

Not all clients are comfortable completing self-monitoring exercises. For many, the focus on symptoms elicits powerful negative emotions. This provides an opportunity to consider the types of cognitions they hold about their illness and to consider using cognitive techniques to challenge these thoughts. Internalized stigma about the illness is extremely common (Perlick et al., 2001; Michalak, 2011), and clinicians can be helpful in coaching a patient toward a more compassionate stance about this illness. For some clients, negative thoughts such as "I'll never be able to control these symptoms" emerge, and again, provide an important target for cognitive techniques. These types of cognitive interventions may need to be instituted before a client can effectively learn to self-monitor for symptoms. That is, self-monitoring should be considered as a supportive tool for learning how to respond to emergent symptoms.

Negative Cognitive Styles

Given the overlap between unipolar and bipolar depression, most manuals provide techniques for challenging overly negative cognition. These include techniques such as identifying automatic thoughts (e.g., negative thoughts that the client may not be aware of but can be accessed by focusing attention on thoughts); questioning negative assumptions (for example, helping clients to elucidate mental "rules" or other beliefs that support automatic thoughts, such as "A person who can't control their emotions is a failure"), and then, cognitive restructuring (helping clients to generate rational alternative thoughts in response to the original negative thought).

Just as with unipolar depression, CBT for bipolar depression often involves scheduling pleasant and rewarding activities so as to break the cycle of withdrawal and lack of reward that can intensify depression. A caveat is that it is important for individuals with BD to avoid overscheduling. With the considerable evidence that disruptions in schedule and sleep can provoke episodes of mania, clients should be coached to implement small, regular changes in their daily activities rather than take on massive endeavors that could interfere with sleep and calm (Lam et al., 2010).

Preventing Manic Episodes and Their Aftermath

Some of the features of mania may make cognitive techniques particularly difficult to apply during that state. As examples, prototypical signs of mania include high confidence and surges of energy. The hypomanic state is often intrinsically satisfying, and the client's insight and concern may dissipate as manic symptoms intensify (Johnson & Fulford, 2008). Clients may also resist attempts to dampen high levels of confidence as they become hypomanic. Given these difficulties, many manuals focus on early recognition and detection, as discussed earlier, so that techniques can be applied before mania becomes severe.

Nonetheless, if clients recognize these early warning signs, it is important for them to have skills for responding. Calling a doctor for a potential medication adjustment is one important response to symptoms, but there is evidence that psychological approaches can supplement pharmacological approaches. Dominic Lam and his colleagues asked persons with BD to identify the strategies they had used to cope with prodromal manic symptoms. Many people described strategies of reducing stimulation and activity, and protecting their sleep. People who endorsed using more strategies to reduce stimulation when they observed prodromal symptoms were less likely to develop mania over time (Lam, Wong, & Sham, 2001). Therapists and clients can collaborate to develop and test strategies for reducing stimulation and promoting calm.

Beyond strategies designed to limit the upward spiral of mania, another core set of skills involves protecting relationships, finances, and workplace function from damage if manic symptoms do develop. As examples, people may want to avoid highly public roles, like giving speeches, on days when they feel their mania is starting to be evident. Dating and meeting new people might be avoided. Many people have ways to limit their spending, such as giving their credit cards and checkbook to a trusted other. Important business decisions can be postponed. Some people designate a trusted friend or family member to be a sounding board for decisions that would involve major resources. Newman and colleagues (2002) suggest the "two-person feedback rule" in which "any patient idea or plan that the therapist cannot safely endorse will be shelved until at least two other people are consulted on the matter" (p. 57). Similarly, they also describe a "48 hours" rule, in which clients are encouraged to wait full two days before acting on any large or risky decisions. During well periods, with a life chart in hand, clients often have a clear sense of the life problems they want to avoid, and a collaborative focus on problem solving in these areas during a well period can be highly beneficial.

Although implementing this type of problem solving can reduce losses consequent to mania, many clients still engage in actions when they are manic that trigger a deep sense of shame in retrospect. People often lose confidence, and internalized stigma about BD is all too common. Overly harsh judgments about actions during manic states are perfectly suited for CBT techniques.

Summary of Clinical Applications

CBT offers a wealth of techniques for the treatment of BD. The chief goals include helping a client understand the disorder and its treatment, promoting an increased awareness of the behaviors and cognitions that might indicate mania, using behavioral activation and cognitive restructuring to reduce depressive symptoms, implementing strategies for reducing incipient manic symptoms through pharmacological and lifestyle adjustments, working with clients to protect their lifestyle in the face of manic symptoms, and reducing shame and self-stigma about the disorder.

RESEARCH ON CBT

Over the past twenty years, a series of randomized controlled trials (RCTs) have been conducted to examine the efficacy of CBT as an adjunct to medication for BD. Early studies indicated that patients found CBT to be helpful (Palmer et al., 2006) and that six weeks of CBT was related to better lithium adherence and lower hospitalization rates compared to medication treatment alone (Cochran & Gitlin, 1988).

In one of the first large-scale RCTs of BD therapy, individual CBT was compared to pharmacological care alone (Lam et al., 2003). Patients in the CBT condition were offered twelve to eighteen sessions of therapy within the first six months and two booster sessions in the second six months of care. CBT included psychoeducation, cognitive interventions, and a focus on regulating levels of activity. Those who received CBT had lower relapse rates (44% versus 75%), fewer days in episode, higher social functioning, and less depression and mania during the first year of follow-up than did the clients in the control group. At the two-year follow-up, significant advantages were seen for CBT in reducing depressive symptoms, but the reductions in manic symptoms as compared to the control condition were not maintained (Lam et al., 2005), suggesting that more intensive maintenance treatment might be warranted.

In a small trial (N = 42) of a broader CBT approach that included cognitive intervention, activity regulation, and sleep intervention (Scott, Garland, & Moorhead, 2001), clients were randomly assigned to CBT or to a six-month wait list condition followed by CBT, and assessments were conducted at six-month and eighteen-month follow-ups. CBT was related to significant improvements in global functioning, depressive symptoms, and depressive relapse rates, but manic symptoms were not reduced significantly compared to the wait list control. Taken together, these early studies indicated that current CBT treatments may be more powerful for depression than mania intervention.

Other researchers have compared CBT to active treatments, such as psychoeducation or supportive therapy, as adjuncts to medication treatment. In one, CBT was related to greater decreases in depressive symptoms as compared to those who received six sessions of group psychoeducation (Zaretsky, Lancee, Miller, Harris, & Parikh, 2008). This effect was not observed in a larger study of 204 clients in which CBT did not differ from group psychoeducation in relapse or symptom severity across an eighteen-month follow-up (Parikh et al., 2012). At an economic level, group psychoeducation (estimated to cost $180 per patient) was significantly more affordable than intensive CBT (estimated to cost $1,200 per patient). Similarly, in a study of seventy-six patients randomly assigned to CBT versus psychoeducation, mood monitoring, and supportive therapy, groups did not differ in relapse rates (Meyer & Hautzinger, 2012). These findings suggest that CBT and other active treatment approaches may achieve comparable results.

Other research has been conducted to examine efficacy, or the generalizability of findings to the general community. In a multicenter trial involving 253 patients across five sites, clients who varied in their episode status were randomly assigned to receive twenty-two sessions of CBT as an adjunct to medication or to receive medication alone (Scott et al., 2006). Overall, those who received CBT did not differ in relapse rates or symptom severity levels during follow-up compared to those who assigned to medication alone. More promising efficacy findings were obtained in the STEP-BD study, which assessed the treatment outcome of 293 persons who were experiencing bipolar depression. Clients were randomly assigned to receive family-focused therapy, interpersonal psychotherapy, CBT, or a control condition of collaborative care as adjuncts to medication management (Miklowitz et al., 2007). Perhaps because this trial focused on depressed patients, patients who received CBT demonstrated more reduction in depressive symptoms than did those assigned to receive collaborative care, supporting the usefulness of CBT for bipolar depression. As with the comparisons against active treatments discussed earlier, outcomes were comparably positive for CBT versus family-focused and interpersonal psychotherapies.

In sum, findings for CBT have not been uniform. Several studies, though, suggest that CBT can be helpful, particularly in the management of bipolar depressive symptoms. Questions remain about whether CBT is beneficial compared to other active forms of treatment. Efficacy in the general community has been supported only when treatment was focused on bipolar depression.

CONCLUSIONS

BD, with its extreme variation in mood, is an ideal focus for the study of cognitions and mood. With over two decades of cognitive research and treatment in BD, a good deal has been learned. Theory and research highlight that bipolar and unipolar depression share remarkable overlap in a profile of overly negative cognitive styles. Accordingly, there is considerable evidence that cognitive-behavioral techniques that have been so well developed for addressing unipolar depression can be applied within BD. Although mania may not involve all facets of thought becoming overly positive, there is evidence that heightened ambition can be observed between episodes and can predict the onset and course of disorder. People often become overly confident during manic episodes, which may intensify the excessive activity and poor judgment that are core manic symptoms.

Several manuals are available that provide tools for addressing cognition and behavior in BD. Clearly, CBT provides an advantage compared to medication alone. Nonetheless, using these techniques for mania prevention requires finesse and skill, and several treatment trials demonstrate that it can be difficult to use cognitive-behavioral techniques to address mania. Successes have been attained using behavioral calming skills as mania encroaches. Finally, mania can all too often have a destructive influence, and CBT can be extremely helpful in addressing the types of negative self-image that can result from these difficult episodes.

Several goals remain a priority for research. First, research could refine understanding of the types of cognition that predict changes in manic symptoms. Multiple features of cognition appear to be involved in manic symptoms, and there is a need for integrative, longitudinal research. Second, given that impairment in executive functioning is often observed in BD and can be observed across mood states (Martinez-Aran et al., 2004; Martino et al., 2008), there is a need for research that considers the effects of such deficits on CBT outcomes. More research is needed on how to tailor CBT approaches for those who do experience problems with neurocognitive functioning. General guidelines for conducting intervention studies focused on neurocognitive variables are now available (Burdick, Ketter, Goldberg, & Calabrese, 2015) and may be helpful for this aim.

Third, there is a need for ongoing research on what types of scaffolding can best help people implement good treatment as manic symptoms unfold. Structuring clinical care so that people with BD have rapid access to a well-trained nurse practitioner, who interfaces closely with the psychiatric team, can reduce relapse and hospitalizations (Bauer et al., 1997; Simon, Ludman Bauer, Unutzer, & Operskalski, 2006). A growing number of researchers are trying to identify automatic systems to detect mania, for example, using actigraphy to monitor increases in movement (Gershon, Ram, Johnson, Harvey, & Zeitzer, 2015; Gonzalez, Tamminga et al., 2014). Although not yet reliable, if such predictors could be identified, automated reminder systems could help. In the meanwhile, some of the best results have emerged from a trial in which people learned behavioral strategies for self-calming in the face of prodromal manic symptoms.

Fourth, most treatment research has focused on BD I. BD II is a natural target for treatment, given that we have such well-developed depression techniques, and depression is part of the diagnostic criteria for BD II. A self-help workbook that incorporates CBT strategies specifically for BD II is now available (Roberts, Sylvia, & Reilly-Harrington, 2014).

Fifth, treatment development should focus on the extremely high rates of comorbidity in BD. Those with BD are as likely to experience anxiety as they are depression, and some recent studies have found that attentional vigilance for threat-relevant images, a major aspect of anxiety-relevant cognition, is observed across all phases of BD (Garcia-Blanco et al., 2014). Early studies suggest that mindfulness-based cognitive-behavioral therapy (MBCBT) may be helpful in reducing comorbid anxiety in BD, even though evidence from a large randomized, controlled trial and other smaller trials indicated that this approach did not significantly reduce depressive or manic symptoms (Meadows et al., 2014; Perich, Manicavasagar, Mitchell, Ball, & Hadzi-Pavlovic, 2013; Williams, 2008). A treatment manual for MBCT in BD is available (Deckersbach, Holzel, Eisner, Lazar, & Nierenberg, 2014).

Notwithstanding the ongoing goals for research and treatment development, this is a period of rich innovation in the bipolar field. A number of clear findings have emerged regarding the role of cognition in BD, and a wealth of treatment techniques have been developed to address these concerns. At the same time, the field has reached a level of maturity, and new work is tackling how to identify the best candidates for CBT, how to refine treatment to provide rapid intervention when manic symptoms emerge, and how to address comorbid conditions.

ACKNOWLEDGMENTS

This work was completed while Andrew Peckham was a doctoral student at the University of California Berkeley

REFERENCES

Alloy, L. B., Abramson, L. Y., Walshaw, P. D., Gerstein, R. K., Keyser, J. D., Whitehouse, W. G., . . . Harmon-Jones, E. (2009). Behavioral approach system (BAS)-relevant cognitive styles and bipolar spectrum disorders: Concurrent and prospective associations. *Journal of Abnormal Psychology, 118,* 459–471.

Alloy, L. B., Bender, R. E., Whitehouse, W. G., Wagner, C. A., Liu, R. T., Grant, D. A., . . . Abramson, L. Y. (2012). High Behavioral Approach System (BAS) sensitivity, reward responsiveness, and goal-striving predict first onset of bipolar spectrum disorders: A prospective behavioral high-risk design. *Journal of Abnormal Psychology, 121,* 339–351.

Alloy, L. B., Reilly-Harrington, N., Fresco, D. M., Whitehouse, W. G., & Zechmeister, J. S. (1999). Cognitive styles and life events in subsyndromal unipolar and bipolar disorders: Stability and prospective prediction of depressive and hypomanic mood swings. *Journal of Cognitive Psychotherapy, 13,* 21–40.

American Psychiatric Association. (2013). *Diagnostic and statistical manual of mental disorders* (5th ed.). Arlington, VA: Author.

Basco, M. R. (2015). *The bipolar workbook: Tools for controlling your symptoms* (2nd ed.). New York: Guilford Press.

Basco, M. R., & Rush, A. J. (2005). *Cognitive-behavioral therapy for bipolar disorder.* New York: Guilford Press.

Bauer, M., McBride, L., Shea, N., Gavin, C., Holden, F., & Kendall, S. (1997). Impact of an easy-access VA clinic-based program for patients with bipolar disorder. *Psychiatric Services, 48,* 491–496.

Beck, A. T. (1976). *Cognitive therapy and the emotional disorders.* New York: Penguin.

Beck, A. T., Colis, M. J., Steer, R. A., Madrak, L., & Goldberg, J. F. (2006). Cognition Checklist for Mania-Revised. *Psychiatry Research, 145,* 233–240.

Beck, A. T., Epstein, N., Harrison, R. P., & Emery, G. (1983). *Development of the*

Sociotropy-Autonomy Scale: A measure of personality factors in depression. Unpublished manuscript, University of Pennsylvania, Philadelphia, PA.

Burdick, K. E., Ketter, T. A., Goldberg, J. F., & Calabrese, J. R. (2015). Assessing cognitive function in bipolar disorder: Challenges and recommendations for clinical trial design. *Journal of Clinical Psychiatry, 76,* e342–e350.

Caponigro, J. M., Lee, E. H., Johnson, S. L., & Kring, A. M. (2012). *Bipolar disorder: A guide for the newly diagnosed.* Oakland, CA: New Harbinger.

Cochran, S. D., & Gitlin, M. J. (1988). Attitudinal correlates of lithium compliance in bipolar affective disorders. *Journal of Nervous and Mental Disease, 176,* 457–464.

Cuellar, A. K., Johnson, S. L., & Winters, R. (2005). Distinctions between bipolar and unipolar depression. *Clinical Psychology Review, 25,* 307–339.

Deckersbach, T., Holzel, B., Eisner, L., Lazar, S. W., & Nierenberg, A. A. (2014). *Mindfulness-based cognitive therapy for bipolar disorder.* New York: Guilford Press.

Dodd, A. L., Mansell, W., Morrison, A. P., & Tai, S. (2011). Extreme appraisals of internal states and bipolar symptoms: The Hypomanic Attitudes and Positive Predictions Inventory. *Psychological Assessment, 23,* 635–645.

Fletcher, K., Parker, G., & Manicavasagar, V. (2013). Cognitive style in bipolar disorder subtypes. *Psychiatry Research, 206,* 232–239.

Fulford, D., Tuchman, N., & Johnson, S. L. (2009). The Cognition Checklist for Mania-Revised (CCL-M-R): Factor-analytic structure and links with risk for mania, diagnoses of mania, and current symptoms. *International Journal Cognitive Therapy, 2,* 313.

Garcia-Blanco, A., Salmeron, L., Perea, M., & Livianos, L. (2014). Attentional biases toward emotional images in the different episodes of bipolar disorder: An eye-tracking study. *Psychiatry Research, 215,* 628–633.

Gershon, A., Ram, N., Johnson, S. L., Harvey, A. G., & Zeitzer, J. M. (2015). Daily actigraphy profiles distinguish depressive and interepisode states in bipolar disorder. *Clinical Psychological Science.* [Epub ahead of print]

Gilbert, P., McEwan, K., Hay, J., Irons, C., & Cheung, M. (2007). Social rank and attachment in people with a bipolar disorder. *Clinical Psychology and Psychotherapy, 14,* 48–53.

Goldberg, J. F., Gerstein, R. K., Wenze, S. J., Welker, T. M., & Beck, A. T. (2008). Dysfunctional attitudes and cognitive schemas in bipolar manic and unipolar depressed outpatients. *Journal of Nervous and Mental Disease, 196,* 207–210.

Gonzalez, R., Tamminga, C. A., Tohen, M., & Suppes, T. (2014). The relationship between affective state and the rhythmicity of activity in bipolar disorder. *Journal of Clinical Psychiatry, 75,* e317–e322.

Hales, S. A., Deeprose, C., Goodwin, G. M., & Holmes, E. A. (2011). Cognitions in bipolar affective disorder and unipolar depression: Imagining suicide. *Bipolar Disorders, 13,* 651–661.

Hollon, S. D., Kendall, P. C., & Lumry, A. (1986). Specificity of depressotypic cognitions in clinical depression. *Journal of Abnormal Psychology, 95,* 52–59.

Holmes, E. A., Geddes, J. R., Colom, F., & Goodwin, G. M. (2008). Mental imagery as an emotional amplifier: Application to bipolar disorder. *Behaviour Research and Therapy, 46,* 1251–1258.

Holmes, E. A., & Mathews, A. (2010). Mental imagery in emotion and emotional disorders. *Clinical Psychology Review, 30,* 349–362.

Jabben, N., Arts, B., Jongen, E. M. M., Smulders, F. T. Y., van Os, J., & Krabbendam, L. (2012). Cognitive processes and attitudes in bipolar disorder: A study into personality, dysfunctional attitudes and attention bias in patients with bipolar disorder and their relatives. *Journal of Affective Disorders, 143,* 265–268.

Jamison, K. R. (1995). *The unquiet mind: A memoir of moods and madness.* New York: Vintage Books.

Johnson, S. L., Carver, C. S., & Gotlib, I. H. (2012). Elevated ambitions for fame among persons diagnosed with bipolar I disorder. *Journal of Abnormal Psychology, 121,* 602–609.

Johnson, S. L., Edge, M. D., Holmes, M. K., & Carver, C. S. (2012). The behavioral activation system and mania. *Annual Review of Clinical Psychology, 8,* 243–267.

Johnson, S. L., & Fingerhut, R. (2004). Negative cognitions predict the course of dipolar depression, not mania. *Journal of Cognitive Psychotherapy, 18,* 149–162.

Johnson, S. L., & Fulford, D. (2008). Development of the treatment attitudes questionnaire in bipolar disorder. *Journal of Clinical Psychology, 64,* 466–481.

Johnson, S. L., & Jones, S. (2009). Cognitive correlates of mania risk: Are responses to success, positive moods, and manic symptoms distinct or overlapping? *Journal of Clinical Psychology, 65,* 891–905.

Johnson, S. L., Morriss, R., Scott, J., Paykel, E., Kinderman, P., Kolamunnage-Dona, R., . . . Bentall, R. P. (2011). Depressive and manic symptoms are not opposite poles in bipolar disorder. *Acta Psychiatrica Scandinavica, 123,* 206–210.

Johnson, S. L., Murray, G., Fredrickson, B., Youngstrom, E. A., Hinshaw, S., Bass, J. M., . . . Salloum, I. (2012). Creativity and bipolar disorder: Touched by fire or burning with questions? *Clinical Psychology Review, 32,* 1–12.

Jones, S. H. (2001). Circadian rhythms, multilevel models of emotion and bipolar disorder—An initial step towards integration? *Clinical Psychology Review, 21,* 1193–1209.

Jones, S., & Day, C. (2008). Self appraisal and behavioural activation in the prediction of hypomanic personality and depressive symptoms. *Personality and Individual Differences, 45,* 643–648.

Jones, S. H., Hayward, P., & Lam, D. H. (1999). *Coping with bipolar disorder: A CBT-informed guide to living with manic depression* (rev. ed.). London: Oneworld.

Jones, S., Hayward, P., & Lam, D. (2009). *Coping with bipolar disorder: A CBT-informed guide to living with manic depression.* Oxford, UK: Oneworld.

Jones, S., Mansell, W., & Waller, L. (2006). Appraisal of hypomania-relevant experiences: Development of a questionnaire to assess positive self-dispositional appraisals in bipolar and behavioural high risk samples. *Journal of Affective Disorders, 93,* 19–28.

Judd, L. L., Akiskal, H. S., Schettler, P. J., Endicott, J., Maser, J., Solomon, D. A., . . . Keller, M. B. (2002). The long-term natural history of the weekly symptomatic status of bipolar I disorder. *Archives of General Psychiatry, 59,* 530–537.

Just, N., Abramson, L. Y., & Alloy, L. B. (2001). Remitted depression studies as tests of the cognitive vulnerability hypotheses of depression onset: A critique and conceptual analysis. *Clinical Psychology Review, e21,* 63–83.

Keller, M. B., Lavori, P. W., Coryell, W., Endicott, J., & Mueller, T. I. (1993). Bipolar I: A five-year prospective follow-up. *Journal of Nervous and Mental Disease, 181,* 238–245.

Kupka, R. W., Altshuler, L. L., Nolen, W. A., Suppes, T., Luckenbaugh, D. A., Leverich, G. S., . . . Post, R. M. (2007). Three times more days depressed than manic or hypomanic in both bipolar I and bipolar II disorder. *Bipolar Disorders, 9,* 531–535.

Lam, D. H., Jones, S. H., & Hayward, P. (2010). *Cognitive therapy for bipolar disorder: A therapist's guide to concepts, methods and practice* (2nd ed.). Chichester, UK: Wiley.

Lam, D., Wong, G., & Sham, P. (2001). Prodromes, coping strategies and course of illness in bipolar affective disorder—a naturalistic study. *Psychological Medicine, 31,* 1397–1402.

Lam, D., Wright, K., & Sham, P. (2005). Sense of hyper-positive self and response to cognitive therapy in bipolar disorder. *Psychological Medicine, 35,* 69–77.

Lam, D., Wright, K., & Smith, N. (2004). Dysfunctional assumptions in bipolar disorder. *Journal of Affective Disorders, 79,* 193–199.

Leahy, R. L. (1999). Decision making and mania. *Journal of Cognitive Psychotherapy, 13,* 83–105.

Leahy, R. L. (2005). Cognitive therapy. In S. L. Johnson & R. L. Leahy (Eds.), *Psychological treatment of bipolar disorder* (pp. 139–161). New York: Guilford Press.

Leahy, R. L., & Beck, A. T. (1988). Cognitive therapy of depression and mania. In A. Georgotas & R. Cancro (Eds.), *Depression and mania* (pp. 517–537). New York: Elsevier.

Lee, R., Lam, D., Mansell, W., & Farmer, A. (2010). Sense of hyper-positive self, goal-attainment beliefs and coping strategies in bipolar I disorder. *Psychological Medicine, 40,* 967–975.

Lex, C., Hautzinger, M., & Meyer, T. D. (2011). Cognitive styles in hypomanic episodes of bipolar I disorder. *Bipolar Disorders, 13,* 355–364.

Lex, C., Meyer, T. D., Marquart, B., & Thau, K. (2008). No strong evidence for abnormal levels of dysfunctional attitudes, automatic thoughts, and emotional information-processing biases in remitted bipolar I affective disorder. *Psychology and Psychotherapy: Theory, Research, and Practice, 81,* 1–13.

Lozano, B. E., & Johnson, S. L. (2001). Can personality traits predict increases in manic and depressive symptoms? *Journal of Affective Disorders, 63,* 103–111.

Lyon, H. M., Startup, M., & Bentall, R. P. (1999). Social cognition and the manic defense: Attributions, selective attention, and self-schema in bipolar affective disorder. *Journal of Abnormal Psychology, 108,* 273–82.

Mansell, W. (2006). The Hypomanic Attitudes and Positive Predictions Inventory (HAPPI): A pilot study to select cognitions that are elevated in individuals with bipolar disorder compared to non-clinical controls. *Behavioural and Cognitive Psychotherapy, 34,* 467–476.

Mansell, W., & Lam, D. (2006). "I won't do what you tell me!": Elevated mood and the assessment of advice-taking in euthymic bipolar I disorder. *Behaviour Research and Therapy, 44,* 1787–1801.

Mansell, W., Morrison, A. P., Reid, G., Lowens, I., & Tai, S. (2007). The interpretation of, and responses to, changes in internal states: An integrative cognitive model of mood swings and bipolar disorders. *Behavioural and Cognitive Psychotherapy, 35,* 515–539.

Mansell, W., Tai, S., Clark, A., Akgonul, S., Dunn, G., Davies, L., . . . Morrison, A. P. (2014). A novel cognitive behaviour therapy for bipolar disorders (Think Effectively About Mood Swings or TEAMS): Study protocol for a randomized controlled trial. *Trials, 15,* 405.

Martínez-Arán, A., Vieta, E., Reinares, M., Colom, F., Torrent, C., Sánchez-Moreno, J., . . . Salamero, M. (2004). Cognitive function across manic or hypomanic, depressed, and euthymic states in bipolar disorder. *American Journal of Psychiatry, 161,* 262–270.

Martino, D. J., Strejilevich, S. A., Scápola, M., Igoa, A., Marengo, E., Ais, E. D., . . . Perinot, L. (2008). Heterogeneity in cognitive functioning among patients with bipolar disorder. *Journal of Affective Disorders, 109,* 149–156.

Meadows, G. N., Shawyer, F., Enticott, J. C., Graham, A. L., Judd, F., Martin, P. R., . . . Segal, Z. (2014). Mindfulness-based cognitive therapy for recurrent depression: A translational research study with 2-year follow-up. *Australian and New Zealand Journal of Psychiatry, 48,* 743–755.

Merikangas, K. R., Akiskal, H. S., Angst, J., Greenberg, P. E., Hirschfeld, R. M. A., Petukhova, M., . . . Kessler, R. C. (2007). Lifetime and 12-month prevalence of bipolar spectrum disorder in the National Comorbidity Survey Replication. *Archives of General Psychiatry, 64,* 543–552.

Meyer, T. D., & Hautzinger, M. (2012). Cognitive behaviour therapy and supportive therapy for bipolar disorders: Relapse rates for treatment period and 2-year follow-up. *Psychological Medicine, 42,* 1429–1439.

Michalak, E. E., Hole, R., Livingston, J. D., Murray, G., Parikh, S. V., Lapsley, S., . . . McBride, S. (2012). Improving care and wellness in bipolar disorder: Origins, evolution and future directions of a collaborative knowledge exchange network. *International Journal of Mental Health Systems, 6,* 16.

Michalak, E., Livingston, J. D., Hole, R., Suto, M., Hale, S., & Haddock, C. (2011). "It's something that I manage but it is not who I am": Reflections on internalized stigma in individuals with bipolar disorder. *Chronic Illness, 7,* 209–224.

Miklowitz, D. J., Otto, M. W., Frank, E., Reilly-Harrington, N. A., Wisniewski, S. R., Kogan, J. N., . . . Sachs, G. S. (2007). Psychosocial treatments for bipolar depression: A 1-year randomized trial from the systematic treatment enhancement program. *Archives of General Psychiatry, 64,* 419–427.

Murray, G., Leitan, N. D., Berk, M., Thomas, N., Michalak, E., Berk, L., . . . Kyrios, M. (2015). Online mindfulness-based intervention for late-stage bipolar disorder: Pilot evidence for feasibility and effectiveness. *Journal of Affective Disorders, 178,* 46–51.

Newman, C. F., Leahy, R. L., Beck, A. T., Reilly-Harrington, N. A., & Gyulai, L. (2002). *Bipolar disorder: A cognitive therapy approach.* Washington, DC: American Psychological Association.

Ng, R. M. K., Di Simplicio, M., & Holmes, E., (2016). Mental imagery and bipolar disorders: Introducing scope for psychological treatment development? *International Journal of Social Psychiatry, 62*(2), 110–113.

NICE. (2014). *Bipolar disorder: The assessment and management of bipolar disorder in adults, children and young people in primary and secondary care. NICE clinical guideline 185.* London: National Institute for Health and Clinical Excellence. Retrieved from *http://guidance.nice.org/uk/cg185.*

Nordentoft, M., Mortensen, P. B., & Pedersen, C. B. (2011). Absolute risk of suicide after first hospital contact in mental disorder. *Archives of General Psychiatry, 68,* 1058–1064.

Otto, M. W., Reilly-Harrington, N. A., Knauz, R. O., Henin, A., Kogan, J. N., & Sachs, G. S. (2008). *Managing bipolar disorder: A cognitive-behavioral approach* [Workbook]. Oxford, UK: Oxford University Press.

Palmer, S., Davidson, K., Tyrer, P., Gumley, A., Tata, P., Norrie, J., . . . Seivewright, H. (2006). The cost-effectiveness of cognitive behavior therapy for borderline personality disorder: Results from the BOSCOT trial. *Journal of Personality Disorders, 20,* 466–481.

Parikh, S. V., Zaretsky, A., Beaulieu, S., Yatham, L. N., Young, L. T., Patelis-Siotis, I., . . . Streiner, D. L. (2012). A randomized controlled trial of psychoeducation or cognitive-behavioral therapy in bipolar disorder: A Canadian network for mood and anxiety treatments (CANMAT) study. *Journal of Clinical Psychiatry, 73,* 803–810.

Patelis-Siotis, I., Young, L. T., Robb, J. C., Marriott, M., Bieling, P. J., Cox, L. C., & Joffe, R. T. (2001). Group cognitive behavioral therapy for bipolar disorder: A feasibility and effectiveness study. *Journal of Affective Disorders, 65,* 145–153.

Peckham, A. D., Johnson, S. L., & Gotlib, I. H. (2016). Attentional bias in euthymic bipolar I disorder. *Cognition and Emotion, 30,* 472–487.

Perich, T., Manicavasagar, V., Mitchell, P. B., Ball, J. R., & Hadzi-Pavlovic, D. (2013). A randomized controlled trial of mindfulness-based cognitive therapy for bipolar disorder. *Acta Psychiatrica Scandinavica, 127,* 333–343.

Perlick, D. A., Rosenheck, R. A., Clarkin, J. F., Sirey, J. A., Salahi, J., Struening, E. L., . . . Link, B. G. (2001). Stigma as a barrier to recovery: Adverse effects of perceived stigma on social adaptation of persons diagnosed with bipolar affective disorder. *Psychiatric Services, 52,* 1627–1632.

Peterson, C., Semmel, A., von Baeyer, C., Abramson, L. Y., Melatsky, G. I., & Seligman, M. E. P. (1982). The attributional style questionnaire. *Cognitive Therapy and Research, 6,* 287–300.

Pompili, M., Gonda, X., Serafini, G., Innamorati, M., Sher, L., Amore, M., . . . Girardi P. (2013). Epidemiology of suicide in bipolar disorders: A systematic review of the literature. *Bipolar Disorders, 15,* 457–490.

Reilly-Harrington, N. A., Alloy, L. B., Fresco, D. M., & Whitehouse, W. G. (1999). Cognitive styles and life events interact to predict bipolar and unipolar symptomatology. *Journal of Abnormal Psychology, 108,* 567–578.

Reilly-Harrington, N. A., Miklowitz, D. J., Otto, M. W., Frank, E., Wisniewski, S. R., & Sachs, G. S. (2010). Dysfunctional attitudes, attributional styles, and phase of illness in bipolar disorder. *Cognitive Therapy and Research, 34,* 24–34.

Roberts, S. M., Sylvia, L. G., & Reilly-Harrington, N. A. (2014). *The bipolar II disorder workbook: Managing recurring depression, hypomania, and anxiety*. Oakland, CA: New Harbinger.

Roy-Byrne, P., Post, R. M., Uhde, T. W., Porcu, T., & Davis, D. (1985). The longitudinal course of recurrent affective illness: Life chart data from research patients at the NIMH. *Acta Psychiatrica Scandinavica, 71*(s317), 1–34.

Schaffer, A., Isometsa, E. T., Tondo, L., Moreno, D. H., Turecki, G., Reis, C., . . . Yatham, L. N. (2015). International Society for Bipolar Disorders Task Force on Suicide: Meta-analyses and meta-regression of correlates of suicide attempts and suicide deaths in bipolar disorder. *Bipolar Disorders, 17,* 1–16.

Scott, J., Garland, A., & Moorhead, S. (2001). A pilot study of cognitive therapy in bipolar disorders. *Psychological Medicine, 31,* 459–467.

Scott, J., Paykel, E., Morriss, R., Bentall, R., Kinderman, P., Johnson, T., . . . Hayhurst, H. (2006). Cognitive-behavioural therapy for severe and recurrent bipolar disorders: Randomised controlled trial. *British Journal of Psychiatry, 188,* 313–320.

Scott, J., & Pope, M. (2003). Cognitive style in individuals with bipolar disorders. *Psychological Medicine, 33,* 1081–1088.

Scott, J., Stanton, B., Garland, A., & Ferrier, I. N. (2000). Cognitive vulnerability in patients with bipolar disorder. *Psychological Medicine, 30,* 467–472.

Simon, G. E., Ludman, E. J., Bauer, M. S., Unutzer, J., & Operskalski, B. (2006). Long-term effectiveness and cost of a systematic care program for bipolar disorder. *Archives of General Psychiatry, 63,* 500–508.

Stange, J. P., Sylvia, L. G., da Silva Magalhães, P. V., Miklowitz, D. J., Otto, M. W., Frank, E., . . . Deckersbach, T. (2013). Extreme attributions predict the course of bipolar depression. *Journal of Clinical Psychiatry, 74,* 249–255.

Swartz, H. A., Frank, E., & Cheng ,Y. (2012). A randomized pilot study of psychotherapy and quetiapine for the acute treatment of bipolar II depression. *Bipolar Disorders, 14,* 211–216.

Tracy, A., Bauwens, F., Martin, F., Pardoen, D., & Mendlewicz, J. (1992). Attributional style and depression: A controlled comparison of remitted unipolar and bipolar patients. *British Journal of Clinical Psychology, 31,* 83–84.

Vallarino, M., Henry, C., Etain, B., Gehue, L. J., Macneil, C., Scott, E. M., . . . Scott, J. (2015). An evidence map of psychosocial interventions for the earliest stages of bipolar disorder. *Lancet Psychiatry, 2,* 548–563.

Van der Gucht, E., Morriss, R., Lancaster, G., Kinderman, P., & Bentall, R. P. (2009). Psychological processes in bipolar affective disorder: Negative cognitive style and reward processing. *British Journal of Psychiatry, 194,* 146–151.

Weissman, A. N., & Beck, A. T. (1978). *Development and validation of the Dysfunctional Attitude Scale: A preliminary investigation.* Paper presented at the annual meeting of the America Educational Research Association, Toronto, Ontario, Canada.

Williams, C. H. (2008). Cognitive behaviour therapy within assertive outreach teams: Barriers to implementation: A qualitative peer audit. *Journal of Psychiatric and Mental Health Nursing, 15,* 850–856.

Wright, K. A., Lam, D., & Brown, R. G. (2008). Dysregulation of the behavioral activation system in remitted bipolar I disorder. *Journal of Abnormal Psychology, 117,* 838–848.

Wright, K., Lam, D., & Newsom-Davis, I. (2005). Induced mood change and dysfunctional attitudes in remitted bipolar I affective disorder. *Journal of Abnormal Psychology, 114,* 689–696.

Zaretsky, A., Lancee, W., Miller, C., Harris, A., & Parikh, S. V. (2008). Is cognitive-behavioural therapy more effective than psychoeducation in bipolar disorder? *Canadian Journal of Psychiatry, 53,* 441–448.

CHAPTER 16

Cognitive Therapy for Psychosis

Anthony P. Morrison
Elizabeth K. Murphy

Psychosis refers to a set of symptoms or experiences that are characterized by losing touch with reality or experiencing or believing things that others do not believe. Schizophrenia, a common form of psychosis, is associated with significant personal, social, and financial costs. Common symptoms include delusional beliefs, hearing voices, or seeing visions, as well as disorganized speech. Current evidence regarding the treatment of psychosis and schizophrenia suggests that several treatment options are likely to be helpful for both management and alleviation of acute distress and symptoms as well as prevention of relapse or recurrence. These options include antipsychotic medication, cognitive therapy, and family intervention. Treatment guidelines for psychosis and schizophrenia in adults and adolescents recommend that people with psychosis should be offered access and choice regarding these treatments (National Institute for Health and Care Excellence, 2014).

Cognitive therapy for psychosis has been developed over the last few decades, although the first case study was published by Beck in 1952. More recently, empirically tested cognitive models of psychotic experiences (Garety, Kuipers, Fowler, Freeman, & Bebbington, 2001; Morrison, 2001) have been used to inform cognitive therapy for people with psychosis; these models have been informed by Beck's original cognitive model of emotional disorders and recent cognitive conceptualizations of anxiety disorders. General cognitive models of psychosis, as well as models of specific symptoms, tend to share several principles, including the importance of life history in the development of current difficulties, and the role of appraisals and responses in the maintenance of psychosis. A model of psychosis will be described in more detail, and the treatment approach that is derived from this model will be outlined, followed by a summary of current research evidence and future directions.

AN INTEGRATIVE COGNITIVE MODEL OF PSYCHOSIS

There are three important principles of this cognitive model of psychosis (Morrison, 2001), (the model is illustrated using a case example in Figure 16.1). First, symptoms of psychosis, such as paranoid thoughts or hearing voices or seeing visions, are conceptualized as essentially normal experiences that any of us could experience under certain circumstances. This normalizing perspective is central to engaging people in cognitive therapy. Second, the goal of cognitive therapy for psychosis is to alleviate the distress and disability associated with psychotic experiences, rather than eliminate such symptoms per se. However, these symptoms may abate as a secondary consequence of reductions in distress. As asserted in Beck's original model, as well as current approaches to anxiety disorders, it is the interpretation of intrusive experiences, or the response to such experiences, that causes distress and disability. Therefore, the treatment targets within cognitive therapy for psychosis are the interpretations of, and responses to, psychotic experiences, but the goals are usually focused on reducing distress or improving quality of life (Morrison, Renton, Dunn, Williams, & Bentall, 2004b). This often will include addressing nonpsychotic problems that are commonly experienced by people with psychosis, such as anxiety disorders, low mood and hopelessness, relationship issues, and stigma. Third, a defining factor in whether someone is given a diagnosis of a psychotic disorder depends on the cultural acceptability or unusual nature of their appraisals. Therefore, if someone misinterprets their racing thoughts or palpitations as a sign of alien control or persecution via telekinesis, he or she will be classified as delusional, whereas misinterpretation of the same sensations as a sign of impending madness or a heart attack will be regarded as indicative of panic disorder. However, as outlined in Beck's theory, the nature of the interpretations that people make is an understandable consequence of their previous experiences, knowledge, and associated beliefs. In summary, we conceptualize psychotic experiences as normal intrusions, and we regard delusional beliefs as understandable when we consider the person's life history and idiosyncratic sociocultural context. It is also assumed that the factors involved in the development and maintenance of symptoms will be similar, regardless of whether an appraisal is unusual or more common or acceptable.

As mentioned, this model suggests that interpretations of intrusions mediate the associated distress and disability. For example, how a person is likely to respond will vary according to whether, upon hearing a voice, the person thinks "The devil is talking to me" or "I must be going crazy," or dismissively, "That was a strange sensation, I must have been overtired" (Kingdon & Turkington, 1994, p. 78). The interpretation of the intrusion influences the individual's choice of cognitive and behavioral responses or coping strategies. If the person fears that something bad will happen, he or she will adopt safety-seeking behaviors to try to avoid it, but this prevents disconfirmation of the interpretation. For example, holding a belief about being monitored and followed may be associated with behaviors such as walking with a hood up, taking back streets, and hiding behind cars. As well as preventing disconfirmation of the belief (since the person may believe he would have been attacked had he not taken these precautions), such behaviors can increase conspicuousness to others. Some cognitive and behavioral responses may also increase the frequency of problematic intrusions. Holding an interpretation of an intrusion as a threat or a sign of madness is likely to be associated with selective attention for similar experiences, heightened self-focus, attempts to suppress the experience, or other counterproductive control strategies that may maintain further difficulties such as hallucinations.

Mood and physiology are also implicated in the maintenance and onset of psychotic experiences. People who experience psychosis are often able to recognize the links between feeling stressed or physiologically aroused with intrusions such as the onset of voices, dissociative experiences, and symptoms such as thought disorder (e.g., disorganized speech). Physiological factors, such as the effects of sleep deprivation or drug use, can also be included in the model as factors that may result in increased intrusions or anomalous experiences.

THE ROLE OF EXPERIENCES AND BELIEFS IN THE DEVELOPMENT OF PSYCHOSIS

Early experiences and the beliefs formed as a result contribute to the development of unusual beliefs and psychotic experiences. Persecutory delusions can be seen as an understandable consequence of genuine experiences of persecution such as bullying, abuse, racism, and other traumatic life events, contributing to negative beliefs such as viewing the self as bad or vulnerable, others as untrustworthy, and the world as dangerous. Culturally unacceptable interpretations of intrusions may also reflect deficits in social knowledge related to poverty and social isolation, or interests in occult or spiritual influences outside of established religions. Metacognitive and procedural beliefs (beliefs about cognition and implicit beliefs that guide cognitive and attentional responses) are also included in the model. For example, past experiences of threatening environments can result in the development of positive beliefs about paranoid ideation as a functional survival strategy ("my paranoia keeps me safe"), but if paranoia is also negatively appraised as uncontrollable or dangerous, this can result in distress and in reliance on potentially unhelpful control strategies (e.g., suppression and avoidance). Implicit procedural beliefs also guide information-processing strategies such as self-focused attention, selective attention for threat-related cues, biased memory recall, confirmation bias, and external attributions for internal mental events. Furthermore, hallucinatory experiences can be a direct response to traumatic life events, such as hearing voices that reflect the content of past abuse. There is increasing evidence that psychosis may emerge as a reaction to trauma (Read, 1997; Varese et al., 2012).

An example of an idiosyncratic case conceptualization based on this model is given in Figure 16.1. The case example is based on a 42-year-old woman ("Jill") who was diagnosed with treatment-resistant schizophrenia. She heard voices and saw associated visions that were threatening, critical, and commanding. Her goal for therapy was to feel less anxious in response to her voices. Jill had a history of traumatic experiences, which were reflected in the voice content, and she had developed negative beliefs about herself as evil, the world as dangerous, and others as untrustworthy. Jill also had positive metacognitive beliefs about the need to be hypervigilant to stay safe, as well as positive beliefs about some of her voices as providing companionship. Such positive beliefs about psychotic experiences can be implicated in the development and maintenance of psychosis (Morrison et al., 2011), consistent with predictions from a metacognitive model (Wells & Matthews, 1994). Overall, her psychotic experiences were associated with feelings of acute anxiety and distress owing to her appraising these experiences as originating from "the Devil," believing in the content of what the voices said, and fearing she was about to be harmed. As a consequence, she avoided going out whenever possible, or she would scan for danger in her environment. She also focused on the voices, appeased the voices' commands to hurt herself (via self-harm), and sometimes shouted at the voices, who would argue back in return.

A COGNITIVE APPROACH TO UNDERSTANDING NEGATIVE SYMPTOMS

Negative symptoms include flat or blunted affect, poverty of thought and speech, avolition, apathy, and anhedonia. These symptoms are commonly

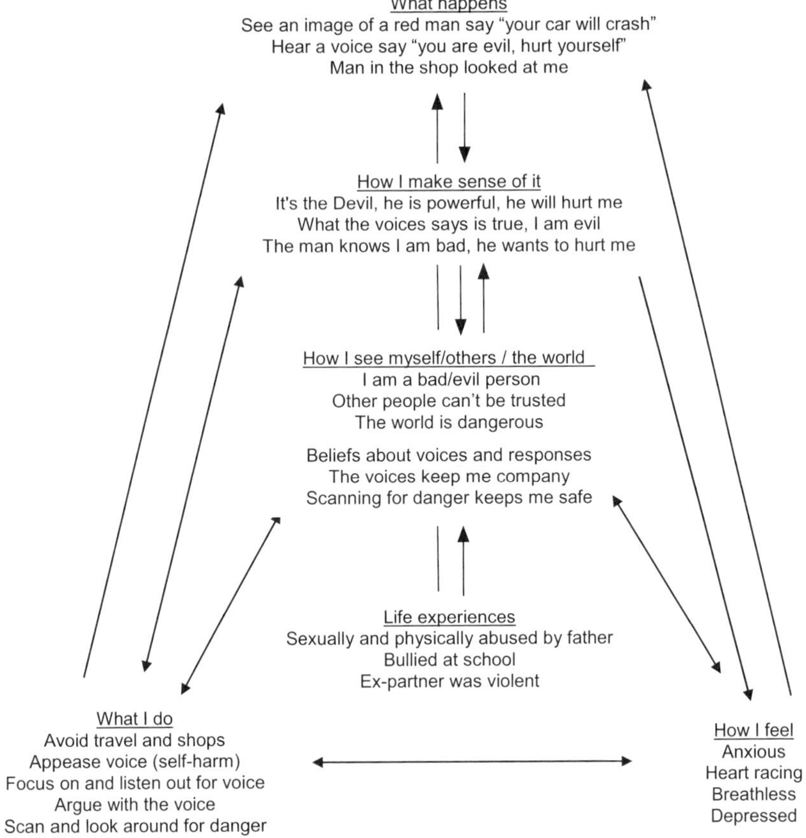

FIGURE 16.1. A case conceptualization of "Jill" based on the cognitive model of psychosis.

assumed to reflect deficits with a neurobiological cause. However, environmental and psychological factors have also been shown to have an impact on the expression of these symptoms, which suggests that they are amenable to formulation and intervention within a cognitive model (Morrison et al., 2004b). Aversive social experiences and stigmatization may lead to the development of asocial beliefs to protect the self from rejection ("I prefer hobbies and leisure activities that do not involve other people"; Grant & Beck, 2010). Conviction in defeatist beliefs about performance (for example, "If you cannot do something, well, there is little point in doing it at all") has also been shown to be associated with diminished goal-oriented behavior (Grant & Beck, 2009). Other factors contributing to the appearance of negative symptoms may include side effects of neuroleptic medication, the effects of institutionalization, social isolation, low self-efficacy beliefs, negative expectancies about pleasure, depression, anxious avoidance, emotional numbing associated with posttraumatic stress disorder (PTSD), or the use of affective flattening as a learned safety behavior (e.g., to avoid hospitalization; Morrison et al., 2004b).

CLINICAL APPLICATION

Cognitive therapy for psychosis follows the same principles as cognitive therapy for other disorders in that interventions are based on an empirically validated cognitive model of psychosis. Other key principles of cognitive therapy include use of a normalizing philosophy, emphasis on collaboration and teamwork, use of structure and educational approaches, including guided discovery and the importance of an active stance, and use of homework.

STAGES AND THE PROCESS OF THERAPY

The following stages outline the process of therapy:

1. Assessment and engagement phase (approximately sessions 1 to 3)
2. Change strategy phase (sessions 4 onward)
3. Longitudinal formulation phase (usually in the latter stages of therapy)
4. Consolidation phase and therapy blueprint (final sessions)

Sessions are usually offered on a weekly basis, for up to sixty minutes, for approximately twenty sessions in total. In practice, the number, the frequency and length of sessions, and the timing of the stages of therapy may vary according to client needs. For example, the longitudinal formulation phase of therapy may be introduced earlier if the client's goal is to understand the development of her problems, or if intervention at the maintenance level has not enabled the client to make changes and, therefore, further formulation is required.

1. Assessment and Engagement

The main intended outcomes of the assessment and engagement phase is to have identified a shared list of problems and goals, and a shared maintenance formulation of the prioritized problem, so that active work on change strategies can begin in the next phase. However, assessment and formulation is a continuous and iterative process throughout therapy. The individual components of the assessment phase include engagement, problem list and goals, cognitive-behavioral assessment of problems, risk assessment, historical assessment, normalizing if appropriate, and development of the shared CBT maintenance formulation.

Engagement and Expectations of Therapy

Patients' attitudes toward therapy can be influenced by previous experiences of mental health services Therefore, clinical experience has taught us to be mindful of how we are perceived in terms of potential power imbalance and the importance of transparency about what they can expect from the process of therapy. Engagement is facilitated by the collaborative nature of cognitive therapy in itself, particularly the principles of normalization and "sitting on a collaborative fence" in a spirit of "let's find out together" rather than directly challenging the client's belief in the initial sessions. Core conditions of warmth and genuineness, combined with a flexibility of approach (e.g., offering the client a break during the session if he requires it, using lay terms rather than technical language), while still maintaining the structure of therapy, also aid in engagement. It is important to be clear and explicit about non-negotiable issues such as the limits to confidentiality and communication with involved workers. It can also be beneficial to clarify expectations of therapy (e.g., who will do the hard work and the likely rate and degree of change). Given these considerations, our experience is that patients who experience psychosis are not generally difficult to engage and that they frequently build strong working alliances.

Identification of Problems and Goals

Cognitive-behavioral assessment begins by asking the client about her concerns in order to develop a shared problem list. Once a comprehensive list of problems has been identified, it is important to collaboratively prioritize the problems and then set goals in relation to these. Prioritization can be decided according to the patient's wishes, the amenability of the problems to change, and the impact that change in one problem area may have on the other difficulties. Goals should be specific, measurable, and proximal. As stated earlier, goals are frequently not related to the psychotic experiences.

Cognitive-Behavioral Assessment

The main aim of cognitive-behavioral assessment is to assess the presenting problem in order to inform a formulation, including assessment of cognitive, behavioral, affective, and physiological components, as well as triggers and mediators of problematic experiences. These components should be elicited in an assessment process that is based on the model, in order to enable the development of an idiosyncratic case conceptualization. This usually begins with an analysis of recent incidents that are related to the prioritized problem(s).

Inquiring about commonly co-occurring difficulties is also advised, such as alcohol and substance misuse, posttraumatic distress, depression, and social anxiety, following which more detailed problem-focused assessment can be carried out as indicated. Other areas to assess include antipsychotic medication and its side effects (types of drugs and dosages) and cognitive deficits in memory and attention (via observation, based on discussion with the patient/carers/staff or formally assessed using neuropsychological tests) in order to guide pacing and length of sessions. This may also inform use of visual or written aids when presenting information, the timing of review sessions, the nature of homework, and the likelihood of success when setting goals. Suicidal ideation and risk can be assessed by inquiring about suicidal ideation and intent, whether a method and timescale have been decided on, any history of self-harm or suicidal behavior, and consideration of the advantages and disadvantages of dying and living, as well as eliciting deterrents (e.g., the effect on family or relation to religious beliefs).

Although more detailed historical assessment of life experiences and associated beliefs may be carried out in the longitudinal formulation phase, it is important to gain an initial understanding of the patient's personal, social, and cultural history, as well as the person's current context. Relevant areas to assess include family life, school experiences with peers and teachers, friendships, sexual relationships, and cultural factors, such as religious influences, eccentric or occult influences, or other idiosyncratic cultural experiences. The latter factors may be important in determining if a symptom is labelled "psychotic." Awareness of a history of difficult and traumatic experiences is of particular relevance to understanding the person's current presentation. Common experiences include unwanted sexual experience, bullying at work or school, and physical assault (Mueser et al., 1998). It can be helpful to ask about these experiences directly, or through presentation of normalizing information prior to asking about these experiences (e.g., after sharing information that such experiences are commonly found in people who hear voices or have unusual beliefs). Read (1997) recommends inquiring about sexual and physical assault in a gradual and sensitive manner by asking general questions (e.g., about the worst and happiest memories from childhood), more specific questions if necessary (e.g., how discipline was enforced at home and school), and finally asking whether the person has had any sexual experiences about which she has felt uncomfortable. It is important to respond to disclosure in a manner that the person feels listened to and safe and that she is not being judged; to check that she has some coping strategies and social support; and to share the possibility that critical voices may get worse in the short term as a result of disclosure.

Self-Report Measures and Structured Interview Tools

Administration of standardized measures is recommended pre- and post-therapy as a minimum, but using measures regularly at review sessions or even using brief measures weekly can be helpful. The Psychotic Symptoms Rating Scales (PSYRATS [Haddock, McCarron, Tarrier, & Faragher, 1999]) is a useful interview tool for assessing dimensions of hallucinations and delusions and monitoring change. Self-report measures to assess psychotic experiences and beliefs include the Beliefs about Voices Questionnaire (BAVQ; Chadwick, Lees, & Birchwood, 2000), which assesses beliefs about and responses to voices (such as engagement and resistance); the Interpretation of Voices Inventory (Morrison et al., 2004a), which assesses positive and negative beliefs about voices; and the Beliefs about Paranoia Scale (Morrison et al., 2005), which assesses metacognitive beliefs about paranoid thinking.

Development of the Maintenance Formulation: Cognitive Models to Understand Cognitive and Behavioral Reactions

A simple linear model of event–appraisal–feeling–response links is usually the first model that is shared with clients to socialize them to the cognitive model (i.e., it is the interpretation of an event or intrusion that results in distress and guides the choice of responses that they make, which may in turn be helpful or unhelpful; see Figure 16.2 for examples).

When developing maintenance formulations of intrusions (e.g., hallucinations, anomalous experiences, bodily sensations, thoughts, images, or memories), we can ask about the trigger to the intrusions, but in these simple linear formulations it is the content of intrusions that forms the "event." As well as formulating intrusive experiences, the "event" can also be an external event (e.g., noises, smells, interactions with people, things said by others, things said on television, or other situations or events that are perceived by the person). The appraisal is how those events are interpreted.

Cognitive Models to Understand Maintenance Links

As the development of the formulation progresses, it is important to help clients identify further maintenance links, for example, regarding the impact of any cognitive-behavioral responses or safety behaviors (e.g., whether they stop the person from disconfirming the interpretation or have an impact on the intrusion itself, and whether emotional responses have a direct impact on intrusions). Similarly, when formulating external stimuli, particularly regarding interactions with people as the triggering event, it can be useful to inquire about links between responses as potentially contaminating the social situation (e.g., certain safety-seeking behaviors, such

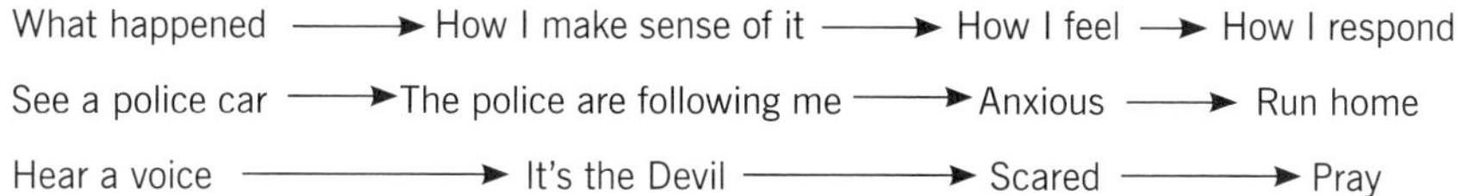

FIGURE 16.2. Linear maintenance formulations.

as avoiding all eye contact or constantly staring at others, are likely to attract attention and negative reactions from others). It can also be useful to socialize clients to information-processing biases such as selective attention, thinking errors, and the biased interpretation of ambiguous material and how these can affect thinking and subsequent occurrence of intrusions.

Normalizing in the Assessment Phase

Patients are often caught between "a rock and a hard place," either believing in their distressing interpretation (e.g., "I am hearing the voice of the devil" or "I am being persecuted") versus believing "I am schizophrenic and mad." Therefore, providing a third, normalizing perspective is important to facilitate engagement, reduce distress, and destigmatize these experiences. Assessment can offer an opportunity to provide normalizing information as symptoms are elicited, such as providing information about the prevalence of hearing voices or unusual beliefs, or famous celebrities who have experienced such symptoms. For example, patients can be informed that 35 to 40% of students have hallucinatory experiences, 10 to 25% of the population hear voices in their lifetime, and 5% of the population hear voices in any one year (Kingdon & Turkington, 1994). Furthermore, up to 70% of people hold beliefs that could be considered delusional in content (Peters, Joseph, & Garety, 1999). Paranoid thinking is extremely common in the general population (Freeman et al., 2011) and is often associated with common experiences such as worry and sleep deprivation.

2. Change Strategy Phase (from Session 4 Onward)

Examples are given next of the common cognitive and behavioral change strategies applied to experiences of psychosis. The choice of strategies is guided by the formulation that has been collaboratively developed and on the basis of negotiation with the patient.

Examining Advantages and Disadvantages

Hallucinatory experiences, distressing unusual beliefs, and the cognitive and behavioral responses to these experiences and beliefs can all be associated with advantages, as well as disadvantages, and may have developed as understandable adaptation to past experiences. For example, paranoid thinking can be a logical response to a childhood that was characterized by interpersonal threat and danger. Similarly, voices may keep the person company if they are socially isolated, as in the case example of "Jill" (Figure 16.1). If people were not distressed by their experiences, then we would not aim to change them; however, people are often ambivalent and identify a mixture of benefits and difficulties. It is, therefore, advisable to help the person to consider both the advantages and disadvantages prior to change strategies, thereby helping them to make an informed choice about whether to change the symptom, belief, or behavior. For example, in Jill's case, advantages and disadvantages were elicited for her voices prior to intervention. The advantages included voices that kept her company and passed the time; compared to the disadvantages of feeling scared of the voices, worrying that the voices could harm her, doing self-harm in response to voices, and not being able to travel due to fear of the voices. This enabled her to make a choice about whether it was worth potentially losing the company of her voices in order to feel less anxious. It may also be important to help the person find other means of achieving the functions or advantages prior to change (for example, improving self-esteem before evaluating a belief about exceptional status or powers, or interventions to reduce social isolation in cases such as Jill's).

Reviewing the Evidence

Verbal reattribution methods can be used to review the evidence supporting and not supporting distressing appraisals. It is important that this be done Socratically rather than attempting to disprove the belief, as this may result in resistance. When working with threat-based appraisals that have been a long-lasting concern (e.g., a voice threatening harm or fears of persecution), it can be helpful to review the cumulative evidence over time (e.g., asking the person how many times the voices have made threats per day, for how many weeks, and for how many years) in order to calculate the probable outcome of the next threat. As further evidence is collected over the course of therapy, for example, following behavioral experiments, the cumulative list can be expanded. In Jill's case, the generation of cumulative evidence helped her to learn that voices often "lied" and that they did not have the power to harm her. This knowledge gave her confidence to test her fears more directly in behavioral experiments.

Alternative Explanations

Generating alternative explanations is useful for evaluating appraisals for which other factors may have had a role. For example, when people have paranoid thoughts (e.g., thinking a cough was a signal for imminent assault), it can be useful to list other (less distressing) reasons for why someone might cough (e.g., smoker, cold, allergy, nervous cough). This is a useful strategy for evaluating interpretations of voices (e.g., whether they come from a demon, are a sign of illness, are the product of an unusual thought process, and are an understandable response to trauma). Pie charts can also be used as a visual summary of the percentage likelihood of each explanation. It is important to help the person to find an explanation that is least distressing for them, even if this differs from our own view. For example, Jill had been in contact with psychiatric services for many years, and she found that viewing her experiences as hallucinations caused by illness/schizophrenia was the least distressing and made most sense for her. Furthermore, the "dual model strategy" (Wells, 1997) or "Theory A/Theory B" (Salkovskis, 1996) can be used to reflect the stance of "sitting on a collaborative fence"—that is, either the problem is real or the problem is their concern that it is real; for example, they are being persecuted by terrorists, or they believe that they are being persecuted by terrorists. In such circumstances, considering the evidence of each perspective and the most helpful responses if that was the case can be helpful.

An Alternative Conceptualization via Longitudinal Formulation

Generation of an alternative conceptualization via longitudinal formulation can also provide an alternative, normalizing explanation for the person's difficulties, as opposed to being stuck between a rock and a hard place (e.g., believing in an actual conspiracy versus seeing oneself as crazy or mad). For example, if the client is able to link his distressing thoughts to his beliefs and early experiences, and to view his difficulties as understandable, this can provide a less distressing explanation. For example, given experiences of assault, and beliefs in the self as vulnerable and others as untrustworthy, it is therefore understandable how one would be susceptible to paranoid thinking.

Normalizing as an Intervention

As well as normalizing in the assessment phase, normalization can be used in an intervention, particularly when the formulation reveals appraisals related to viewing oneself as abnormal, weird, or bad for having unusual experiences. As well as normalizing the prevalence of voices or unusual beliefs and highlighting famous hearers of voices (e.g., Beethoven, Anthony Hopkins, Brian Wilson, Zoe Wannamaker, Joan of Arc, and Winston Churchill), information can also be provided on common triggers for psychotic experiences (trauma and abuse, drug use, isolation, sensory deprivation, bereavement, sleep deprivation—e.g., Kingdon & Turkington, 1994).

Internally Generated Explanations for Voices

When considering less distressing explanations for voices, it can be useful to consider whether voices might be internally generated. Strategies include presenting information in a neutral manner about research showing that the patients' voice boxes move when they hear voices (see Bentall, 2003) and that talking to yourself in your mind (subvocalization) can inhibit voices. Behavioral experiments using subvocalization (e.g., asking the person to read or count backwards in her head) can also be used to observe the effect on voices. Analysis of voice content in relation to their thoughts or concerns can also facilitate reattribution to an internal source. If voices are ego-dystonic, presenting information on intrusive thoughts that is relevant to the content of their voices (such as blasphemous, violent, or sexual thoughts, images, and impulses) can help to normalize unwanted thoughts and voices.

Imagery Modification

Imagery is an important feature of psychotic disorders. For example, distressing images of being attacked are often associated with paranoid beliefs (Morrison et al., 2002). Similar to work in anxiety disorders (Hackmann, 1997), imagery modification techniques can be used to help modify distressing content or to increase the person's sense of control over the images. Examples of such techniques include treating the image as a video (fast forward, rewind, freeze frame, and eject it) or introducing a rescuer to the image and introducing humor (e.g., incorporating a cartoon character). It can be useful to ask about appraisals of images (e.g., people may have metacognitive beliefs that having an image of something means that it is likely to happen). These can be evaluated by examining the evidence and carrying out behavioral experiments with more positive images (e.g., generating an image of winning the lottery to see if it affects the outcome).

Questionnaires and Surveys

Questionnaires and surveys can be useful for gaining alternative perspectives or to gather evidence on a patient's beliefs and concerns, to normalize certain experiences, thoughts, or responses (e.g., by asking others if they have experienced anything similar), and to generate ideas for coping or alternative responses based on other people's experiences. For example, Jill came to believe that she was an "evil" child and deserved to be punished for some misbehavior, that is, shouting back at her parents. We, therefore, conducted a survey to ask others their opinions on whether they thought a child who shouts at her parents was evil, to state whether they themselves had ever shouted at their parents, and to cite any other examples of ways they had misbehaved when younger, to help her to reevaluate her belief that she was evil.

Behavioral Strategies

Behavioral techniques are based on a cognitive formulation with the aim of testing interpretations and appraisals.

Behavioral Experiments

Behavioral experiments offer a means of going out into the world to test the reality of one's concerns. It is important to collaboratively design the experiment with the patient, to identify the prediction, to define the predicted outcome in concrete, observable, measurable terms, to identify the safety behaviors to be reversed for true exposure to test the belief, and to summarize the results as related to the case formulation. Experiments to test the usefulness of specific responses can also be both beneficial and informative—for example, evaluating the effects of thought suppression on the occurrence of unwanted thoughts by asking a client to compare suppression and acceptance of target thoughts, or evaluating the impact of internal versus external focus of attention on mood and physiology by comparing deliberate attentional strategies.

Behavioral Experiments Specific to Psychosis

VOLITION, CONSEQUENCES OF VOICES, AND DISOBEYING THE VOICES

If patients appraise their voices as powerful and omnipotent (Chadwick & Birchwood, 1994), then they may have distressing beliefs about the consequences of disobeying voices (e.g., beliefs that the voices will harm them or others). It is important to devise experiments that allow patients to test out their concerns in a way that they feel comfortable. After initial normalization and verbal reattribution to help weaken the belief, it is recommended that experiments be graded in a hierarchical manner (with more challenging experiments saved for later in the therapy). With regard to testing the power of voices to harm, it can be helpful to question the mechanism regarding how a voice could cause harm. The therapists should use themselves as the initial target in testing this out (e.g., testing whether the voices have the power to throw an object, to break the therapist's finger in the session, cause a nosebleed during the session). For example, Jill believed that the voices had the power to harm by being able to physically move objects. She agreed to an initial in-session behavioral experiment that involved asking the voices to prove their power by throwing a cup at the therapist. Jill then had the confidence to reduce her own safety behaviors in response to the voices until she was ultimately no longer distressed by their presence.

THOUGHT-BROADCAST EXPERIMENTS

For patients who have concerns that others can hear their thoughts, experiments can be devised to purposely send out thoughts that would cause an observable and measurable reaction in others (e.g., getting on the bus or going into a busy shop and thinking "bomb"). Experiments can also be carried out using audio recording equipment to test out whether thoughts, or voices, can be detected and potentially heard by others.

If I Show Weakness, I Will Be Attacked

This is a common belief of paranoid patients. Weakness can be operationalized and then demonstrated by the therapist—for example, going onto a busy street and lying down or shaking. The therapist may have to model this first before the client feels safe to experiment with it.

The Reactions of Others

Fears of stigma, social anxiety, and social isolation are common difficulties for people experiencing psychosis. Behavioral experiments can help test concerns about other people's reactions (e.g., purposefully going into a shop and chatting at the checkout in order to test fears such as "normal people will think I am mad and refuse to talk to me.").

Activity Scheduling

Activity scheduling can be used to test the accuracy of cognitions linked to the avoidance of activity and maintenance of distress, such as low expectancies of pleasure from activity ("I won't enjoy it"), concerns about failure ("If I try something new, I'll mess it up"), or fears that activity will worsen voices or symptoms. Activity recording or scheduling, as well as ratings of enjoyment, achievement, or frequency of symptoms, can be used to test out the patient's cognitions.

Action Plans

Cognitive therapy is not about convincing patients that situations are better than they seem, but rather about balanced and accurate thinking. If upon gathering further evidence it becomes apparent that there is truth in the individual's distressing interpretation, then action plans can be used to solve problems that have been identified. This can involve breaking tasks down into smaller chunks, problem solving, identifying others in the environment who may be able to offer assistance (such as residential or social care staff, friends, or relatives), and using role plays to rehearse strategies to deal with difficult situations (for example, how to respond politely, but assertively, to exploitative neighbors).

3. Longitudinal Formulation Phase (Latter Half of Therapy)

Longitudinal formulations are used to develop an historical understanding of the development of the patient's difficulties. They are also useful for the purpose of relapse prevention since core beliefs and underlying assumptions may be vulnerability factors for future episodes of psychosis. The longitudinal formulation phase usually occurs toward the end of therapy after change strategies have been implemented at the maintenance level. However, longitudinal formulation may be introduced earlier in therapy, depending on the patient's goals. For example, the patient may want to tell his story and to understand why his difficulties have developed ("why me?"). Another indication for the use of longitudinal formulation earlier in therapy is to address "stuck points" when interventions at the maintenance level of formulation have been unsuccessful.

The longitudinal formulation phase involves assessment of early experience and identification of declarative (core beliefs) and assumptions, which are sometimes referred to as schematic beliefs (Beck, 1976)—that is, knowledge structures that guide information processing and behavior. Core beliefs include unconditional beliefs about the self, world, or others (e.g., "I am bad"), and maladaptive assumptions often take the form of conditional "if–then statements" (e.g., if I am not liked by everyone, then I am unlovable). Procedural beliefs that influence choice of control strategies (Wells & Matthews, 1994), including beliefs about the advantages or disadvantages of cognitive and behavioral responses, are also part of the longitudinal model of psychosis.

Schema Change Methods

Schema change methods used in affective disorders can also be applied to working with people experiencing psychosis. These methods are relevant given the nature of difficult early life experiences and negative beliefs that are commonly found in this group. Strategies include the prejudice metaphor (Padesky, 1993) to socialize clients to how negative beliefs about the self (e.g., "I am bad") serve as a kind of self-prejudice in which information that contradicts their belief is often ignored, distorted, or treated as an exception. Collaborative exploration of the advantages and disadvantages of core beliefs, rules, or assumptions is advised, including examination of short-term versus long-term utility of these beliefs, particularly as these beliefs may have developed as an adaptation to difficult early-life experiences. For example, examination of the advantages and disadvantages of Jill's negative belief "I am evil" enabled her to realize that challenging her negative belief may result in feelings of anger toward those who had told her she was evil during childhood. Jill still chose to question this belief so that she could feel better about herself. Beck (1976) describes how assumptions ("if–then") or rule statements ("I should, I must") can be explored and questioned using the Socratic technique and how behavioral experiments can be used to further test problematic assumptions (e.g., "acting as if" the belief did not exist in order to test the outcome of alternative behaviors). Other techniques include the historical test of a belief (Padesky, 1994), which involves breaking the patient's life down into chunks (e.g., in five-year segments) and recording experiences that appear to support the negative belief and also recording experiences that do not support the belief, as well as questioning and reevaluating the supporting evidence. Pie charts are particularly useful for evaluating beliefs that reflect inappropriate conclusions regarding responsibility for past events (e.g., challenging self-blame for abuse, which is a common experience among people with psychosis). Continua methods (Padesky, 1994) can be used to introduce the notion of relativity regarding negative core beliefs by creating rating scales with reference points based on extreme examples (e.g., ratings of being unlovable relative to Hitler).

Other methods include positive data logs to repeatedly record evidence in support of an alternative, less negative belief the patient would like to hold; and surveys to normalize or collect alternative perspectives on the evidence that the patient identifies as supporting their negative belief; and imagery modification relating to distressing childhood memories. Jill found survey responses to be particularly useful in helping her to question whether her childhood behavior was truly evidence of being evil, or whether it was, in fact, completely understandable. Schema change methods can also be applied to evaluating the content of voices (e.g., if someone hears a voice telling her that she is worthless, bad, or evil). Finally, worksheets and flashcards are particularly useful for people with psychotic experiences (as they may have problems with memory due to medication, preoccupation with psychotic experiences or cognitive deficits) to document original and alternative core beliefs, summarize the evidence that supports the alternative, and give instructions for more helpful behavioral responses.

4. Consolidation Phase (Final Sessions)

The aim of the final few sessions is to develop a therapy blueprint for the maintenance of gains and relapse prevention. The therapy blueprint can include information on the goals of therapy, the outcome of therapy in terms of progress toward these goals, a copy of the formulation, a summary of useful strategies, and a collaborative plan of action for the maintenance of gains.

With respect to relapse prevention, it is important to normalize setbacks and to decatastrophize potential relapse. A plan for relapse prevention can involve identification of potential stressors or triggers in future, identification of warning signs of potential relapse, a plan for early intervention in response to these signs, as well as a list of resources and professional contacts if needed. The longitudinal formulation provides a starting point for identifying historical stressors or triggers, as well as exploration of past incidences of relapse. It is often easier for the patient to recognize links between physiological state and onset of symptoms (e.g., sleep disturbance, medication changes, drug or alcohol consumption, physical illness). However, it is also relevant to identify the events that preceded these physiological factors (e.g., changes to housing arrangement, associated worry and anxiety followed by sleep disturbance) to inform plans for action. The maintenance formulation of cognitive and behavioral responses to stressors can also be used to identify potential vulnerabilities for relapse (e.g., staying in bed and being inactive and maintaining social isolation, and experiencing sleep disturbance and rumination, and maintaining low mood). The formulation can subsequently be used to consider alternative, more helpful strategies.

RESEARCH

Considerable evidence supports the cognitive model of psychosis, including systematic reviews and meta-analyses that demonstrate the role of adverse life events in the development of psychotic experiences (Varese et al., 2012), the role of metacognitive beliefs in psychosis (Sellers, Varese, Wells, & Morrison, 2016), and the importance of appraisals (Mawson, Cohen, & Berry, 2010) and responses (Tully, Wells, & Morrison, 2016). There is also an extensive research literature demonstrating the validity of the continuum approach (van Os, Linscott, Myin-Germeys, Delespaul, & Krabbendam, 2009) and, therefore, the applicability of a normalizing approach to conceptualizing psychotic experiences. There is clear evidence from clinical trials and meta-analyses that cognitive therapy has a small to moderate effect size when considered in relation to overall psychiatric symptoms (Jauhar et al., 2014; Turner, van der Gaag, Karyotaki, & Cuijpers, 2014; Wykes, Steel, Everitt, & Tarrier, 2008), as well as specific positive symptoms (van der Gaag, Valmaggia, & Smit, 2014) and negative symptoms (Grant, Huh, Perivoliotis, Stolar, & Beck, 2012). Recent evidence suggests that cognitive therapy may also be promising as a treatment for people who have chosen not to take medication (Morrison et al., 2014). However, several important research questions remain unanswered. For example, for whom does cognitive therapy for psychosis work best? Is there a group of people who may experience unwanted effects or harm? Is an individually tailored, formulation-driven treatment required, or can brief interventions or group approaches be as effective? There is also some debate about whether primary outcomes should be symptoms, functioning, quality of life, or subjectively defined recovery (Thomas, 2015) and whether CT for people with psychosis can be most effective when it targets specific symptoms, such as command hallucinations (Birchwood et al., 2014), or specific processes, such as worry (Freeman et al., 2015). We also need to know the relative efficacy of cognitive therapy in a direct head-to-head comparison with antipsychotic medication and whether it works for people who have exhausted all the pharmacological treatment options (i.e., they have not responded to clozapine, which is the last line of antipsychotic medications). The research studies currently being conducted should address these questions (e.g., Pyle et al., 2016).

CONCLUSIONS

There have been significant developments in the understanding and treatment of psychosis from a cognitive-behavioral perspective. There are empirically tested models that have led to an empirically supported treatment (cognitive therapy), which is recommended in the treatment guidelines for psychosis and schizophrenia in numerous countries. There are challenges in terms of providing equitable and rapid access to this treatment and in training and disseminating this approach, but efforts are currently being made to ensure that more people with psychosis have access to this treatment as an additional option to antipsychotic medication. Future research challenges include identifying those for whom it works best and those who may not benefit from it and showing what the essential elements are (including whether a fully compliant, model-driven, formulation-based approach is required for all).

REFERENCES

Beck, A. T. (1952). Successful outpatient psychotherapy of a chronic schizophrenic with a delusion based on borrowed guilt. *Psychiatry, 15,* 305–312.

Beck, A. T. (1976). *Cognitive therapy and the emotional disorders.* New York: International Universities Press.

Bentall, R. P. (2003). *Madness explained: Psychosis and human nature.* London: Penguin Books.

Birchwood, M., Michail, M., Meaden, A., Tarrier, N., Lewis, S., Wykes, T., . . . Peters, E. (2014). Cognitive behaviour therapy to prevent harmful compliance with command hallucinations (COMMAND): A randomised controlled trial. *The Lancet Psychiatry, 1*(1), 23–33.

Chadwick, P., & Birchwood, M. (1994). The omnipotence of voices: A cognitive approach to auditory hallucinations. *British Journal of Psychiatry, 164,* 190–201.

Chadwick, P., Lees, S., & Birchwood, M. (2000). The revised Beliefs about Voices Questionnaire (BAVQ-R). *British Journal of Psychiatry, 177,* 229–232.

Freeman, D., Dunn, G., Startup, H., Pugh, K., Cordwell, J., Mander, H., . . . Kingdon, D. (2015). Effects of cognitive behaviour therapy for worry on persecutory delusions in patients with psychosis (WIT): A parallel, single-blind, randomised controlled trial with a mediation analysis. *The Lancet Psychiatry, 2*(4), 305–313.

Freeman, D., McManus, S., Brugha, T., Meltzer, H., Jenkins, R., & Bebbington, P. (2011). Concomitants of paranoia in the general population. *Psychological Medicine, 41*(5), 923–936.

Garety, P. A., Kuipers, E., Fowler, D., Freeman, D., & Bebbington, P. E. (2001). A cognitive model of the positive symptoms of psychosis. *Psychological Medicine, 31,* 189–195.

Grant, P. M., & Beck, A. T. (2009). Defeatist beliefs as a mediator of cognitive impairment and negative symptoms in schizophrenia. *Schizophrenia Bulletin, 35,* 798–806.

Grant, P. M., & Beck, A. T. (2010). Asocial beliefs as predictors of asocial behavior in schizophrenia. *Psychiatry Research, 177*(1), 65–70.

Grant, P. M., Huh, G. A., Perivoliotis, D., Stolar, N. M., & Beck, A. T. (2012). Randomized trial to evaluate the efficacy of cognitive therapy for low-functioning patients with schizophrenia. *Archives of General Psychiatry, 69*(2), 121–127.

Hackmann, A. (1997). The transformation of meaning in cognitive therapy. In M. Power & C. R. Brewin (Eds.), *Transformation of meaning in psychological therapies.* Chichester, UK: Wiley.

Haddock, G., McCarron, J., Tarrier, N., & Faragher, E. B. (1999). Scales to measure dimensions of hallucinations and delusions: The psychotic symptoms rating scales (PSYRATS). *Psychological Medicine, 29,* 879–889.

Jauhar, S., McKenna, P. J., Radua, J., Fung, E., Salvador, R., & Laws, K. R. (2014). Cognitive-behavioural therapy for the symptoms of schizophrenia: Systematic review and meta-analysis with examination of potential bias. *British Journal of Psychiatry, 204*(1), 20–29.

Kingdon, D. G., & Turkington, D. (1994). *Cognitive-behavioural therapy of schizophrenia.* Hove, UK: Erlbaum.

Mawson, A., Cohen, K., & Berry, K. (2010). Reviewing evidence for the cognitive model of auditory hallucinations: The relationship between cognitive voice appraisals and distress during psychosis. *Clinical Psychology Review, 30*(2), 248–258.

Morrison, A. P. (2001). The interpretation of intrusions in psychosis: An integrative cognitive approach to hallucinations and delusions. *Behavioural and Cognitive Psychotherapy, 29,* 257–276.

Morrison, A. P., Beck, A. T., Glentworth, D., Dunn, H., Reid, G., Larkin, W., . . . Williams, S. (2002). Imagery and psychotic symptoms: A preliminary investigation. *Behaviour Research and Therapy, 40,* 1063–1072.

Morrison, A. P., Gumley, A. I., Ashcroft, K., Manousos, R., White, R., Gillan, K., . . . Kingdon, D. (2011). Metacognition and persecutory delusions: Tests of a metacognitive model in a clinical population and comparisons with non-patients. *British Journal of Clinical Psychology, 50*, 223–233.

Morrison, A. P., Gumley, A. I., Schwannauer, M., Campbell, M., Gleeson, A., Griffin, E., . . . Gillan, K. (2005). The beliefs about paranoia scale: Preliminary validation of a metacognitive approach to conceptualising paranoia. *Behavioural and Cognitive Psychotherapy, 33*, 153–164.

Morrison, A. P., Nothard, S., Bowe, S. E., & Wells, A. (2004a). Interpretations of voices in patients with hallucinations and non-patient controls: A comparison and predictors of distress in patients. *Behavioral Research Therapy, 42*, 1315–1323.

Morrison, A. P., Renton, J. C., Dunn, H., Williams, S., & Bentall, R. P. (2004b). *Cognitive therapy for psychosis: A formulation-based approach*. London: Brunner-Routledge.

Morrison, A. P., Turkington, D., Pyle, M., Spencer, H., Brabban, A., Dunn, G., . . . Hutton, P. (2014). Cognitive therapy for people with schizophrenia spectrum disorders not taking antipsychotic drugs: A single-blind randomised controlled trial. *The Lancet, 383*, 1395–1403.

Mueser, K. T., Goodman, L. B., Trumbetta, S. L., Rosenberg, S. D., Osher, F. C., Vidaver, R., . . . & Foy, D. W. (1998). Trauma and posttraumatic stress disorder in severe mental illness. *Journal of Consulting and Clinical Psychology, 66*, 493–499.

National Institute for Health and Care Excellence. (2014). *Psychosis and schizophrenia in adults: Treatment and management*. London: NICE.

Padesky, C. A. (1993). Schema as self-prejudice. *International Cognitive Therapy Newsletter, 5/6*, 16–17.

Padesky, C. A. (1994). Schema change processes in cognitive therapy. *Clinical Psychology and Psychotherapy, 1*, 267–278.

Peters, E. R., Joseph, S. A., & Garety, P. A. (1999). Measurement of delusional ideation in the normal population: Introducing the PDI (Peters et al. Delusions Inventory). *Schizophrenia Bulletin, 25*, 553–576.

Pyle, M., Norrie, J., Schwannauer, M., Kingdon, D., Gumley, A., Turkington, D., . . . Morrison, A. P. (2016). Design and protocol for the Focusing on Clozapine Unresponsive Symptoms (FOCUS) trial: A randomised controlled trial. *BMC Psychiatry, 16*(1), 1–12.

Read, J. (1997). Child abuse and psychosis: A literature review and implications for professional practice. *Professional Psychology: Research and Practice, 28*, 448–456.

Salkovskis, P. M. (1996). The cognitive approach to anxiety: Threat beliefs, safety-seeking behavior, and the special case of health anxiety and obsessions. In P. M. Salkovskis & M. Paul (Eds.), *Frontiers of cognitive therapy* (pp. 48–74). New York: Guilford Press.

Sellers, R., Varese, F., Wells, A., & Morrison, A. P. (2016). A meta-analysis of metacognitive beliefs as implicated in the self-regulatory executive function model in clinical psychosis. *Schizophrenia Research*. [Epub ahead of print]

Thomas, N. (2015). What's really wrong with cognitive behavioral therapy for psychosis? [Opinion]. *Frontiers in Psychology, 6*(323).

Tully, S., Wells, A., & Morrison, A. P. (2017). An exploration of the relationship between use of safety-seeking behaviours and psychosis: A systematic review and meta-analysis. *Clinical Psychology and Psychotherapy.*

Turner, D. T., van der Gaag, M., Karyotaki, E., & Cuijpers, P. (2014). Psychological interventions for psychosis: A meta-analysis of comparative outcome studies. *American Journal of Psychiatry, 171*(5), 523–538.

van der Gaag, M., Valmaggia, L. R., & Smit, F. (2014). The effects of individually tailored formulation-based cognitive behavioural therapy in auditory hallucinations and delusions: A meta-analysis. *Schizophrenia Research, 156*(1), 30–37.

van Os, J., Linscott, R. J., Myin-Germeys, I., Delespaul, P., & Krabbendam, L. (2009). A systematic review and meta-analysis of the psychosis continuum: Evidence for a psychosis pronenesspersistence-impairment model of psychotic disorder. *Psychological Medicine, 39*(2), 179–195.

Varese, F., Smeets, F., Drukker, M., Lieverse, R., Lataster, T., Viechtbauer, W., . . . Bentall, R. P. (2012). Childhood adversities increase the risk of psychosis: A meta-analysis of patient-control, prospective- and cross-sectional cohort studies. *Schizophrenia Bulletin, 38*(4), 661–671.

Wells, A. (1997). *Cognitive therapy for anxiety disorders.* London: Wiley.

Wells, A., & Matthews, G. (1994). *Attention and emotion: A clinical perspective.* London: LEA.

Wykes, T., Steel, C., Everitt, B., & Tarrier, N. (2008). Cognitive behavior therapy for schizophrenia: Effect sizes, clinical models, and methodological rigor. *Schizophrenia Bulletin, 34,* 523–537.

CHAPTER 17

Advances in Cognitive-Behavioral Therapy for Substance Use Disorders and Addictive Behaviors

Bruce S. Liese
Jessica C. Tripp

It has been more than two decades since the publication of our text *Cognitive Therapy of Substance Abuse* (Beck, Wright, Newman, & Liese, 1993). Certainly, our most exciting advance over these years is reflected in the title of this chapter; we have shifted our focus from exclusively "substance abuse" to the broad spectrum of "addictive behaviors." When our text was published, one year prior to publication of the fourth edition of the *Diagnostic and Statistical Manual of Mental Disorders* (DSM-IV; American Psychiatric Association, 1994), the word "addiction" was still considered a lay term. Back then, "behavioral addictions" were nowhere to be found in the DSM. At that time, which was considered the height of the cocaine epidemic, we focused exclusively on chemical addictions. However, over the years we have learned that addictions extend well beyond consumption of chemical substances to include an array of behaviors (e.g., gambling and Internet gaming). Now it is widely accepted that individuals who struggle with chemical and behavioral addictions have common cognitive features (e.g., Fortune & Goodie, 2012; Goodie & Fortune, 2013;

Grant, Potenza, Weinstein, & Gorelick, 2010; Merrill, Read, & Barnett, 2013; Shorey, Anderson, & Stuart, 2012).

Another advance (also reflected in the title of this chapter) has been to shift our emphasis from cognitive therapy to cognitive-*behavioral* therapy (e.g., Liese, 2014). The first author (BSL) recalls a discussion with Dr. Aaron Beck at a restaurant in the early 1990s, when Dr. Beck explained that he hoped to see "the end of cognitive therapy." Naturally, this came as a surprise to BSL, who asked, "Why on Earth would you want an end to cognitive therapy?" Dr. Beck's response was humble and forthright. He said, "I just want therapists to do good therapy. Someday we'll refer to all *good therapy* simply as *psychotherapy*." The point here is that Dr. Beck was more interested in formulating good therapy than branding his own therapy. Hence, we have moved away from the brand name cognitive therapy (CT) toward the generic cognitive-behavioral therapy (CBT). It should be noted that Beck's daughter, Judy Beck (a highly respected scholar in her own right), refers to her own work now as cognitive behavior therapy (J. S. Beck, 2011).

So what is an addiction? The definition of addiction depends on your source. In fact, this term has been included in DSM only since 2013. According to DSM-5 (American Psychiatric Association, 2013), an addiction involves cognitive, behavioral, and affective symptoms; intense activation of the brain's reward system; social impairment; risky behavior; continued use despite associated problems; and lowered levels of self-control, likely reflecting impairments of brain inhibitory mechanisms. This most recent edition of DSM (APA, 2013) includes other noteworthy changes from its predecessor. For example, rather than dividing addictions into two categories, abuse and dependence, substance use disorders (SUDs) and addictions are considered to be on a continuum from mild (2–3 symptoms), to moderate (4–5 symptoms), to severe (6 or more symptoms). Craving, defined as strong urges to use, has been added. Additionally, gambling disorder has been included as the first behavioral addiction, and Internet gaming disorder is included as another potential behavioral addiction in the "Conditions for Further Study" section (APA, 2013, pp. 795–798).

Various researchers have focused their efforts on studying the full range of chemical and behavioral addictions. Perhaps most notable of these is Howard Shaffer, who introduced the addiction syndrome (Shaffer et al., 2004; Shaffer, LaPlante, & Nelson, 2012). The addiction syndrome is characterized by complex patterns that underlie all addictive processes. Rather than viewing each addiction (e.g., cocaine, alcohol, opioids, nicotine, gambling) as unique and separate, all addictions are regarded as having similar distal (past) and proximal (recent) antecedents, as well as consequences (e.g., expressions, manifestations, and sequelae). In other words, there are different manifestations of the addiction syndrome, but all reflect similar underlying processes. Evidence for the addiction syndrome includes shared neurobiological elements (e.g., the brain's reward system is similarly activated by both addictive substances and behaviors), shared psychosocial elements (e.g., individuals with addictions tend to have similar psychological problems), and shared experiences (e.g., the course of addictive behaviors tends to be similar across addictions). The addiction syndrome provides a broad conceptualization of addiction that focuses on commonalities between the various addictive processes. According to this model, certain behaviors and chemicals have the potential to produce desirable, robust, reliable, and subjective *shifts* (Shaffer et al., 2012, p. xxxi). As in DSM-5, it is assumed that both chemical and behavioral *shifters* similarly activate the brain's reward centers.

Addictive behaviors adversely affect millions of people. Alcohol is the most widely consumed potentially addictive substance (besides caffeine), with slightly over half of adult Americans reporting past month use. The National Survey on Drug Use and Health (NSDUH, 2015) reported that in 2014, 6.2% of all respondents were heavy alcohol users. Approximately 10.2% of Americans reported using an illicit drug in the past month (primarily marijuana and nonmedical prescription pain relievers). Tobacco use has slightly decreased since prior years but is still present in 66.9 million Americans ages 12 or older. Rates of behavioral addictions generally appear to be lower. Approximately 1% of the adult population has a severe gambling problem (Kessler et al., 2008), but 6 to 9% of young adults experience problems related to gambling (Barnes, Welte, Hoffman, & Tidwell, 2010). Internet gaming disorder is under consideration as an addictive behavior in DSM-5; prevalence rates vary in Europe and North America but may be as high as 8% for males and 5% for females in Asian countries (DSM-5, 2013).

What are the consequences of SUDs and addictive behaviors? There are many shared biological, psychological, and social consequences of different types of addictive behaviors. However, each addictive behavior may lead to unique consequences that warrant mentioning. Excessive alcohol consumption is one of the highest contributors to disease burden. Long-term consequences include liver disease (e.g., cirrhosis), heart disease, cancer, hepatitis, and pancreatitis. Short-term consequences of excessive alcohol consumption may include accidents, injuries, and academic or occupational difficulties. Excessive gambling may lead to financial problems and overwhelming debt. Individuals who smoke cigarettes experience a variety of medical illnesses, including but not limited to pulmonary and heart disease. Intravenous drug use may lead to infections (e.g., sepsis) and ultimately death.

Although marijuana is largely considered to be a "safe" substance in comparison to alcohol and other drugs, it is not without negative effects. Short-term consequences include difficulty thinking, problem solving, and impaired memory, while the long-term consequences may be impaired academic functioning for those who used heavily during adolescence (Meier et al., 2012). Other physical ailments may include breathing problems, increased heart rate, and child developmental delay for those who were exposed to marijuana in utero (National Institute on Drug Abuse [NIDA], 2016).

Mark Griffiths is another researcher who focuses on mechanisms underlying chemical and behavioral addictions. Griffiths (2005) describes six components of addiction that include (1) salience, (2) mood modification, (3) tolerance, (4) withdrawal, (5) conflict, and (6) relapse. *Salience* refers to the high degree of importance placed on the addictive behavior by the addicted person. The addictive behavior may become the most significant activity in life, dominating thoughts, feelings, and behaviors. Addicted individuals may spend most of their time engaging in addictive behaviors or thinking about future opportunities to do so. *Mood modification* occurs when the addictive behavior or substance use creates a subjective experience of momentary satisfaction (the "high"), which may eventually lead to self-medication in attempts to feel better, happier, or less depressed. *Tolerance* occurs when individuals require increasing amounts of a behavior or substance to attain former desired effects (e.g., requiring increased amounts of cocaine to achieve the same high or increasing the bet amount in gambling). *Withdrawal* symptoms are the psychological and physiological states that occur after discontinuing the activity or substance. It is important to note that physical withdrawal symptoms may occur in both substance and behavioral addictions. For example, in one study of pathological gamblers, 65% reported at least one physical symptom such as headaches, upset stomach, or loss of appetite while attempting to decrease or discontinue gambling (Rosenthal & Lesieur, 1992). *Conflict* refers to both *inter*personal and *intra*personal struggles resulting from addictive behaviors. Interpersonal difficulties may occur between addicted individuals and those around them, and intrapersonal conflict may occur when individuals are distressed about the consequences that result from their addictive behaviors. *Relapse* occurs when the individual reverts to previous patterns of addiction activity, violating a commitment to reduce or abstain from that activity. Griffiths (2005) asserts that the presence of all six components is necessary for a behavior to be defined as an addiction, and if the behavior does not interfere with one's functioning, it is likely not an addiction.

CBT MODEL OF SUDs AND ADDICTIVE BEHAVIORS

Our basic cognitive-behavioral model of SUDs and addictive behaviors (Figure 17.1) has not changed much over the last twenty-four years. In fact, our work with thousands of addicted individuals across diverse addictive behaviors has continually validated this model. We regularly observe that SUDs and addictive behaviors are maintained by self-reinforcing cycles of thoughts, feelings, and behaviors. The pattern is simple: following triggers that may be internal or external, learned addiction-related thoughts and beliefs are activated. These thoughts and beliefs contribute to urges and cravings to engage in addictive behaviors. And despite opportunities to abstain, addicted individuals continue to engage in their self-defeating behaviors, often with permission-granting thoughts that lead to lapse and relapse cycles.

A fictitious case example of binge eating (often characterized as addictive behavior) will help to illustrate our model. "Mary" is a 55-year-old divorced woman who lives alone and works at a factory job where she makes just enough money to pay her bills. Mary has struggled with addictions her whole life. At the present time, she only struggles with binge eating, though in the past she has been addicted to marijuana, alcohol, cocaine, cigarettes, gambling, and shopping. Figure 17.2 reflects Mary's typical thoughts, feelings, and behaviors associated with binge eating and her prior addictions. In Mary's case, external triggers like being alone, and internal emotional triggers such as loneliness, boredom, and despair activate addiction-related thoughts such as "I can't stand it," "I want to feel better," and "It'll taste so good." Mary's beliefs that overeating provides relief from loneliness lead her to experience urges to eat and craving for her favorite foods. Not included in this basic model but pertinent to Mary's beliefs are the distal antecedents that involve her relationship with food as a child. Growing up with unpredictably angry parents, Mary learned to view food as a source of comfort and fulfillment (more on the development of cognitive-behavioral patterns in the next section). After having these thoughts, Mary can choose to abstain from overeating (e.g. "I know I shouldn't be eating right now"), but she overrides this restrictive thought with permission by saying "What

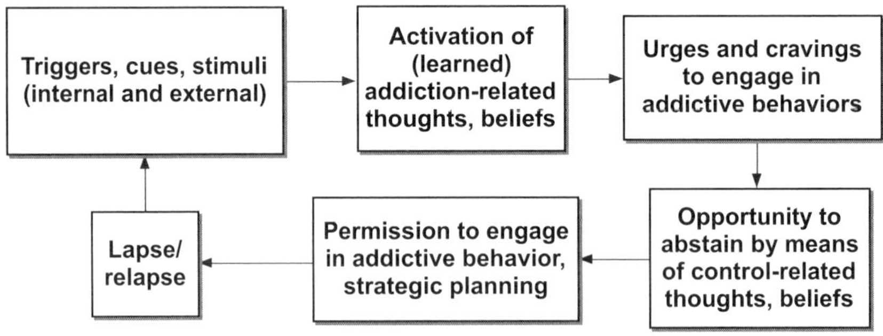

FIGURE 17.1. Basic CBT model of SUDs and addictive behaviors.

the heck. It doesn't matter anyway." Mary then engages in the instrumental behavior of driving to the grocery store and stocking up on her favorite junk foods (pizzas, chips, and ice cream). Finally, she binge eats all of the purchased food and then feels an even greater sense of despair.

This model is readily applied to other SUDs and addictive behaviors, including cigarette smoking, excessive drinking, problem gambling, and more. Figure 17.3 illustrates the fictitious case example of "Brian," who is addicted to marijuana. Brian regularly parties with friends who smoke marijuana. The sights, sounds, and smells of partying naturally trigger intense craving as Brian observes his friends getting high. Despite a desire to quit or cut down his marijuana consumption, he experiences automatic thoughts such as "I'd love to get stoned" and "Time to party." These thoughts cause strong craving for marijuana, but after having these thoughts Brian always has the option to abstain as he reminds himself, "I know I shouldn't be smoking weed." Brian instead gives himself permission to get high, thinking "No big deal" and "I can stop whenever I want." Brian proceeds to smoke several joints with his friends at the party.

In 1998, we introduced the developmental CBT model of substance use disorders and addictive behaviors (Liese & Franz, 1998). Since the introduction of this model, we have made some subtle modifications, somewhat influenced by the work of Shaffer et al. (2004, 2012), reflecting our greater understanding of distal and proximal antecedents. As can be seen in Figure 17.4, distal antecedents include neurobiological and psychosocial early-life experiences. These distal antecedents lead to cognitive, behavioral, and

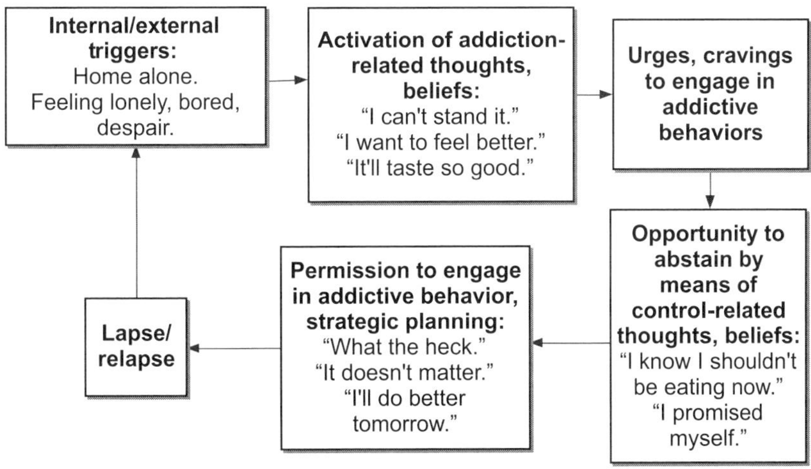

FIGURE 17.2. Cognitive-behavioral model of binge eating and the case of Mary.

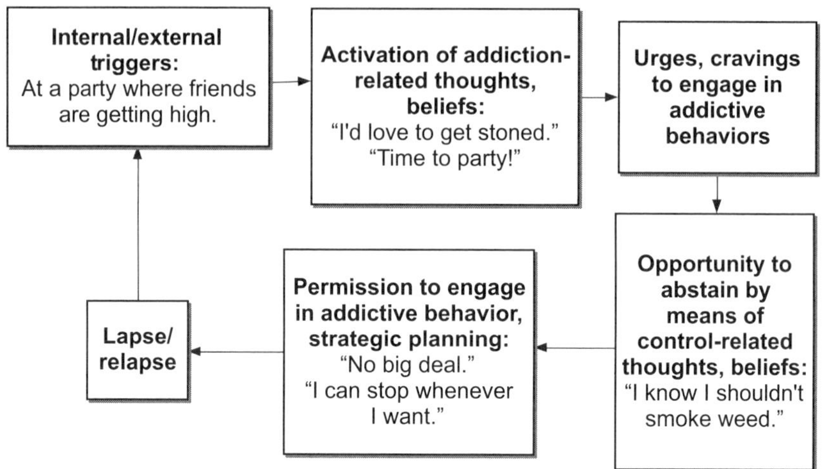

FIGURE 17.3. Cognitive-behavioral model of marijuana addiction and the case of Brian.

affective vulnerabilities to addiction. Most individuals who are exposed to and experiment with addictive substances and behaviors do not develop addictions. However, those who are cognitively, behaviorally, and affectively vulnerable to addictions go on to develop thoughts and beliefs that perpetuate addictive behaviors. As mentioned earlier, Mary struggled with various addictive behaviors for most of her life. These likely functioned as compensatory strategies to deal with maladaptive cognitive, behavioral, and affective processes that developed in her volatile home environment. It should also be mentioned here that Mary has an extensive family history of problems related to substance misuse, making it likely that she is genetically at risk for addictions. No doubt, all of these distal antecedents have led Mary to pursue instant gratification wherever she might find it.

CLINICAL APPLICATION OF CBT FOR SUDs AND ADDICTIVE BEHAVIORS

When we first began treating people with SUDs and addictive behaviors, we focused primarily on individual therapy. Then in the late 1990s another advance occurred: we began to develop *group* CBT for SUDs and addictive behaviors (Liese, Beck, & Seaton, 2002; Wenzel, Liese, Beck, & Friedman-Wheeler, 2012). Our first experiences with group CBT convinced us that both individual and group CBT were beneficial for people with addictions. Patients found each modality to be helpful, and many chose to participate

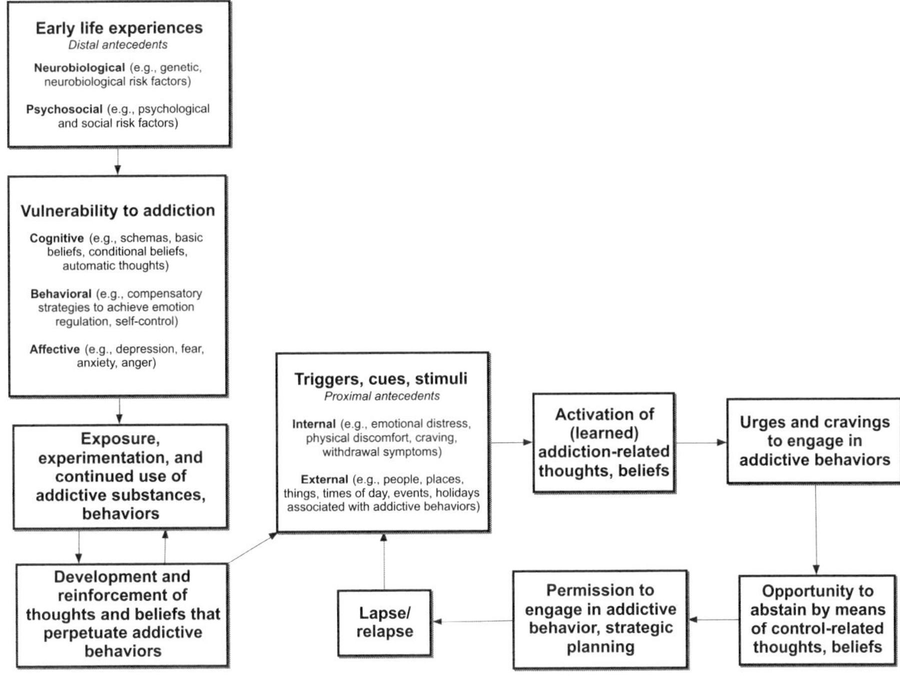

FIGURE 17.4. The developmental CBT model of SUDs and addictive behaviors.

in group and individual CBT concurrently, describing them as complementary. In this section, we discuss the clinical application of CBT for SUDs and addictive behaviors in both individual and group settings.

Cognitive-behavioral therapy for SUDs and addictive behaviors has five important components. While individual and group therapy for addictions differ in some important ways, both emphasize the importance of these components: (1) structure, (2) collaboration, (3) case conceptualization, (4) psychoeducation, and (5) specific techniques. Individual CBT sessions follow a carefully designed structure that includes the following elements: agenda setting, mood check, bridging from the last session (including any homework assigned), prioritizing and discussing agenda items, assigning new homework, feedback, and closure. At the beginning of each session, the therapist and patient work together to establish an agenda. Therapists ask questions like "What do you want to put on our agenda?" or "What would you like to work on today?" After generating a list of agenda items, they choose the items most important to the patient and discuss them with the intention of problem solving. It is important for patients to provide and prioritize agenda items for several reasons. First, doing so increases the likelihood that essential issues and concerns are discussed in each session. Second, it sets the stage for sessions that will be well structured. And third, asking patients for agenda items shows that patients are ultimately responsible for identifying and articulating their problems. Following agenda setting, therapists conduct a brief mood check to determine how the patient feels. This is particularly important since addictive behaviors often function to regulate emotions. Homework is another important component of cognitive therapy. Patients are reminded that they are only in therapy one of many hours per week, and their time outside of therapy is their opportunity to fully acquire and practice skills discussed in session. As with setting the agenda, homework assignments are chosen in a collaborative manner, with therapist and patient working together to determine appropriate assignments that continue the work begun in session. At the end of sessions, therapists are encouraged to summarize and elicit feedback by asking, "What have you gotten out of today's session?"

Group CBT for addictions is structured differently from individual CBT. Group CBT sessions average ninety minutes in length. Ideally, groups consist of five to eight members, and enrollment is open (i.e., "rolling"). Group members are welcome to concurrently pursue approaches that have been helpful in the past (e.g., individual psychotherapy, 12-step programs, SMART Recovery, and other mutual help programs). Individual members' goals are variable, with some members seeking help with abstinence, others seeking to reduce the harm associated with their addictive behaviors, and still others seeking new skills (e.g., emotion regulation, interpersonal communication, and impulse control strategies).

The elements of group CBT for addictions include facilitator introductions, member introductions, a presentation of problem-solving strategies (based on group member needs), the assignment of homework, and closure. Facilitators introduce themselves at the beginning of each group, providing reminders of group purpose, structure, and rules (e.g., regarding confidentiality). Following facilitator introductions, group members introduce themselves to the rest of the group. In addition to their names, group members describe their addictive behaviors, including the status of these behaviors. They discuss their goals for therapy, and in doing so they reveal their stage of readiness to change (Norcross, Krebs, & Prochaska, 2011). For example, a member who states "I am taking steps to stop smoking" might be considered in the preparation stage of change, while a member who states "I might eventually cut down on my drinking, but not yet" might be considered in the contemplation stage of change. It is likely that personal goals and readiness to change will vary *between* members and *within* members. For example, some group members may only be contemplating abstinence from gambling but maintaining years of abstinence from alcohol and cocaine. At the same time, other group members will likely still be engaged in their addictive behaviors, and some might even report that they don't yet need to change any behaviors (e.g., "I'm here because my wife is threatening divorce and I may learn something"). As a result, facilitators should be prepared to use harm-reduction strategies, skill-building strategies or abstinence-related strategies with patients.

Because cognitive-behavioral therapy tends to be more structured and goal-oriented than other types of therapy, it is important for therapists and patients to work in *collaboration* with one another throughout individual and group therapy. During individual therapy, collaboration involves the development of strong one-on-one relationships, while in group therapy this process is more complex. In the group context, the therapist must collaborate with individual group members and simultaneously facilitate collaboration between members.

Wishing to be helpful, some therapists urge patients to make changes before they are ready to do so. Insisting that patients change likely does more to alienate them than facilitate change. A common misconception of CBT is that change techniques are more important than collaboration, but in fact a collaborative relationship is the foundation on which therapy succeeds. Disregard for collaboration at the beginning of therapy will likely lead to patient dissatisfaction, disengagement from therapy, and dropout (Liese & Beck, 1996). Empathy is essential to collaboration in therapy. For example, consider a patient who presents in therapy with heavy drinking related to comorbid depression. A therapist who has difficulty understanding how depression can lead to addictive symptoms might blame the patient for relapse or for having difficulty practicing new skills. A high degree of empathy helps therapists better understand the kinds of thoughts that lead to relapses (e.g., "I'll never really feel better, so I may as well keep drinking") and difficulty completing homework (e.g., "I'm too hung over and depressed to get out of bed today. I'll just tell my therapist I couldn't get it done"). It is not uncommon for therapists to become frustrated with patients' addictive behaviors, relapses, and other self-destructive behaviors, especially if they are unfamiliar with addictive processes. It is essential for therapists to have a foundational knowledge of addictive behaviors and genuinely empathize with patients.

Also important to the collaborative process is setting mutual goals for therapy. Many patients initiate therapy hoping to change certain behaviors without realizing they are not ready to make these changes. Therapists are encouraged to work with patients to create appropriate and achievable goals. Although therapists might believe that abstinence from the substance or behavior is best for patients, it is important for therapists to "meet patients where they're at" in their readiness to change. This is not to imply that therapists have no say in helping the patient increase readiness, but therapists should be prepared to witness lapses and relapses without reacting negatively. Techniques such as motivational interviewing or harm reduction are appropriate when patients continue to engage in addictive behaviors despite negative health, psychological, or social consequences. However, as with any negotiation in therapy, the goal-setting process might lead to ruptures in the alliance (Safran, Muran, & Eubanks-Carter, 2011). These ruptures might result from differences between therapists' and patients' beliefs about the appropriateness of each other's goals. Therapists should pay close attention to rupture markers (e.g., patient anger, dissatisfaction, or withdrawal) and attempt to thoroughly discuss and effectively repair ruptures. Ruptures may actually create opportunities to strengthen the therapeutic alliance and help patients make even further gains—as long as they are satisfactorily repaired (Safran et al., 2011; Stiles et al., 2004).

Also important to CBT for treating SUDs and addictions is the *case conceptualization*. Therapists should take all necessary steps to understand patients' presenting problems, current life issues, and developmental history in order to have a greater understanding of the processes contributing to current addictive behaviors. Essential to this process is therapist empathy in that therapists might misconstrue or ignore important information without empathetic listening. Therapists should convey the case conceptualization directly to patients in order to provide them with a clear understanding of the various processes contributing to their addictive behaviors (e.g., maladaptive thoughts, traumatic childhood experiences, current relationship difficulties). This conveying of information provides a greater sense of collaboration between therapists and patients and helps patients feel empowered to change by providing a greater understanding of the processes contributing to their addictive behaviors.

The case conceptualization helps therapists make decisions about the choice and timing of interventions. While some therapists are most concerned with targeting proximal (current) addiction triggers, thoughts, feelings, and behaviors, it is important to be cognizant of distal factors (i.e., childhood and past experiences) that contribute to current addictive behaviors. Take for example Mary, who grew up in an emotionally abusive home where she was told, "You are stupid." When Mary first experimented with drugs as an adolescent, she learned that she did not feel stupid while she was high on marijuana or other drugs. She also found that eating her favorite foods effectively distracted her from emotional distress. Drug use and food consumption were therefore influenced by her distal experiences. Important background information like this should not be ignored in conceptualizing her case. When Mary recognizes that she overeats in an effort to find comfort (as she learned to do as a child), she better understands that she needs to find comfort in healthier ways.

Comorbid disorders including depression, anxiety, personality disorders, and schizophrenia are common among individuals with SUDs and addictive behaviors. However, rather than treat the comorbid disorder as a separate entity, it is important for clinicians to treat all psychological problems concurrently. While some disorders such as schizophrenia or bipolar disorder typically require pharmacotherapy, other disorders including depression, personality disorders, and anxiety are likely to respond well to CBT alone. Integrating the comorbid disorder into the case conceptualization helps clinicians understand how the disorder is contributing to the patient's addictive behaviors. Many addicted individuals report that they are using drugs to "self-medicate." Hence, acquiring skills to cope with emotional distress is especially important for patients who report that they are self-medicating. For example, individuals with social anxiety who use alcohol in social situations to reduce anxiety will likely benefit from interventions that challenge thoughts related to fear of social judgment. As they are able to challenge thoughts and beliefs that lead to anxiety, the need to self-medicate with alcohol likely decreases.

As is true regarding collaboration, case conceptualization is more complex in group therapy than individual therapy. In addition to conceptualizing individual group members, therapists must conceptualize group dynamics (e.g., cohesiveness, conflict, modeling, etc.) and then address these dynamics.

Also important for treating SUDs and addiction is *psychoeducation*, the deliberate facilitation of learning and skill acquisition. The process of psychoeducation is sometimes referred to as socialization because its aim is to profoundly influence how patients view themselves, their personal worlds, their relationships, and their future. Some examples of psychoeducation include discussing the general CBT model, the positive and negative effects of substance use, and how substance use may affect thoughts, feelings, and behaviors. Patients with addictive behaviors often struggle with personal issues for years prior to entering CBT, and many have engaged in other types of treatment (e.g., 12-step programs) that are not CBT-based. Clinicians are encouraged to work collaboratively as they orient patients to the CBT approach and to be patient with those who have difficulty understanding various concepts (e.g., schemas, basic beliefs, and automatic thoughts). Therapy is less effective when therapists and patients cannot understand each other's views, and therefore clinicians should regularly check patients' understanding—especially during sessions that are highly education-oriented. Ultimately, the goal of CBT for SUDs and addictions is to create a learning environment where skills are acquired and applied in the "real world" so the therapist is no longer needed.

A strongly emphasized concept in CBT is that *thoughts influence feelings and behaviors* (i.e., "You *are* what you *think*"). Many patients enter therapy blaming external circumstances for their problems or emotional difficulties, and it is important for therapists to emphasize that emotions are largely influenced by patients' own internal processes. For example, patients who continually attribute emotions and behaviors to external causes (e.g., "He hurt my feelings" or "I started drinking because everyone else at the party was drinking") should be reminded that their emotions and behaviors are best understood as products of their own thoughts and beliefs. This will help patients in future high-risk situations to ask themselves, "What am I thinking that's causing me to feel the way I do?" and "What are the thoughts leading to my addictive behaviors?"

Techniques are structured activities designed to facilitate skill development. Examples of techniques include the daily thought record, advantages–disadvantages analysis, scaling, functional analysis, and more. In some ways, these techniques are easier to teach in a group CBT setting because they can be learned from direct instruction or vicariously, as group members watch each other develop important skills. As previously mentioned, techniques are considered to be the "tools" that patients are taught and encouraged to practice during the course of therapy. It is hoped that they put these skills to use so that they will no longer need the therapist's help and can conduct, for example, an advantages–disadvantage analysis on their own.

As mentioned earlier, the five main components of CBT (structure, collaboration, case conceptualization, psychoeducation, and techniques) work in conjunction with each other. For example, an accurate case conceptualization facilitates timely and effective psychoeducation, structure, and the appropriate application of techniques. At the same time, when shared with patients, it facilitates a more collaborative relationship. When therapy is well structured and collaborative, the case is well conceptualized, psychoeducation is effectively presented, and techniques are timely and customized to patients' needs, patients tend to believe, "This therapy makes sense and is likely to help me."

RESEARCH ON CBT FOR SUDs AND ADDICTIVE BEHAVIORS

Cognitive-behavioral therapy for individuals with SUDs and addictions, including alcohol and illicit drug use disorders, has been shown to have significant effects in various meta-analyses (e.g., Magill & Ray, 2009). In the largest meta-analysis of randomized controlled trials (RCTs) for substance use disorders, Magill and Ray found that CBT had statistically significant effects compared to other treatment approaches. They reported that 58% of subjects receiving CBT did better than subjects in the comparison condition and that 79% of subjects treated with CBT did better than subjects receiving no treatment. Reflecting the chronic nature of addictions, they also found that effects for CBT diminished over time, with lower effects at six- to nine-month follow-ups and much lower effects at twelve months. These findings are analogous to research on chronic medical conditions (e.g., diabetes), where symptoms worsen when treatment is discontinued. Magill and Ray also found that women benefited more from CBT than men, and CBT for marijuana use disorder demonstrated larger effect sizes than effect sizes found when treating other substance use disorders. And finally, no differences in effects were found between individual and group CBT modalities for treating addictions. It has been hypothesized that CBT leads to long-term and lasting changes due to its emphasis on skill development that may at first lead to abstinence but may also apply to a wide variety of co-occurring issues (Carrol & Onken, 2005). Another meta-analysis found relapse prevention, a CBT treatment that focuses on immediate and distal mechanisms that lead to relapse, effective in treating several substance use disorders, including alcohol, smoking, and polysubstance disorders (Irvin, Bowers, Dunn, & Wang, 1999). Another study demonstrated that despite initially revealing less significant effects than a contingency management treatment, CBT had more durable effects one year posttreatment (Epstein, Hawkins, Covi, Umbritch, & Preston, 2003).

CBT has also been shown to be effective in treating nicotine dependence (Webb, de Ybarra, Baker, Reis, & Carey, 2010; Marks & Sykes, 2002) and Internet gaming disorder (Young, 2013). Several studies have used CBT in addition to pharmacotherapy (e.g., nicotine replacement therapy) in treating nicotine dependence. For example, Marks and Sykes's (2002) randomized controlled trial of CBT with economically disadvantaged individuals found that one in five smokers who received CBT was fully abstinent twelve months postintervention. The authors also found that CBT was significantly more efficacious and cost effective than health education or advice alone. Webb and colleagues' (2010) RCT of group-based CBT for smoking cessation among African Americans found that in comparison to general health education, CBT showed higher abstinence over time.

Although Internet gaming disorder has yet to be examined in RCTs, a preliminary study found that after receiving twelve weeks of CBT for Internet addiction, 95% of participants were able to manage their symptoms and 78% kept those gains after six months (Young, 2013).

Compulsive buying might be well understood as an addictive behavior, though it is not currently characterized as such in DSM-5. It is easily argued that compulsive buying warrants further research and treatment, given the economic burden and psychological suffering often associated with it. Although there are no known RCTs that have examined CBT for compulsive buying, a preliminary trial found group CBT to be superior to a telephone guided self-help condition (Müller, Arikian, Zwaan, & Mitchell, 2013). Overall, CBT appears to be an effective treatment for a wide range of SUDs and addictive behaviors.

As previously discussed, addictive behaviors frequently co-occur with other psychological disorders. The prevalence of SUDs among individuals with a mood disorder or anxiety disorder is approximately 20% and 15%, respectively (Grant et al., 2004). The presence of a psychological disorder increases the risk of future nicotine, alcohol, or drug dependence

(Swendsen et al., 2010). Addictive behaviors may also increase one's risk for future mental illness, as they may lead to trauma exposure and negative side effects of the substances or behaviors. The DSM-5 also contains several "substance-induced" disorders (e.g., substance-induced mood disorder, psychotic disorder, sleep disorder), which are a direct result of substance use. RCTs have demonstrated that CBT for co-occurring disorders is effective in treating both disorders simultaneously. For example, one study found that integrated CBT for comorbid depression and substance dependence showed more substantial decreases in substance use over time compared to a 12-step facilitation treatment (Lydecker et al., 2010). Another study found that CBT for depression demonstrated greater decreases in substance use and depressive symptoms and negative consequences from using over time compared to a usual care group (Hunter et al., 2012). It is not uncommon for CBT to be offered in conjunction with other interventions for individuals with comorbid disorders. For example, CBT may be combined with mindfulness meditation for individuals with comorbid anxiety or depression. Integrated CBT (ICBT) for comorbid posttraumatic stress disorder (PTSD) and substance use that included mindful relaxation and flexible thinking demonstrated reductions in PTSD symptoms and produced better outcomes in toxicology screens than the other two conditions (individual addiction counseling and standard care; McGovern et al., 2015). Those in the ICBT condition also self-reported less illicit drug use than the standard care group.

CONCLUSIONS

In this chapter, we have described advances in cognitive-behavioral therapy for SUDs and addictive behaviors. Over the years we have made some changes to our approach, but most of these changes reflect advances in the field of addiction psychology. For example, in the past it had been thought that addictions must involve the ingestion of *substances* (e.g., alcohol, nicotine, marijuana, opioids), but recently experts have agreed that *behaviors* can be addictive (e.g., gambling, Internet gaming). Furthermore, it is now well understood that chemical and behavioral addictions can be equally refractory and devastating.

Almost twenty years ago, we published a chapter outlining lessons learned while providing cognitive therapy to people with SUDs and addictive behaviors (Liese & Franz, 1998). It should not come as a surprise that many of the lessons learned back then are still pertinent today. For example, when treating people with SUDs and addictions, we are continually reminded that addictive behaviors function as compensatory strategies for individuals who have not developed effective coping skills. Therefore, a substantial component of therapy must involve skill building (e.g., emotion regulation, impulse control, interpersonal skills). We continue to understand that CBT consists of interrelated components that are all important (i.e., structure, collaboration, case conceptualization, psychoeducation, and techniques); none should be overlooked or minimized in treating SUDs and addictions. We regularly find that relationship ruptures are common when treating people with addictive behaviors. Ruptures may result when therapists become frustrated with patients or patients become frustrated with therapists—especially when they do not agree on goals or a time frame for making changes. It is essential for therapists to understand how these ruptures occur and to resolve them in ways that enable the therapeutic relationship to grow. Finally, given the pervasiveness of addictive behaviors and their comorbidity with other psychological conditions, all therapists should be open to participating in the diagnosis and treatment of SUDs and addictive behaviors (Liese & Reis, 2016).

Over a quarter-century ago, Dr. Beck wrote a now classic *American Psychologist* article as a thirty-year retrospective of cognitive therapy (Beck, 1991). The last two sentences of his article are poignant: "At this point in time, cognitive therapy is no longer fledgling and has demonstrated its capacity to fly under its own power. How far it will fly remains to be seen" (p. 374). We feel fortunate to have been in the right place at the right time with Dr. Beck, applying CBT to such an important and salient mental health issue. We are now confident in the value of CBT for treating SUDs and addictive behaviors and, like Beck back in 1991, we look forward to seeing how far it will fly.

REFERENCES

American Psychiatric Association. (1994). *Diagnostic and statistical manual of mental disorders* (4th ed.). Washington, DC: Author.

American Psychiatric Association. (2013). *Diagnostic and statistical manual of mental disorders* (5th ed.). Arlington, VA: Author.

Barnes, G. M., Welte, J. W., Hoffman, J. H., & Tidwell, M. O. (2010). Comparisons of gambling and alcohol use among college students and noncollege young people in the United States. *Journal of American College Health, 58*(5), 443–452.

Beck, A. T. (1991). Cognitive therapy: A 30-year retrospective. *American Psychologist, 46*(4), 368–375.

Beck, A. T., Wright, F. D., Newman, C. F., & Liese, B. S. (1993). *Cognitive therapy of substance abuse.* New York: Guilford Press.

Beck, J. S. (2011). *Cognitive behavior therapy: Basics and beyond* (2nd ed.). New York: Guilford Press.

Carroll, K. M., & Onken, L. S. (2005). Behavioral therapies for drug abuse. *American Journal of Psychiatry, 162*(8), 1452–1460.

Epstein, D. H., Hawkins, W. E., Covi, L., Umbricht, A., & Preston, K. L. (2003). Cognitive-behavioral therapy plus contingency management for cocaine use:

Findings during treatment and across 12-month follow-up. *Psychology of Addictive Behaviors, 17*(1), 73–82.

Fortune, E. E., & Goodie, A. S. (2013). Cognitive distortions as a component and treatment focus of pathological gambling: A review. *Psychology of Addictive Behaviors, 26*(2), 298–310.

Goodie, A. S., & Fortune, E. E. (2013). Measuring cognitive distortions in pathological gambling: Review and meta-analysis. *Psychology of Addictive Behaviors, 27*(3), 730–743.

Grant, B. F., Stinson, F. S., Dawson, D. A., Chou, P., Dufour, M. C., Compton, W., . . . Kaplan, K. (2004). Prevalence and co-occurrence of substance use disorders and independent mood and anxiety disorders: Results from the National Epidemiologic Survey on Alcohol and Related Conditions. *Archives of General Psychiatry, 61*(8), 807–816.

Grant, J. E., Potenza, M. N., Weinstein, A., & Gorelick, D. A. (2010). Introduction to behavioral addictions. *American Journal of Drug Abuse, 36*(5), 233–241.

Griffiths, M. E. (2005). A "components" model of addiction within a biopsychosocial framework. *Journal of Substance Use, 10*(4), 191–197.

Grilo, C. M., Masheb, R. M., Wilson, G. T., Gueorguieva, R., & White, M. A. (2011). Cognitive-behavioral therapy, behavioral weight loss, and sequential treatment for obese patients with binge-eating disorder: A randomized controlled trial. *Journal of Consulting and Clinical Psychology, 79*(5), 675–685.

Hunter, S. B., Witkiewitz, K., Watkins, K. E., Paddock, S. M., & Hepner, K. A. (2012). The moderating effects of group cognitive-behavioral therapy for depression among substance users. *Psychology of Addictive Behaviors, 26*(4), 906–916.

Irvin, J. E., Bowers, C. A., Dunn, M. E., & Wang, M. C. (1999). Efficacy of relapse prevention: A meta-analytic review. *Journal of Consulting and Clinical Psychology, 67*(4), 563–570.

Kessler, R. C., Hwang, I., LaBrie, R., Petukhova, M., Sampson, N. A., Winters, K. C., . . . Schaffer, H. J. (2008). DSM-IV pathological gambling in the National Comorbidity Survey Replication. *Psychological Medicine, 38*(9), 1351–1360.

Liese, B. S. (2014). Cognitive-behavioral therapy for people with addictions. In S. L. A. Straussner (Ed.), *Clinical work with substance abusing clients* (3rd ed., pp. 225–250). New York: Guilford Press.

Liese, B. S., & Beck, A. T. (1996). Back to basics: Fundamental cognitive therapy skills for keeping drug-dependent individuals in treatment. In L. S. Onken, J. D. Blain, & J. J. Boren (Eds.), *Beyond the therapeutic alliance: Keeping drug dependent individuals in treatment* (pp. 210–235). Washington, DC: U.S. Government Printing Office.

Liese, B. S., Beck, A. T., & Seaton, K. (2002). The cognitive therapy addictions group. In D. W. Brook & H. I. Spitzer (Eds.), *Group psychotherapy of substance abuse* (pp. 37–57). New York: Haworth Medical Press.

Liese, B. S., & Franz, R. A. (1998). Treating substance use disorders with cognitive therapy: Lessons learned and implications for the future. In P. Salkavskis (Ed.), *Frontiers of cognitive therapy* (pp. 470–508). New York: Guilford Press.

Liese, B. S., & Reis, D. J. (2016). Failing to diagnose and failing to treat an addicted client: Two potentially life threatening clinical errors. *Psychotherapy, 53*(3), 342–346.

Lydecker, K. P., Tate, S. R., Cummins, K. M., McQuaid, J., Granholm, E., & Brown, S. A. (2010). Clinical outcomes of an integrated treatment for depression and substance use disorders. *Psychology of Addictive Behaviors, 24*(3), 453–465.

Magill, M., & Ray, L. A. (2009). Cognitive-behavioral treatment with adult alcohol and illicit drug users: A meta-analysis of randomized controlled trials. *Journal of Studies on Alcohol and Drugs, 70*(4), 516–527.

Marks, D. F., & Sykes, C. M. (2002). Randomized controlled trial of cognitive behavioural therapy for smokers living in a deprived area of London: Outcome at one-year follow-up. *Psychology, Health and Medicine, 7*(1), 17–24.

McGovern, M. P., Lambert-Harris, C., Xie, H., Meier, A., McLeman, B., & Saunders, E. (2015). A randomized controlled trial of treatments for co-occurring substance use disorders and post-traumatic stress disorder. *Addiction, 110*(7), 1194–1204.

Meier, M. H., Caspi, A., Ambler, A., Harrington, H., Houts, R., Keefe, R. E., . . . Moffitt, T. E. (2012). Persistent cannabis users show neuropsychological decline from childhood to midlife. *Proceedings of the National Academy of Sciences of the United States of America, 109*(40), E2657–E2664.

Merrill, J. E., Read, J. P., & Barnett, N. P. (2013). The way one thinks affects the way one drinks: Subjective evaluations of alcohol consequences predict subsequent change in drinking behavior. *Psychology of Addictive Behaviors, 27*(1), 42–51.

Müller, A., Arikian, A., Zwaan, M., & Mitchell, J. E. (2013). Cognitive-behavioural group therapy versus guided self-help for compulsive buying disorder: A preliminary study. *Clinical Psychology Psychotherapy, 20*(1), 28–35.

National Institute on Drug Abuse (NIDA). (2016). DrugFacts: Marijuana. Retrieved from *www.drugabuse.gov/publications/drugfacts/marijuana.*

Norcross, J. C., Krebs, P. M., & Prochaska, J. O. (2011). Stages of change. *Journal of Clinical Psychology, 67*(2), 143–154.

Rosenthal, R., & Lesieur, H. (1992). Self-reported withdrawal symptoms and pathological gambling. *American Journal of the Addictions, 1,* 150–154.

Safran, J. D., Muran, J. C., & Eubanks-Carter, C. (2011). Repairing alliance ruptures. *Psychotherapy, 48*(1), 80–87.

Shaffer, H. J., LaPlante, D. A., LaBrie, R. A., Kidman, R. C., Donato, A. N., & Stanton, M. V. (2004). Toward a syndrome model of addiction: Multiple expressions, common etiology. *Harvard Review of Psychiatry, 12*(6), 367–374.

Shaffer, H. J., LaPlante, D. A., & Nelson, S. E. (2012). *APA addiction syndrome handbook: Vol. 1. Foundations, influences, and expressions of addiction.* Washington, DC: American Psychological Association.

Shorey, R. C., Anderson, S., & Stuart, G. L. (2012). Gambling and early maladaptive schemas in a treatment-seeking sample of male alcohol users: A preliminary investigation. *Addictive Disorders and Their Treatment, 11*(4), 173–182.

Stiles, W. B., Glick, M. J., Osatuke, K., Hardy, G. E., Shapiro, D. A., Agnew-Davies, R., . . . Barkham, M. (2004). Patterns of alliance development and the rupture–repair hypothesis: Are positive relationships U-shaped or V-shaped? *Journal of Counseling Psychology, 51*(1), 81–92.

Swendsen, J., Conway, K. P., Degenhardt, L., Glantz, M., Jin, R., Merikangas, K. R., . . . Kessler, R. C. (2010). Mental disorders as risk factors for substance use, abuse and dependence: Results from the 10-year follow-up of the National Comorbidity Survey. *Addiction, 105*(6), 1117–1128.

Webb, M. S., de Ybarra, D. R., Baker, E. A., Reis, I. M., & Carey, M. P. (2010). Cognitive-behavioral therapy to promote smoking cessation among African American smokers: A randomized clinical trial. *Journal of Consulting and Clinical Psychology, 78*(1), 24–33.

Wenzel, A., Liese, B. S., Beck, A. T., & Friedman-Wheeler, D. G. (2012). *Group cognitive therapy of addictions.* New York: Guilford Press.

Young, K. S. (2013). Treatment outcomes using CBT-IA with Internet-addicted patients. *Journal of Behavioral Addictions, 2*(4), 209–215.

CHAPTER 18

Cognitive Therapy for Anxiety

David A. Clark

Everyone experiences mild to moderate anxiety and worry at least occasionally. Although anxiety, worry, and their underlying basic emotion, fear, are ubiquitous to the human condition, millions of individuals struggle with more extreme forms of fear and anxiety referred to as the "anxiety disorders." Threat is the core feature of both fear and anxiety, with fear being a more automatic emotion response to imminent danger, and anxiety a more diffuse, generalized tension and preparation for anticipated future negative outcomes (American Psychiatric Association, 2013).

Fear, as a universal emotion, is the affect at the heart of anxiety (Barlow, 2002). In the original cognitive theory of anxiety, Beck and colleagues considered fear the appraisal of actual or potential danger in a specific situation and anxiety as the emotional response evoked by fear (Beck, Emery, & Greenberg, 1985). More recently, D. A. Clark and Beck (2010) defined anxiety as

> a complex cognitive, affective, physiological and behavioral response system (i.e., threat mode) that is activated when anticipated events or circumstances are deemed to be highly aversive because they are perceived to be unpredictable, uncontrollable events that potentially threaten the vital interests of an individual. (p. 5)

The cognitive perspective assumes a continuity between normal and abnormal anxiety and fear, with fear distinguished by (1) the presence of maladaptive and biased cognitive processes, (2) greater interference in daily functioning, (3) elevated distress and persistence, (4) reliance on maladaptive coping and safety seeking, and (5) hypersensitivity to threat and danger cues (D. A. Clark & Beck, 2010).

With the publication of DSM-5, changes were made in the anxiety disorder classification scheme (APA, 2013). Separation anxiety disorder and selective mutism were added to the class of anxiety disorders, and obsessive–compulsive disorder (OCD) and posttraumatic stress disorder (PTSD) were moved to separate classification categories. However, five disorders—specific phobia (SP), social anxiety disorder (SAD), panic disorder (PD), agoraphobia (AG), and generalized anxiety disorder (GAD)—continue to form the core of the DSM-5 anxiety disorder classification and are the most common types of anxiety seen in clinical settings.

The anxiety disorders constitute the most prevalent form of mental health problem, affecting hundreds of millions of people globally. Estimates of the twelve-month prevalence of any type of anxiety disorder range from a low of 2.4% in Shanghai, China, to 18.2% in the United States (Kessler, Chiu, Demler, & Walters, 2005; WHO World Mental Health Surveys, 2004). Approximately twice as many women experience an anxiety disorder, with anxiety often persisting over many years at the clinical or subclinical symptom level (Craske, 2003; McLean, Asnaani, Liz, & Hofmann, 2011). Individuals with multiple anxiety disorders and those with SAD and AG may experience a more chronic course (Hendriks, Spiujker, Licht, Beekman, & Penninx, 2013). Presence of an anxiety disorder is associated with significant functional impairment and reduced quality of life (Olatunji, Cisler, & Tolin, 2007). Most anxiety disorders begin in late childhood to early adulthood and are associated with significant treatment-seeking delay often lasting many years (Kessler, Berglund, Demler, Jin, Merikangas, & Walters, 2005; Wang et al., 2005). Most individuals with an anxiety disorder have another coexisting disorder, with major depression, substance use disorder, and another anxiety disorder most common (Brown, Campbell, Lehman, Grisham, & Mancill, 2001; Kessler, Chiu, Demler, & Walters, 2005). The vast majority of individuals with anxiety disorders fail to seek treatment, despite the development of highly effective treatments such as cognitive therapy and exposure-based interventions (Johnson & Coles, 2013). In fact, cognitive therapy (CT) or cognitive-behavioral therapy (CBT), is now considered an empirically established first-line treatment for many anxiety disorders (e.g., Chambless et al., 1998; NICE, 2011).

This chapter provides an overview of the cognitive-behavioral perspective on the anxiety disorders. It begins by delineating the core psychological features of clinical anxiety and how each feature is expressed in the specific anxiety disorders. Next the cognitive model of anxiety is presented along with an evaluation of the empirical support for various constructs in the model. This is followed by a consideration of the treatment implications of the model. The chapter concludes with the ongoing debate about the necessity and sufficiency of cognitive interventions for the anxiety disorders as well as a consideration of future directions for cognitive research and treatment of anxiety.

CORE CLINICAL FEATURES OF ANXIETY

Several core features of anxiety guide psychological theory, research, and treatment of these disorders. Like other perspectives on anxiety, the cognitive model addresses each of these constructs in its conceptualization and treatment approach.

Exaggerated Threat

A central feature of the anxiety disorders is the presence of an information-processing bias for threat (e.g., Mathews & MacLeod, 1994). This takes the form of overestimating the probability and severity of threat or danger, as well as a biased assumption that the potential harm may be closer in time and location (Craske, 2003). Riskind (1997) argued that clinical anxiety is also characterized by an exaggerated sense that threat or danger is looming, that is, temporally accelerating toward the person faster than would be expected. Together these processes cause the anxious individual to be hypervigilant for threat cues. In SAD, the exaggerated threat involves the possibility of negative evaluation by others; in GAD, the threat is that of future negative life experiences; and in PD it is a specific inexplicable physical sensation such as the sudden occurrence of heart palpitations or shortness of breath.

Heightened Physiological Arousal

It has long been noted that elevated autonomic arousal is a prominent symptom of clinical anxiety (Barlow, 2002; Gray, 1987). However, more recent research indicates that physiological arousal may be more characteristic of panic attacks and less evident in other anxiety disorders such as GAD, blood/injury phobias, or anxiety more generally (Brown, Chorpita, & Barlow, 1998; Longley, Watson, Noyes, & Yoder, 2006). Nevertheless, panic attacks are often present in SAD, SP, and AG, so that elevated physiological arousal may be an important, albeit secondary, feature of certain anxiety disorders. Because of the prominence of autonomic arousal, various relaxation-based interventions have been used to treat anxiety with varying degrees of success. The rationale is that by dampening down the hyperaroused sympathetic nervous system, anxiety will subside. However, in CBT, relaxation strategies are considered optional and not the most effective way to deactivate the threat-based system that is hypervalent in anxiety. This is because relaxation could become a safety cue that individuals use to curtail the anxious state, which then undermines the processing of disconfirming evidence that their feared consequence is unrealistic.

High Negative Affect

Anxiety involves the higher-order negative emotion state or general distress termed *negative affect* (NA; Mineka, Watson, & L. A. Clark, 1998). Individuals with anxiety disorders tend to experience more NA, with significant correlations between the construct and anxious symptoms and disorders (e.g., Watson & Naragon-Gainey, 2014). However, high NA is common to anxiety and depression, and so it may be one of the common factors that account for the high comorbidity among the emotional disorders (Mineka et al., 1998). Because anxious feelings are highly unpleasant, individuals are so motivated to avoid or at least minimize their anxiousness that anxiety reduction itself can be a significant reinforcement (Gray, 1987). More recently, distress tolerance—that is, "the capacity to effectively manage emotional states" (p. 106)—has been linked to anxiety sensitivity as an individual difference variable that may amplify the intensity and persistence of clinical anxiety (Schmidt, Mitchell, Keough, & Riccardi, 2011).

Safety-Seeking and Avoidance

Finally, the strategies used to minimize or eliminate anxiety are considered important contributors to the etiology and maintenance of the disorder. Because of their importance in early learning theories of fear and anxiety, elimination of escape, avoidance, and other safety-seeking behaviors has been a critical focus of behavior therapy. In fact, avoidance is such a prominent symptom feature of anxiety that it is included in the DSM-5 diagnostic criteria of SAD, AG, SP, and, to a lesser extent, PD (APA, 2013). The pervasiveness of avoidance is considered one indicator of the severity of the anxiety disorder (Barlow, 2002). In addition to active avoidance of fear stimuli, defensive reactions may be present such as withdrawal, freezing, aggression, and appeasement or submission responses (Marks, 1987). Avoidance of external situational triggers is most common, especially in AG, but practically any cue associated with anxiety can be avoided such as physical sensations, activity, certain feeling states, thoughts, images, or memories, and the like (Barlow, 2002).

Safety-seeking behaviors refer to a broad range of responses that anxious individuals employ to manage anxiety because they believe these actions reduce the likelihood of an anticipated danger (Salkovskis, 1991). Examples of safety-seeking include the person with AG who can manage a grocery store when accompanied by a trusted friend but experiences a panic attack if entering the situation alone; the individual with PD who is less anxious knowing her benzodiazepine medication is in her purse; or the person with SAD who wears extra clothing to conceal sweating in social situations.

Cognitive accounts of anxiety argue that safety-seeking and avoidance contribute to anxiety persistence because they prevent exposure to disconfirming evidence that the threatening outcome will not occur (i.e., Salkovskis, 1996). Thus, reduction of avoidance and safety-seeking responses is an important ingredient of CBT for anxiety. Current inhibitory learning models argue that safety-seeking behaviors can interfere in the development of inhibitory associations and so should be phased out when doing exposure-based therapy (Craske et al., 2014). However, the antitherapeutic effects of safety-seeking have been questioned and by extension their role in the persistence of anxiety (i.e., see Rachman, Radomsky, & Shafran, 2008). In a recent meta-analysis of twenty-three CBT outcome studies that compared presence versus absence of safety-seeking behaviors, there was a slight advantage for exposure without safety-seeking, although the findings were so mixed that the authors concluded that the removal or addition of safety-seeking during exposure had minimal therapeutic impact (Meudlers, Daele, Volders, & Vlaeyen, 2016). A systematic literature review indicated that restorative safety-seeking that does not interfere with threat confrontation does not hinder the effectiveness of exposure, but preventive safety-seeking that reduces the intensity of contact with a threat stimulus does weaken exposure (Goetz, Davine, Siwiec, & Lee, 2016). In sum, the role of avoidance and safety-seeking in anxiety is still a matter of considerable debate. At the very least, the current research indicates that therapists may want to be less dogmatic about the complete elimination of all safety-seeking when treating the anxiety disorders.

THE COGNITIVE MODEL OF ANXIETY

Daily living involves exposure to myriad threats, dangers, risks, ambiguities, and uncertainties that vary in their personal significance and intensity. It has long been observed that people differ greatly in their emotional response and ability to cope with life's difficulties and problems. It is a basic premise of the cognitive perspective that individual differences in the propensity to experience anxiety resides in how individuals process or understand threat and danger. In fact, the various cognitive models of anxiety are based on the proposition that the type and intensity of emotion are determined by how the situation is appraised (Ehring, 2014). Anxiety occurs when individuals exhibit a bias to evaluate situations as a significant threat to personal vital resources, whereas depression occurs when there is a negative bias to appraise experiences as a loss of access to vital resources

(Beck & Haigh, 2014). The following overview presents the basic tenets of the cognitive perspective on anxiety disorders but is based primarily on the cognitive model of anxiety first formulated by Beck and colleagues in *Anxiety Disorders and Phobias: A Cognitive Perspective* (1985) and later elaborated and refined by D. A. Clark and Beck (2010). Although varying in emphasis, many of the cognitive constructs found in the Beck model are fundamental processes in the disorder-specific CBT models proposed for SAD, PD, and GAD (i.e., D. M. Clark, 1986; Rapee & Heimberg, 1997; Wells, 2006).

Automatic Attentional Bias for Threat

An attentional bias for threat and danger at both the automatic (subliminal) and strategic (supraliminal) levels of information processing is a robust phenomenon that characterizes trait anxiety and its disorders (for reviews, see Bar-Haim, Lamy, Bakermans-Franenburg, Pergamin, & van Ijzendoorn, 2007; D. A. Clark & Beck, 2010; de Jong, 2014; Mathews & MacLeod, 2005). For example, in spider phobia, the individual immediately detects a small spider web in the far corner as she walks to the front door of her house. Unconsciously, her visual scanning has picked out the small web. Once detected, she becomes very aware of the web and begins to intentionally search for the presence of a spider, thinking how terrified she'll feel if a spider is found. In the Beck model, the preconscious attentional threat bias is the product of schema activation that serves a self-protective adaptation function focused on ensuring survival of the individual (Beck & Haigh, 2014). In anxiety, these schemas take the form of preexisting beliefs and assumptions about danger, vulnerability, and the need for safety, security, and comfort. When feeling anxious, individuals believe that they will be overcome with a particular threat or danger ("Something terrible could happen to me"), that they are helpless to deal with it ("I can't stand to feel this way"), and that they need to reestablish a state of safety and security as quickly as possible ("I need to calm down, relax"). To provide protection, evaluations of threat and danger must be quick and efficient—thus the need for a system of automatic information processing. However, in the anxiety disorders, threat-mode activation becomes hypervalent so that a preconscious attentional bias becomes dominant; the result is an automatic tendency to selectively attend to the threat value of stimuli. Various experimental studies using the emotional Stroop test, dot probe detection, stimulus identification, and eye-tracking methodologies have shown that individuals with an anxiety disorder automatically attend to threat rather than neutral stimuli (see review by Bar-Haim et al., 2007; D. A. Clark & Beck, 2010). In their meta-analysis of eye-tracking studies, Armstrong and Olatunji (2012) concluded that anxious but not depressed individuals show a strong orienting bias toward threat, suggesting that hypervigilance for threat is specific to anxiety. The consistent finding of selective attentional threat bias over diverse experimental methodologies provides strong empirical support for the importance of cognitive processes in the pathogenesis of anxiety.

A closer examination of threat attentional bias reveals that time and anxiety level influence selective processing. For instance, attentional bias in anxiety may be biphasic. In the early stages of attentional processing (i.e., <500 msec), high-trait-anxious individuals exhibit attentional preference for highly threatening stimuli but attentional avoidance of threat at longer, supraliminal stimulus durations (Cisler & Koster, 2010). Moreover, the attentional problem in anxiety may not be limited to facilitated detection of threat, but also difficulty disengaging from threat stimuli (see Ouimet, Gawronski, & Dozois, 2009). Also, level of anxiety influences threat bias, with high-trait-anxious individuals showing facilitated threat at 100 msec, whereas low-trait-anxious persons exhibit attentional avoidance at 200 msec (e.g., Sagliano, Trojano, Migliozzi, & D'Olimpio, 2014). There is mixed evidence on whether attentional bias in anxiety is specific to the threat content characteristic of different anxiety disorders, or whether it is related to the general valence of the stimulus (D. A. Clark & Beck, 2010). The facilitated threat bias in high-trait-anxious individuals is consistent with the cognitive model's view that threat processing is more readily activated in vulnerable individuals due to preexisting hypervalent threat schemas. The model also predicts that content specificity may not be evident until the latter, more elaborative stage of threat processing. It should also be noted that content specificity is difficult to measure because of the high rate of comorbidity in the anxiety disorders.

There has been considerable interest in determining whether threat attentional bias can be directly modified by training individuals to attend away from threat cues. Labeled *attentional bias modification* (ABM), this approach determines whether attentional threat bias is a causal factor in anxiety and whether training anxious individuals to attend away (avoid) from threat stimuli might have therapeutic value (MacLeod & Mathews, 2012). Probes are presented in the location of only threat words or images (attend training) or only in the location of neutral stimuli (avoid training) over hundreds of trials. Various studies have shown that individuals can be trained to attend to or away from threat stimuli, with training effects associated with an increase or decrease in anxious symptoms, respectively (see MacLeod & Mathews, 2012, for review). This research provides strong evidence that attentional threat bias may play a causal role in the etiology of anxiety.

Naturally, there has been considerable interest in determining the therapeutic benefits of ABM. In one of the classic outcome studies, individuals with generalized social phobia completed 128 trials of attending away from disgust (i.e., threat) faces (Amir et al., 2009). Postassessment analysis revealed that ABM facilitated attentional disengagement from threat, reduced symptom severity, and achieved clinically significant change in 50% of cases. However, a recent meta-analysis of forty-three controlled outcome studies of ABM found only a small overall effect size for anxiety symptoms at posttreatment (Mogoaşe, David, & Koster, 2014). Thus, the therapeutic benefits of ABM remain largely unknown.

Elaborative Threat Appraisal

The cognitive model posits that evaluation of threat and safety also occurs at later stages of information processing when slower, more controlled, and elaborative information processing takes place at the fully conscious level (D. A. Clark & Beck, 2010). Whereas the initial preconscious attentional threat bias elicits the immediate fear response, this later more strategic processing of threat, vulnerability, and safety is responsible for the more sustained state of anxiety found in clinical disorders. If this reappraisal of the situation leads to the conclusion that significant threat and danger remain elevated, while the probability of effective coping and the attainment of safety are low, then a state of anxious anticipation persists. The cognitive model, then, considers conscious and deliberate appraisals of threat and secondary appraisals of personal coping resources and safety-seeking critical to the pathogenesis of anxiety.

The strongest empirical support for strategic processing of threat comes from experimental research on interpretation bias. These studies present ambiguous vignettes that could be interpreted in a threatening or neutral manner. Various studies have found that high-trait-anxious individuals are more likely to make threatening interpretations to ambiguous primes or scenarios than low-anxious individuals (see de Jong, 2014). Moreover, evidence that manipulation of interpretation bias can increase or reduce anxious symptoms again suggests a causal role in the production of anxiety. In one study, individuals with social anxiety who were trained to make positive interpretations of an ambiguous social scenario exhibited less negative interpretation bias and had lower social anxiety symptoms at one week follow-up (Mobini et al., 2014). In a second outcome study, individuals with generalized social anxiety who received training to endorse benign interpretations and reject threatening interpretations to ambiguous social scenarios displayed a significant reduction in threat interpretations and anxiety symptoms at postassessment and three-month follow-up (Amir & Taylor, 2012). Finally, a meta-analysis by Hallion and Ruscio (2011) concluded that the cognitive bias modification effect may be greater for interpretation than attentional bias, although once again the authors concluded that the effect sizes on symptom change were modest at best.

Threat Schema Activation

According to the cognitive model, the information-processing biases in anxiety are the product of underlying knowledge structures involving the individual's beliefs or understanding about the world, self, and survival. The knowledge structures or schemas most relevant to anxiety involve themes relevant to the preservation and well-being of the organism and so strive to maximize safety and minimize danger (D. A. Clark & Beck, 2010). The beliefs and assumptions most relevant to anxiety involve ideas about the individual's sense of vulnerability or helplessness as well as the extent of internal and external dangers that threaten the vital interests of the individual. In the cognitive model, vulnerability to anxiety is the result of preexisting maladaptive schemas about danger and helplessness that remain latent until activated by a situation, cue, or stimulus relevant to the person's anxious concerns. The strength of association between a particular stimulus and threat-related schemas will determine how readily the primal threat mode is activated (see also Ouimet et al., 2009). Once activated, threat-mode schemas dominate the information-processing system, determining how information is processed and how the individual responds to the anxiety experience. For example, an individual with panic disorder detects an unexpected shortness of breath and thinks, "I'm not getting enough air. I can't breathe." Immediately, beliefs about suffocation and dying are activated, and all the individual can think about is getting out of the situation and to a safe place where he can breathe properly. He's convinced that unless he escapes, he'll suffocate. Other more benign explanations for why he feels breathless are not considered because the schema, "I'm suffocating," completely determines how information is processed at that moment.

Empirical support for threat-related schematic vulnerability for anxiety comes mainly from self-report measures of beliefs and assumptions in which highly anxious individuals exhibit greater item endorsement than low-anxious individuals (for reviews see D. A. Clark & Beck, 2010; Ehring, 2014). Because many of the Anxiety Sensitivity Index (ASI; Reiss, Peterson, Gursky & McNally, 1986) items assess beliefs about feeling anxious, research indicating that ASI scores are significantly elevated in anxiety can be taken as further support for the cognitive view of threat-schema activation in anxiety. However, self-report measures of beliefs have inherent weaknesses, and so experimentally based indices of schematic representation provide a stronger empirical base. One of the more interesting approaches is a task borrowed from experimental cognitive psychology called the Implicit Association Task (IAT). The IAT is a reaction time measure of how quickly individuals sort words denoting attribute categories (e.g., positive, negative) according to two target categories (me, not-me). Individuals with social anxiety who were administered the IAT generated more automatic or implicit associations of a weak or vulnerable self, weaker associations of calmness, and more associations with threat cues than did nonanxious controls (Glashouwer, Vroling, de Jong, Lange, & de Keijser, 2013; Wong, Morrison, Heimberg, Goldin, & Gross, 2014). Together these results are consistent with the concept of schematic representation of threat and vulnerability in anxiety, but its causal status and the effects of treatment remain in question.

Avoidance, Safety-Seeking, and Maladaptive Coping

The cognitive model recognizes that avoidance, safety-seeking, and maladaptive coping strategies are critical features of anxiety, as discussed previously. However dysfunctional responses to anxiety are considered consequences of exaggerated threat appraisals, dysfunctional beliefs in personal vulnerability and uncontrollability, inadequate processing of safety information, and deficiency in constructive or problem-oriented thinking (D. A. Clark & Beck, 2010). Two assertions are prominent in the cognitive view of safety-seeking and avoidance. The first is the disconfirmation assumption, which states that anxiety persists because avoidance and safety-seeking block access to disconfirming evidence showing that the threat and danger are unrealistic (Salkovskis, 1991). Second, dysfunctional beliefs about safety and avoidance ensure continued reliance on strategies that ironically contribute to the persistence of anxiety.

As noted previously, evidence that presence of safety-seeking behavior, and even some avoidance, always undermines the effectiveness of exposure has come under question. If certain types of safety-seeking responses, such as those that are restorative in nature, do not hinder the effectiveness of CBT, and if some degree of escape and avoidance can be tolerated without disruption to treatment effectiveness, then this calls into question the validity of the disconfirmation hypothesis. However, Craske et al. (2014) argue that exposure therapy will be maximized when exposure experience violates the anxious individual's threat-based expectancies and when safety behaviors are removed. In the most recent review of safety behavior effects, Blakey and Abramowitz (2016) concluded that safety behaviors have been associated with poorer treatment outcomes. Moreover, they review evidence that safety behaviors such as distraction might interfere with the processing of disconfirming evidence. In sum, we can say that generally, safety behavior and avoidance contribute to the persistence of anxiety, and this may be in part due to failure to process disconfirming evidence (Helbig-Lang & Petermann, 2010). And yet, a distinction must be made between safety-seeking (and avoidance) and adaptive coping with anxiety. In their review, Parrish, Radomsky, and Dugas (2008) state that anxiety-neutralizing behaviors have the potential to be counterproductive, although anxiety-control strategies don't necessarily undermine treatment effectiveness. In other words, distraction, neutralization, and even safety behaviors might actually facilitate treatment effectiveness if the strategy increases self-efficacy, does not tax attentional resources, enables approach behavior and integration of disconfirming evidence, and does not lead to misattribution of safety as the antidote for fear and anxiety (Parrish et al., 2008).

One way to address the debate over the detrimental effects of safety-seeking is to determine whether beliefs about safety and tolerance of anxiety might mediate the effects of safety behaviors on anxiety reduction. The cognitive model predicts that safety-seeking might be most detrimental for clients who believe anxiety is intolerable, and that safety-seeking, escape, and avoidance are the only effective means to deal with an unbearable emotional state. There is some evidence that catastrophic beliefs play a role in the persistence of safety behaviors (see Parrish et al., 2008). Also, in SAD dysfunctional beliefs about the assumed effectiveness of safety behaviors in reducing anxiety as well as increased use of post-event processing are factors in the negative effects of safety-seeking (see Piccirillo, Dryman, & Heimberg, 2016). Despite evidence of an association between dysfunctional beliefs of threat and safety-seeking, the causal role of beliefs has not been established, nor is it known whether belief content mediates the effects of safety-seeking and avoidance on treatment effectiveness.

COGNITIVE THERAPY OF ANXIETY

Cognitive therapy (or CBT) is a complex, multicomponent treatment approach to fear and anxiety. Over the years, numerous clinician handbooks have been published that explain how to deliver CBT to anxiety more generally, or the various specific anxiety disorders (e.g., Beck et al., 1985; D. A. Clark & Beck, 2010; Leahy, 2009, 2017). This section focuses on the two main ingredients in CBT for anxiety, while recognizing that other elements such as case formulation, psychoeducation, homework assignment, and relapse prevention are important to the effectiveness of treatment.

Cognitive Restructuring

Cognitive restructuring (CR) consists of various interventions that focus on change in the exaggerated, maladaptive appraisals and beliefs considered critical in the etiology and maintenance of anxiety and its disorders. Exaggerated appraisals of threat, self-schemas of vulnerability or helplessness, and beliefs about safety-seeking and avoidance are targeted for change. In CBT for anxiety, four CR strategies are most commonly used in the treatment of anxiety disorders.

The first strategy involves examining the evidence. Once the client's exaggerated appraisals and beliefs about threat, danger, and vulnerability have been identified, therapists and clients collaborate on *examining competing evidence* that confirms or disconfirms their expectancies of the elevated probability and severity of threat. For example, CBT of PD involves gathering evidence that the occurrence of unexpected heart palpitations signifies the imminent threat of a myocardial infarct. The intent of evidence gathering is to help the client deeply process disconfirming information about their anxious threat.

A second CR strategy uses guided discovery to help the anxious client develop *an alternative perspective* on the anxious threat and vulnerability that is more balanced and realistic. The alternative perspective is not simply an affirmation of self-reassurance (i.e., "Oh, it's probably not a heart attack"), but rather a genuine, realistic explanation for the threat and its outcome (e.g., "I often get unexpected heart palpitations when I feel stressed and they always disappear once I get distracted").

A third CR strategy is *cost-benefit analysis* in which the therapist and client explore the immediate and long-term advantages and disadvantages of adopting the threat-based interpretation of their anxiety or the alternative perspective (e.g., "What's the cost vs. benefit of assuming your heart palpitations signal a heart attack vs. a physical reaction to stress"?).

A fourth common CR strategy is *de-catastrophizing*. With this intervention, clients articulate their worst case scenario and then use a problem-solving approach to develop a plan for dealing with the imagined catastrophe. Often, CBT therapists encourage clients to engage in repeated and sustained exposure to the catastrophic scenario as a type of imaginal exposure exercise. In addition, taking a problem-solving approach to the various coping strategies that could be used to deal with the catastrophe challenges the client's beliefs in his or her personal vulnerability. Sometimes confronting the catastrophe provides disconfirming evidence for the anxious concern. Recently, a client with generalized anxiety reported a frequent worry about running out of money whenever he encountered an unexpected expense. As we worked through the details of his worst case scenario, he realized it was highly improbable, if not almost impossible, that he would completely deplete his financial resources. Thus, the disconfirming evidence became so overwhelming that he could not even imagine or problem-solve the worst case scenario.

Exposure-Based Behavioral Experiments

Cognitive approaches to anxiety have always recognized that exposure-based intervention is critical for effective treatment (i.e., Beck et al., 1985). It is beyond the scope of the present chapter to review the compelling treatment outcome research on the effectiveness of exposure for all types of fear and anxiety (e.g., see Abramowitz, Deacon, & Whiteside, 2011; Ougrin,

2011). However, the function of exposure in CBT differs from its function in other approaches to anxiety such as the inhibitory learning perspective (Craske et al., 2014). In cognitive therapy, exposure exercises are conducted to provide disconfirming, experiential evidence against the client's anxious appraisals and beliefs, and to provide supportive evidence of the more realistic view of threat, danger, and vulnerability. In CBT, the therapist assigns repeated, graded exposure to fear stimuli, but emphasis is placed on helping clients deeply process the disconfirming aspects of the exposure experience. There has been considerable debate about the additive benefits of incorporating a cognitive perspective on exposure (see the following discussion). However, from a cognitive perspective, it makes little sense to offer a therapy that would deprive clients the opportunity to test out their faulty beliefs and appraisals through exposure-based experiences. It is well recognized that performance-based strategies are the most potent means to achieve lasting change.

CONCLUSIONS

Over the last several decades, the cognitive perspective has significantly increased our understanding of the psychology and treatment of anxiety. We now have efficacious treatments for anxiety and its disorders that integrate both cognitive and behavioral interventions to achieve significant, long-lasting reduction in anxious symptoms. Moreover, cognitive theories and research have greatly expanded our knowledge of the etiology, maintenance and recovery from pathological anxiety. Despite considerable advances in theory, research, and treatment, many fundamental issues remain for future investigation. This chapter concludes with several major questions that remain about the cognitive basis and treatment of anxiety.

Debate continues on whether maladaptive cognition is a cause or consequence of anxiety. As discussed previously, there is an impressive amount of experimental evidence that automatic and controlled cognitive processes have a causal effect on anxiety. However, we cannot assume an etiological role for dysfunctional cognition based solely on experimental studies of causality. More longitudinal and high-risk behavioral research is needed to determine whether biased information processing and dysfunctional beliefs play a significant role in the onset of clinical anxiety. In fact, studies on OCD, still considered an anxiety disorder by many, indicate that changes in cognition do not mediate symptom change and may occur after symptom reduction (e.g., Su, Carpenter, Zandberg, Simpson, & Foa, 2016; Woody, Whittal, & McLean, 2011). This, of course, does not bode well for the etiological status of cognitive constructs. Other variables such as inhibitory learning and maladaptive emotion regulation have been proposed as vulnerability and mediating factors in onset and recovery from anxiety.

Despite several decades of phenomenal growth in cognitive-clinical research on anxiety, researchers are still piecing together the exact mechanisms of cognitive dysfunction and their interaction. For example, it is still unclear whether the main cognitive problem in anxiety is facilitated processing of threat, delayed threat disengagement, and/or faulty processing of safety information. Most likely, cognitive dysfunction is some combination of all three processes, but their modus operandi and temporal sequence still need to be worked out.

Similar to all the affective disorders, questions continue on the relative importance of common versus specific factors in the pathogenesis and treatment of anxiety. Cognitive content specificity, for example, may be less apparent in anxiety, with threat-related cognitions more indicative of negative affect (see D. A. Clark & Beck, 2010). Within the treatment literature, there has been considerable interest in transdiagnostic CBT, with initial comparison studies indicating that transdiagnostic treatment for anxiety can be as effective as disorder-specific CBT (Newby, McKinnon, Kuyken, Gilbody, & Dalgleish, 2015).

Since the beginning of cognitive therapy of anxiety in the late 1980s, the question of cognitive mediation has dominated the field. In their critical review of the topic, Teachman, Beadel, and Steinman (2014) concluded that cognitive mechanisms can explain and even maximize the effectiveness of CBT for anxiety. However, others continue to question whether treatment ingredients that focus directly on cognitive change (i.e., cognitive restructuring) add any significant effect beyond exposure therapy alone. For example, a recent meta-analysis of CBT components for anxiety disorders found no statistically significant difference in treatment effectiveness between behavior therapy, which consisted of exposure, desensitization, relaxation, and the like, and CBT, which included behavioral components as well as cognitive restructuring, reappraisal, and the like (Adams, Brady, Lohr, & Jacobs, 2015). The authors concluded that targeting cognitive processes in treatment of anxiety may not be necessary, and so therapists should offer the simpler and equally effective behavioral treatment. There are many methodological and analytic challenges with treatment component analysis ensuring that the debate over the clinical utility of cognitive interventions will not be resolved in the foreseeable future.

Finally, the emergence of newer therapy approaches to anxiety, such as mindfulness and acceptance and commitment therapy (ACT), has again challenged the widespread acceptance of CBT for anxiety. To date, there appears to be no significant difference in outcome between these "third-wave" therapies and conventional CBT. In fact, the third-wave therapies may be less effective than standard cognitive and behavioral treatment (e.g., Kocovski, Fleming, Hawley, Hutu, & Antony, 2013; Newby et al., 2015; Öst, 2014). Whatever new directions appear on the horizon, the growth of new ideas in theory, research, and treatment speaks to the continued vitality of the cognitive-behavioral approach to anxiety.

REFERENCES

Abramowitz, J. S., Deacon, B. J., & Whiteside, S. P. H. (2011). *Exposure therapy for anxiety: Principles and practice*. New York: Guilford Press.

Adams, T. G., Brady, R. E., Lohr, J. M., & Jacobs, W. J. (2015). A meta-analysis of CBT components for anxiety disorders. *The Behavior Therapist, 38*(4), 87–97.

American Psychiatric Association (APA). (2013). *Diagnostic and statistical manual of mental disorders* (5th ed.). Arlington, VA: Author.

Amir, N., Beard, C., Taylor, C. T., Klumpp, H., Elias, J., Burns, M., & Chen, X. (2009). Attention training in individuals with generalized social phobia: A randomized controlled trial. *Journal of Consulting and Clinical Psychology, 77,* 961–973.

Amir, N., & Taylor, C. T. (2012). Interpretation training in individuals with generalized social anxiety disorder: A randomized controlled trial. *Journal of Consulting and Clinical Psychology, 80,* 497–511.

Armstrong, T., & Olatunji, B. O. (2012). Eye tracking of attention in the affective disorders: A meta-analytic review and status. *Clinical Psychology Review, 32,* 704–723.

Bar-Haim, Y., Lamy, D., Bakermans-Franenburg, M. J., Pergamin, L., & van IJzendoorn, M. H. (2007). Threat-related attentional bias in anxious and nonanxious individuals: A meta-analytic study. *Psychological Bulletin, 133,* 1–24.

Barlow, D. H. (2002). *Anxiety and its disorders: The nature and treatment of anxiety and panic*. New York: Guilford Press.

Beck, A. T., Emery, G., & Greenberg, R. L. (1985). *Anxiety disorders and phobias: A cognitive perspective*. New York: Basic Books.

Beck, A. T., & Haigh, E. A. P. (2014). Advances in cognitive theory and therapy: The generic cognitive model. *Annual Review of Clinical Psychology, 10,* 1–24.

Blakey, S. M., & Abramowitz, J. S. (2016). The effects of safety behavior during exposure therapy for anxiety: Critical analysis from an inhibitory learning perspective. *Clinical Psychology Review, 49,* 1–15.

Brown, T. A., Campbell, L. A., Lehman, C. L., Grisham, J. R., & Mancill, R. B. (2001). Current and lifetime comorbidity of the DSM-IV anxiety and mood disorders in a large clinical sample. *Journal of Abnormal Psychology, 110,* 585–599.

Brown, T. A., Chorpita, B. F., & Barlow, D. H. (1998). Structural relationships among dimensions of the DSM-IV anxiety and mood disorders and dimensions of negative affect, positive affect, and autonomic arousal. *Journal of Abnormal Psychology, 107,* 179–192.

Chambless, D. L., Baker, M. J., Baucom, D. H., Beutler, L. E., Calhoun, K. S., Crits-Christoph, P., . . . Woody, S. R. (1998). Update on empirically validated therapies II. *Clinical Psychologist, 51,* 3–16.

Cisler, J. M., & Koster, E. H. W. (2010). Mechanisms of attentional bias towards threat in anxiety disorders: An integrative review. *Clinical Psychology Review, 30,* 203–216.

Clark, D. A., & Beck, A. T. (2010). *Cognitive therapy of anxiety disorders: Science and practice*. New York: Guilford Press.

Clark, D. M. (1986). A cognitive approach to panic. *Behaviour Research and Therapy, 24,* 461–470.

Craske, M. G. (2003). *Origins of phobias and anxiety disorders: Why more women than men?* Amsterdam, The Netherlands: Elsevier.

Craske, M. G., Treanor, M., Conway, C., Zbozinek, T., & Vervliet, B. (2014). Maximizing exposure therapy: An inhibitory learning approach. *Behaviour Research and Therapy, 58*, 10–23.

de Jong, P. J. (2014). Information processing. In P. Emmelkamp & T. Ehring (Eds.), *The Wiley handbook of anxiety disorders: Vol. I. Theory and research* (pp. 125–147). Chichester, UK: Wiley Blackwell.

Ehring, T. (2014). Cognitive theory. In P. Emmelkamp & T. Ehring (Eds.), *The Wiley handbook of anxiety disorders: Vol. I. Theory and research* (pp. 104–124). Chichester, UK: Wiley Blackwell.

Glashouwer, K. A., Vroling, M. S., de Jong, P. J., Lange, W.-G., & de Keijser, J. (2013). Low implicit self-esteem and dysfunctional automatic associations in social anxiety disorder. *Journal of Behavior Therapy and Experimental Psychiatry, 44*, 262–270.

Goetz, A. R., Davine, T. P., Siwiec, S. G., & Lee, H.-J. (2016). The functional value of preventive and restorative safety behaviors: A systematic review of the literature. *Clinical Psychology Review, 44*, 112–124.

Gray, J. A. (1987). *The psychology of fear and stress* (2nd ed.). Cambridge, UK: Cambridge University Press.

Hallion, L. S., & Ruscio, A. M. (2011). A meta-analysis of the effect of cognitive bias modification on anxiety and depression. *Psychological Bulletin, 137*, 940–958.

Helbig-Lang, S., & Petermann, F. (2010). Tolerate or eliminate?: A systematic review on the effects of safety behavior across anxiety disorders. *Clinical Psychology: Science and Practice, 17*, 218–233.

Hendriks, S. M., Spiujker, J., Licht, C. M. M., Beekman, A. T. F., & Penninx, W. J. H. (2013). Two-year course of anxiety disorders: Different across disorders or dimensions. *Acta Psychiatrica Scandinavica, 128*, 212–221.

Johnson, E. M., & Coles, M. E. (2013). Failure and delay in treatment-seeking across anxiety disorders. *Community Mental Health Journal, 49*, 668–674.

Kessler, R. C., Berglund, P., Demler, O., Jin, R., Merikangas, K. R., & Walters, E. E. (2005). Lifetime prevalence and age-of-onset distributions of DSM-IV disorders in the National Comorbidity Survey Replication. *Archives of General Psychiatry, 62*, 593–602.

Kessler, R. C., Chiu, W. T., Demler, O., & Walters, E. E. (2005). Prevalence, severity, and comorbidity of 12-month DSM-IV disorders in the National Comorbidity Survey Replication. *Archives of General Psychiatry, 62*, 617–627.

Kocovski, N. L., Fleming, J. E., Hawley, L. L., Huta, V., & Antony, M. M. (2013). Mindfulness and acceptance-based group therapy versus traditional cognitive behavioral group therapy for social anxiety disorder: A randomized controlled trial. *Behaviour Research and Therapy, 51*, 889–898.

Leahy, R. L. (2009). *Anxiety free: Unravel your fears before they unravel you.* Carlsbad, CA: Hay House.

Leahy, R. L. (2017). *Cognitive therapy techniques: A practitioner's guide* (2nd ed.). New York: Guilford Press.

Longley, S. L., Watson, D., Noyes, R., & Yoder, K. (2006). Panic and phobic anxiety: Association among neuroticism, physiological hyperarousal, anxiety sensitivity, and three phobias. *Journal of Anxiety Disorders, 20*, 718–739.

Macleod, C., & Mathews, A. (2012). Cognitive bias modification: Approaches to anxiety. *Annual Review of Clinical Psychology, 8*, 189–217.

Marks, I. M. (1087). *Fears, phobias, and rituals: Panic, anxiety and their disorders*. New York: Oxford University Press.

Mathews, A., & MacLeod, C. (1994). Cognitive approaches to emotion and emotional disorders. *Annual Review of Psychology, 45*, 25–50.

Mathews, A., & MacLeod, C. (2005). Cognitive vulnerability to emotional disorders. *Annual Review of Clinical Psychology, 1*, 167–195.

McLean, C. P., Asnaani, A., Liz, B. T., & Hofmann, S. G. (2011). Gender differences in anxiety disorders: Prevalence, course of illness, comorbidity and burden of illness. *Journal of Psychiatric Research, 45*, 1027–1035.

Meudlers, A., Daele, T. V., Volders, S., & Vlaeyen, J. W. S. (2016). The use of safety-seeking behavior in exposure-based treatment for fear and anxiety: Benefit or burden? A meta-analytic review. *Clinical Psychology Review, 44*, 144–156.

Mineka, S., Watson, D., & Clark, L. A. (1998). Comorbidity of anxiety and unipolar mood disorders. *Annual Review of Psychology, 49*, 377–412.

Mobini, S., Mackintosh, B., Illingworth, J., Gega, L., Langdon, P., & Hoppitt, L. (2014). Effects of standard and explicit cognitive bias modification and computer-administered cognitive-behaviour therapy on cognitive bias and social anxiety. *Journal of Behavior Therapy and Experimental Psychiatry, 45*, 272–279.

Mogoașe, C., David, D., & Koster, E. H. W. (2014). Clinical efficacy of attentional bias modification procedures: An updated meta-analysis. *Journal of Clinical Psychology, 70*, 1133–1157.

National Institute of Clinical Excellence (NICE). (2011). Common mental health problems: Identification and pathways to care (NICE guidelines [CG123]). Retrieved August 12, 2016, from *www.nice.org.uk/guidance/cg123/chapter/1-Guidance*.

Newby, J. M., McKinnon, A., Kuyken, W., Gilbody, S., & Dalgleish, T. (2015). Systematic review and meta-analysis of transdiagnostic psychological treatments for anxiety and depressive disorders in adulthood. *Clinical Psychology Review, 40*, 91–110.

Olatunji, B. O., Cisler, J. M., & Tolin, D. F. (2007). Quality of life in the anxiety disorders: A meta-analytic review. *Clinical Psychology Review, 27*, 572–581.

Öst, L.-G. (2014). The efficacy of Acceptance and Commitment Therapy: An updated systematic review and meta-analysis. *Behaviour Research and Therapy, 61*, 105–121.

Ougrin, D. (2011). Efficacy of exposure versus cognitive therapy in anxiety disorders: Systematic review and meta-analysis. *BMC Psychiatry, 11*, 1–12.

Ouimet, A. J., Gawronski, B., & Dozois, D. J. A. (2009). Cognitive vulnerability to anxiety: A review and an integrative model. *Clinical Psychology Review, 29*, 459–470.

Parrish, C. L., Radomsky, A. S., & Dugas, M. J. (2008). Anxiety-control strategies: Is there room for neutralization in successful exposure treatment? *Clinical Psychology Review, 28*, 1400–1412.

Piccirillo, M. L., Dryman, M. T., & Heimberg, R. G. (2016). Safety behaviors in adults with social anxiety: Review and future directions. *Behavior Therapy, 47*, 675–687.

Rachman, S., Radomsky, A. S., & Shafran, R. (2008). Safety behaviour: A reconsideration. *Behaviour Research and Therapy, 46,* 163–173.

Rapee, R. M., & Heimberg, R. G. (1997). A cognitive-behavioral model of anxiety in social phobia. *Behaviour Research and Therapy, 35,* 741–756.

Reiss, S., Peterson, R. A., Gursky, D. M., & McNally, R. J. (1986). Anxiety sensitivity, anxiety frequency and the prediction of fearfulness. *Behaviour Research and Therapy, 24,* 1–8.

Riskind, J. H. (1997). Looming vulnerability to threat: A cognitive paradigm for anxiety. *Behaviour Research and Therapy, 35,* 685–702.

Sagliano, L., Trojano, L., Katja, A., Migliozzi, M., & D'Olimpio, F. (2014). Attentional biases toward threat: The concomitant presence of difficulty of disengagement and attentional avoidance in low trait anxious individuals. *Frontiers in Psychology, 5,* Article 685, 1–7.

Salkovskis, P. M. (1991). The importance of behavior in the maintenance of anxiety and panic: A cognitive account. *Behavioural Psychotherapy, 19,* 6–19.

Salkovskis, P. M. (1996). The cognitive approach to anxiety: Threat beliefs, safety-seeking behavior, and the special case of health anxiety and obsessions. In P. M. Salkovskis (Ed.), *Frontiers of cognitive therapy* (pp. 48–74). New York: Guilford Press.

Schmidt, N. B., Mitchell, M., Keough, M., & Riccardi, C. (2011). Anxiety and its disorders. In M. J. Zvolensky, A. Bernstein, & A. A. Vujanovic (Eds.), *Distress tolerance: Theory, research, and clinical applications* (pp. 105–125). New York: Guilford Press.

Su, Y.-J., Carpenter, J. K., Zandberg, L. J., Simpson, H. B., & Foa, E. B. (2016). Cognitive mediation of symptom change in exposure and response prevention for obsessive-compulsive disorder. *Behavior Therapy, 47,* 474–486.

Teachman, B. A., Beadel, J. R., & Steinman, S. A. (2014). Mechanisms of change in CBT treatment. In P. Emmelkamp & T. Ehring (Eds.), *The Wiley handbook of anxiety disorders: Vol. II. Clinical assessment and treatment* (pp. 824–839). Chichester, UK: Wiley Blackwell.

The WHO World Mental Health Survey Consortium. (2004). Prevalence, severity, and unmet need for treatment of mental disorders in the World Health Organization World Mental Health Surveys. *Journal of the American Medical Association, 291,* 2581–2590.

Wang, P. S., Berglund, P., Olfson, M., Pincus, H. A., Wells, K. B., & Kessler, R. C. (2005). Failure and delay in initial treatment contact after first onset of mental disorders in the National Comorbidity Survey Replication. *Archives of General Psychiatry, 62,* 603–613.

Watson, D., & Naragon-Gainey, K. (2014). Personality, emotions, and the emotional disorders. *Psychological Science, 2,* 422–442.

Wells, A., (2006). The metacognitive model of worry and generalized anxiety disorder. In G. C. I. Davey & A. Wells (Eds.), *Worry and its psychological disorders: Theory, assessment and treatment* (pp. 179–216). Chichester, UK: Wiley.

Wong, J., Morrison, A. S., Heimberg, R. G., Goldin, P. R., & Gross, J. J. (2014). Implicit associations in social anxiety disorder: The effects of comorbid depression. *Journal of Anxiety Disorders, 28,* 537–546.

Woody, S. R., Whittal, M. L., & McLean, P. D. (2011). Mechanisms of symptom reduction in treatment of obsessions. *Journal of Consulting and Clinical Psychology, 79,* 653–664.

CHAPTER 19

Specialized Cognitive-Behavioral Therapy for Obsessive–Compulsive Disorder

Debbie Sookman

Obsessive–compulsive disorder (OCD) is a leading cause of disability worldwide (World Health Organization, 2008). Affecting approximately 3% of the population through the lifespan, OCD is recognized as a major mental illness from which sufferers experience impaired functioning across domains on par with major physical illnesses and schizophrenia (Koran, Thienemann, & Davenport, 1996; Bystritsky et al., 2001). This disorder is commonly associated with depression, hopelessness, high levels of distress, as well as serious psychosocial dysfunction and reduced quality of life secondary to symptoms (Hollander, Stein, Fineberg, & Legault, 2010). Multisphere impairment often occurs in basic self-care and parenting, intrafamilial and social functioning, and capacity for school or work. Severity and chronicity of illness are associated with high health care costs and hospitalizations. Approximately 25% of these latter cases attempt suicide (Kamath, Reddy, & Kandavel, 2007).

In the fifth edition of the *Diagnostic and Statistical Manual of Mental Disorders* (DSM-5, (American Psychiatric Association, 2013), OCD and related disorders are a separate classification, no longer classified with anxiety disorders. This development represents major progress in diagnosis, reflecting convergent research that indicates OCD is distinctive in terms of psychopathology and treatment requirements. Treatment for OCD is a specialized field. There is considerable heterogeneity of symptom subtypes that require specific interventions (e.g., Sookman, Abramowitz, Calamari, Wilhelm, & McKay, 2005).

The causes of OCD remain poorly understood. Genomewide association studies have been inconsistent or require replication (Stewart et al., 2013). Several brain structures and functions have been implicated in OCD, and the heterogeneity of symptoms appears to be represented by a diversity of neural substrates. It is not clear if these changes are the cause or the effect of symptoms. Further, differences on neuroimaging with OCD patients compared with normals may be a question of magnitude, consistent with the finding that normal individuals experience a wide range of similar intrusive thoughts but appraise these thoughts differently. Importantly, several studies have reported that functional abnormalities on neuroimaging improve or resolve with cognitive-behavioral therapy (CBT) alone (for review, see Thorsen, van den Heuvel, Hansen, & Kvale, 2015).

CLINICAL SYMPTOMS OF OCD

Obsessions are repetitive intrusive thoughts, images, or urges experienced as involuntary and distressing. Commonly reported sensations include "not just right" and sense of incompleteness (Summerfeldt, 2007) as well as sensorial experiences (Simpson & Reddy, 2014). Rituals are repetitive behaviors such as washing or checking, or mental acts such as repeating or replacing words or images, carried out in response to obsessions in order to reduce distress and/or to prevent occurrence of a feared event (e.g., becoming ill). Rituals are not connected realistically to feared events (e.g., counting to prevent harm to a loved one) or are clearly excessive (e.g., prolonged hand washing and showering). Repugnant obsessions include blasphemous or sexual thoughts and/or thoughts of harming others. The content of obsessions tends to be those that are contrary to the moral values of the individual (Rachman, 2003). Patients report catastrophic (mis)appraisals of their intrusive thoughts as well as their emotions (e.g., "the fact that I am afraid around knives proves that I am a dangerous person"); distrust of their memory, integrity, and morality; strong feelings of guilt, shame, and self-doubt; and fear that they are vulnerable, dangerous, bad, weird, or going crazy. Concealment, avoidance, and cognitive and behavioral rituals perpetuate misappraisals. Commonly reported information-processing distortions include "Thought Action Fusion" (e.g., "having a bad thought is the same as acting on it"; Shafran & Rachman, 2004), and emotional reasoning (e.g., "I feel scared, so I must be in danger"; Arntz, Rauner, &

van den Hout, 1995). Mild to moderate illness entails symptoms one to three hours daily; however, many individuals experience incessant intrusive thoughts and rituals that are pervasive and incapacitating. For example, very severely ill patients who fear contamination may report bathing in bleach, bleeding, and sleeping in the bathtub because they feel they cannot complete their washing rituals; checkers (individuals with checking rituals) may report remaining paralyzed in one spot at home for many hours in order to feel "just right"—with serious impairments in self-care as well as medical sequelae. In most cases, insight is retained; that is, at least upon quiet reflection the individual recognizes that his or her beliefs and fears are unrealistic. Estimated occurrence of poor insight is 14 to 31% of patients, associated with greater symptom severity, higher comorbidity, and worse treatment outcomes (Jacob, Larson, & Storch, 2014).

OCD SUBTYPES AND COMORBIDITY

The heterogeneity of presenting OCD symptoms and associated comorbidities calls for broad-spectrum diagnostic acumen. Symptom dimensions include contamination/cleaning, doubt about harm/checking, symmetry/ordering, and unacceptable thoughts/mental rituals (Williams, Mugno, Franklin, & Faber, 2013). The estimated prevalence of symptom subtypes includes checking (79.3%), ordering (57.0%), moral concerns (43.0%), sexual/religious concerns (30.2%), contamination (25.7%), harming (24.2%), concerns about illness (14.3%), and other concerns (19.0%), with 81% of respondents endorsing multiple symptoms (Ruscio, Stein, Chiu, & Kessler, 2010). There is evidence that mental contamination is a subtype distinctive from contact contamination, with or without fears of illness (Rachman, Coughtrey, Shafran, & Radomsky, 2015). Perceived threats associated with mental contamination are primarily interpersonal, related thoughts and/or memories, and fear of "morphing" or taking on the characteristics of another person. Past experiences of violation or betrayal are commonly reported prior to symptom onset, and excessive washing is described as an attempt to *get rid of the danger and the feeling*. Musical obsessions are an understudied phenomenon (Taylor et al., 2014). Early-life factors such as perinatal difficulties, physical abuse, negative emotionality, and personality or conduct problems predict the incidence of OCD for some individuals (Grisham et al., 2011). It has been hypothesized that some individuals develop abrupt onset of OCD symptoms and tic disorders related to an autoimmune process following group A beta-hemolytic streptococcal infection (Pediatric Autoimmune Neuropsychiatric Disorders [PANDAS], reviewed by Leckman et al., 2010). However, reliable support for alternative treatments (additional to initial antibiotics) for suspected cases of PANDAS is lacking.

With respect to obsessive–compulsive related disorders, the highest comorbidity is found with tic disorders (17%) and body dysmorphic disorder (BDD, 8–37%; Phillips, 2000). Patients with BDD report poorer insight and greater overvalued ideation and may be less responsive during cognitive therapy to consider alternate meanings of obsessions and to resist rituals. Mood disorder is the most frequent comorbidity (approximately 27%), characterized by earlier age of onset and greater severity of symptoms (Denys, Tenney, Van Megan, de Geus, & Westenberg, 2004). This is distinguished from depression secondary to disabling symptoms that generally remits following successful treatment for OCD (Veale, Freeston, Krebs, Heyman, & Salkovskis, 2009). Comorbidity with anxiety disorders is estimated at 12.8%; approximately 36 % of OCD patients meet the criteria for comorbid personality disorders characterized by lower functioning compared with OCD without personality disorders (Denys et al., 2004). Importantly, evidence-based practice is to treat OCD directly as soon as possible following symptom onset, and most comorbidities can be treated concurrently. Comorbid psychotic disorder (differentiated from poor insight and overvalued ideas) is relatively uncommon and requires pharmacotherapy. Patients with significant substance abuse such as alcohol or street drugs, which are impediments to sustained learning during CBT, require prior or concurrent treatment. The heterogeneity and complexity of OCD symptoms underlie the need for commensurate conceptual and intervention models that can be flexibly tailored on an individualized basis guided by available research.

CONCEPTUAL MODELS

Among the theoretical models important in the development of treatment strategies for OCD are those described by Salkovskis (1985, 1989); Salkovskis, Shafran, Rachman, and Freeston (1999); and Rachman (1998, 2003). This pioneering work focused initially on the importance of patients' appraisals of intrusions related to responsibility. Rachman (1998, 2003) proposed that specific intrusions develop into obsessions if they are considered personally significant and harmful and that the essential problem in OCD is that people interpret their thoughts as signifying that they are bad, crazy, or dangerous. The Obsessive Compulsive Cognitions Working Group (e.g., OCCWG, 2003) identified several domains of dysfunctional beliefs characteristic of OCD, culminating in the development of two gold standard measures of cognition in OCD, the Interpretation of Intrusions Inventory and the Obsessive Beliefs Questionnaire: inflated responsibility, overimportance of thoughts, control of thoughts, overestimation of threat, intolerance of uncertainty, and perfectionism. Some OCD patients do not endorse these beliefs at dysfunctional levels—for example, washers who *just can't stand the feeling* of contamination without fear of illness or those whose distress is disgust-related. Metacognitive theory focuses specifically on monitoring, interpreting, and regulating the content and processes of cognition (Wells, 2000), and research supports the importance of addressing "high-level" cognitive and emotional processes (Beck, 1996). For example, Solem et al. (2009) reported that change in metacognitions was a better predictor of posttreatment symptom levels compared with change in beliefs about responsibility and perfectionism.

There is strong theoretical support among leaders in the CBT field for consideration of schema-based models in cross-diagnostic conceptualization and treatment planning (Beck, 1976, 1996; Beck & Haigh, 2014).

> Cognitive schemas, defined as internally stored representations of stimuli, ideas, or experiences . . . control information-processing systems. . . . When a schema is activated, corresponding meaning is derived from the belief and interacts with other cognitive, affective, motivational, and behavioral systems. . . . When the bias exceeds the built-in adaptive level, it increases the probability of an individual experiencing a subclinical or clinical disorder. (Beck & Haigh, 2014, p. 3)

The important concept of emotional schemas (Leahy, 2002; Leahy, Tirch, & Napolitano, 2011) refers to the person's experience and regulation of emotions as central to the development and maintenance of psychopathology. Individuals who experience their emotions as dangerous or uncontrollable may be risk aversive and especially fearful of exposure and response prevention (ERP) or behavioral experiments. There is evidence for the efficacy of schema-based approaches in treating depression (Carter et al., 2013) and personality disorders (Dickhaut, & Arntz, 2014). Pertinent to early childhood schemas, Salkovskis et al. (1999) proposed several pathways to the development of dysfunctional responsibility beliefs in OCD, including childhood experiences with excessive or too little responsibility, rigid rules, and incidents in which action or inaction contributed to misfortune to self or others. Vulnerability schemas may be a central mechanism underlying emotional experience and appraisals of danger characteristic of several OCD subtypes (Sookman, Pinard, & Beck, 2001; Rachman, 2006). Wilhelm, Berman, Keshaviah, Schwartz, and Steketee (2015) reported that cognitive changes in maladaptive beliefs about perfectionism and certainty as well as maladaptive schemas related to dependency and incompetence significantly mediated improved treatment response and preceded behavioral symptom reduction for OCD patients treated with cognitive therapy.

Figure 19.1 shows the conceptual model for OCD developed by Sookman, Pinard, and Beauchemin (1994), which encompasses evidence-based factors that maintain symptoms as well as their hypothetical interaction with core schemas (identity structure) for use in case conceptualization, intervention planning, and assessment of treatment response.

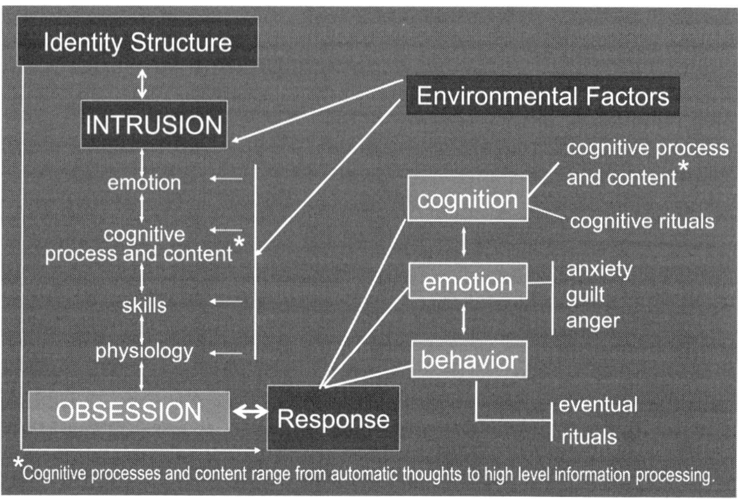

FIGURE 19.1. Transformation of an intrusion. Adapted from Sookman, Pinard, and Beauchemin (1994, p. 179).

Symptom-maintaining factors are operationalized and targeted as precisely as possible for each case. Patients' responses to intrusions range from appraisals and beliefs to more complex cognitive and emotional processes (Beck & Clark, 1997). Sookman and colleagues developed several interventions for CBT treatment-resistant samples based on this model. These interventions include a cognitive therapy protocol to help patients to tolerate, modulate, reappraise, and distance from symptom-related experiences such as intrusions and strong feelings, for practice during behavioral interventions and homework (Sookman & Pinard, 1999). In addition, a relapse prevention strategy, corrective strategic processing,[1] which is designed to strengthen self-directed maintenance of improvement, has also been proposed (Sookman & Pinard, 2007).

Figure 19.2 elaborates that aspect of the model pertaining to "identity structure" (adapted from Guidano & Liotti, 1985). Varied schemas are hypothesized to interact at a tacit level (beyond immediate accessibility to awareness) and to influence explicit information processing, emotional retrieval and experience, and behavioral responses. As Beck and Clark (1997) elaborated, much normal autonomic information processing is ongoing beyond accessibility to awareness. The CBT theoretical

[1]In developing this clinical strategy specifically for OCD, we built upon the conceptual and treatment model of OCD proposed by Sookman et al. (1994); the general information-processing model of anxiety proposed by Beck and Clark (1997); and the model of vulnerability schemas in OCD proposed by Sookman et al. (2001).

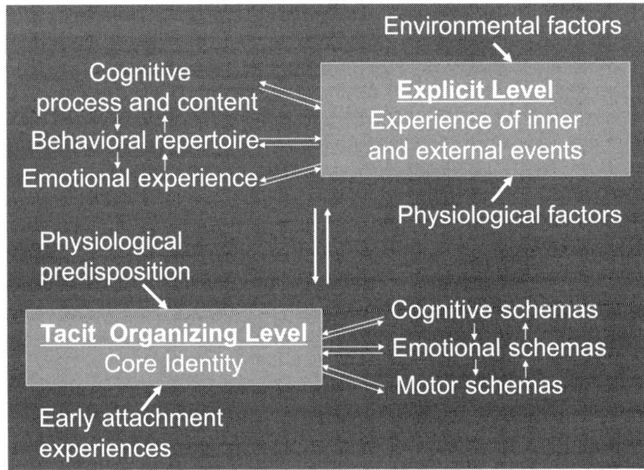

FIGURE 19.2. Identity structure. Adapted from Sookman, Pinard, and Beauchemin (1994, p. 178).

conceptualization of tacit builds on the concept of schemas whose processes and content are transformed through development (Piaget, 1960).

Sookman, 2016 (pp. 114–115) noted:

> A common characteristic of patients who do not respond well to specialty CBT is the intransigent quality of their symptom-related appraisals and beliefs despite apparent contradictory life events. "I know I'm exaggerating the probability something bad will happen, but I still **feel** I'm in danger." Schema-based interventions for OCD . . . are intended to expand upon standard CT methods described above; to improve collaboration with and accommodation during ERP, behavioral experiments, and skills interventions; and to enhance generalization and maintenance of change . . . schemas comprising beliefs, emotions, and memories about threat may underlie intransigent beliefs about threat related to symptoms. . . . These schemas may contribute to risk aversion and difficulty engaging fully in behavioral interventions . . . modification of the structure and content of dysfunctional schemas may be necessary to forestall recurrence of symptoms for some individuals (Beck, 1996; Beck & Haigh, 2014). . . . Inclusion of schemas in the context of evidence-based protocols for OCD may be viewed as encompassing the individual's broader learning history that can contribute to current information processing. This addition may be particularly helpful if focusing solely on current maintaining factors does not result in optimal re-learning and symptom reduction. Concepts from attachment and developmental theory are integrated in conceptualization and treatment planning, thereby broadening the theoretical basis for case conceptualization and intervention (e.g., Sookman & Steketee, 2010; Rachman et al., 2015).

Schemas that do not accommodate adequately to new experience may contribute to intransigence of dysfunctional patterns (Rosen, 1989). In this approach, the *upward arrow technique* described by Sookman and Pinard (1999) is used for select patients to link schemas and related developmental experiences with current symptoms, to reduce the potential effects of dysfunctional schemas on intransigent patterns, and to improve willingness to risk exposure to situations that activate symptoms (see Figure 19.3). Graduated behavioral experiments are designed to disconfirm maladaptive emotional responses, expectations, and core beliefs, and new skills are taught and practiced (for elaboration, see Sookman, 2016).

Although much progress has been made by addressing maintaining factors during CBT for OCD, Salkovskis et al. (1999) observed "Our experience is that, in some cases, there are general and enduring belief factors which may have made the patient prone to developing OCD, and which do not fully change in the course of treatment, and that it can be helpful to identify and deal with these" (p. 1069). More recently, Rachman et al. (2015) reported a promising conceptual and treatment approach for mental contamination that involves "imagery rescripting" (changing the image's content, outcome, and meaning) and other specific strategies to target beliefs,

T: Would you like to risk some "imperfection" without doing rituals, see what you feel, how others respond, how you can learn to cope, using these important reappraisals? (behavioral experiment is planned)

P: As we've discussed in other sessions, I'd like to feel it's not my fault, not my defect. My father had low self-esteem himself and everyone thought he was perfectionistic. Maybe my father's standards were too high, most of the time what I do is good enough, mistakes are not the end of the world and don't reflect on me basically as a person...if only I could feel this is true... I'd like to trust myself without all this checking.

T: We could try to reappraise your experiences with your parents, like we've done for your intrusive thoughts and your feelings in difficult situations now.

P: I check things over and over to make sure there are no mistakes. I do this now more than ever...I've tried to be perfect all my life, I guess so no one can find fault with me, so I don't have to feel upset like that again...

T: I understand this has caused you a lot of emotional pain, and even affected the way you feel about yourself.... How do you feel these past experiences, and the meaning they have to you, may be related to your OCD symptoms?

P: I felt bad about myself and very upset. Nothing I did was good enough for him, even though I tried...I'm just not good enough... something serious is missing in me...I'm an inferior person (patient cries).

T: How did this make you feel?

P: My father was very critical of me. The only way I could earn his respect was by getting only A's in school, by not making mistakes. Never make a fool of yourself in front of others!

FIGURE 19.3. Upward arrow illustration. Copyright © 2016 from *Specialized Cognitive Behavior Therapy for Obsessive–Compulsive Disorder: An Expert Clinician Guidebook*, by Debbie Sookman. Adapted by permission from Taylor and Francis Group, LLC, a division of Informa, PLC.

emotions, and memories related to developmental experiences. Veale, Page, Woodward, and Salkovskis (2015) described a single-case experimental design using imagery rescripting for twelve OCD cases with distressing intrusive images considered to be emotionally linked to memories of past aversive events. Specialized schema-based interventions for OCD may be helpful as an augmenting strategy for patients who do not respond to optimally delivered evidence-based CBT. Further research is required to examine these approaches particularly with treatment-resistant samples.

RESEARCH AND CLINICAL APPLICATIONS

The aim of treatment for OCD, as for other disorders, is recovery of symptoms and restoration of multidimensional quality of life for as many patients as possible. The first-line evidence-based psychotherapeutic treatment of choice for OCD is specialized CBT, including ERP (NICE, 2005; APA, 2007; Koran & Simpson, 2013).[2] Analyses of thirty-seven randomized, controlled trials from 1993 to 2014 have shown that approximately 65% of patients report substantial reduction in symptoms following CBT (average of about 50% improvement, with stronger results reported more recently) maintained at follow-up on average of fifteen months (for review, see Ost, Havnen, Hansen, & Kvale, 2015). Most experts recommend that cognitive therapy (CT) and behavioral experiments be combined with ERP in CBT evidence-based approaches for OCD. Several studies have demonstrated the efficacy of both ERP and CT in reducing symptoms and beliefs (Olatunji et al., 2013). Dropout rates have been reported to be lower with cognitive interventions (Foa et al., 2005; Wilhelm et al., 2009). Individuals with OCD report varied emotional responses and complex metacognitive dysfunction that may be difficult to ameliorate with exposure alone (Foa & McNally, 1996). Cognitive therapy involves helping the patient to identify and modify subtype-specific appraisals, emotional responses, and information processing in response to intrusions, other inner experience, as well as external events perceived as threatening. ERP entails helping individuals to confront what they (unrealistically) fear while resisting urges to ritualize and to reduce avoidance and maladaptive safety behaviors such as interpersonal reassurance seeking (Craske, Treanor, Conway, Zbozinek, & Vervliet, 2014; Salkovskis & Kobori, 2015). Behavioral experiments are

[2]"Third-wave" CBT is characterized by focus on mindfulness and "acceptance" of inner experience, skills to improve observing and accepting inner experience, and change in behavior consistent with the person's objectives or values. Although promising approaches have been reported, they would require further examination with OCD and are therefore not elaborated in this chapter. Comparison of third-wave interventions with "treatment" conditions demonstrated to be ineffective for OCD (e.g., relaxation) does not answer the question of whether these interventions add significantly (or are at least equivalent) to the efficacy of optimally delivered evidence-based CBT.

planned to disconfirm symptom-related beliefs and feelings while optimizing probability of success (e.g., to demonstrate the effect of repeated checking on memory and attention). Cognitive therapy precedes and is combined with ERP and behavioral experiments in feared situations, during sessions and homework, in order to achieve synergistic emotionally meaningful relearning. Recently, Bream, Challacombe, Palmer, and Salkovskis (2017) elaborated on the authors' treatment approach for OCD that aims to modify the meaning to patients of their experiences, considered to be a central contributor to symptom maintenance. Decisions about session location, frequency, and intensity should be individualized and evidence-based. There have been numerous studies on optimal procedural variants of CBT for OCD (for review, see Sookman, 2016), that will require ongoing examination in the context of refined or new approaches. Adherence to homework, and family or significant other involvement to reduce accommodation to symptoms, are important predictors of positive outcome (Simpson, Marcus, Zuckoff, Franklin, & Foa, 2012; Lebowitz, Panza, & Bloch, 2016). "Remote" CBT for OCD has shown promise for dissemination to remote regions and requires further examination (e.g., Wootton, 2016).

Importantly, patients with different OCD subtypes respond differently to specific CBT interventions. For example, a specialized CBT approach developed for obsessions improved the response of this subtype (Freeston et al., 1997). Treatment of mental contamination requires adaptions in conceptualization and intervention such as focus on interpersonal experiences, thoughts, or memories of betrayal that differ from interventions indicated for fear of contamination from external stimuli such as germs (Rachman et al., 2015). Treatment for checking involves targeting associated difficulties such as memory distrust (Alcolado & Radomsky, 2015) and advocating a phase of specific safety behaviors as needed in order to optimize reappraisals during exposure (Radomsky, Shafran, Coughtrey, & Rachman, 2010; Levy & Radomsky, 2014). At present, there remains a lag between development of these innovative approaches and methodologically adequate controlled outcome studies to examine their efficacy (for review and clinical illustrations of specialty CBT for OCD subtypes, see Sookman, 2016).

Development and management of the therapeutic relationship are of course integral to treatment, and effective symptom change during CBT predicts a positive therapeutic relationship. Development of a collaborative therapeutic alliance is fostered from initial contact in combination with specific interventions required to achieve change for specific OCD symptoms. Many patients require therapist-assisted behavioral interventions for feared situations administered in their natural environments, with therapist modeling of normal behavior and emotional modulation, highlighting the importance of technical as well as relational factors. These factors include a therapeutic relationship that fosters trust, normalization of the patient's inner experience, a culturally sensitive empathic and collaborative process, speaking in the developmentally adapted "language" of each person, and active depathologizing impacts on self-esteem.

Current practice guidelines recommend either cognitive-behavioral therapy, including ERP, or serotonin reuptake inhibitors (SRIs) as first-line treatment for OCD (APA, 2007; Koran & Simpson, 2013). SRIs (i.e., clomipramine and selective SRIs) are the only medications approved to treat OCD (APA, 2007; Koran & Simpson, 2013). However, current research indicates that few patients achieve minimal symptoms with SRIs alone (Simpson, Huppert, Petkova, Foa, & Liebowitz, 2006; Bloch et al., 2013). CBT combined with pharmacological treatment is no more effective than CBT alone for OCD symptoms (Foa et al., 2005; Romanelli, Wu, Gamba, Mojtabai, & Segal, 2014). Improvement is more sustained with ERP compared with medication, and adding ERP to medication substantially improves response rate (compared with adding a antipsychotic to an SRI) and reduces susceptibility to relapse compared with medication alone (Simpson et al., 2013; Foa et al., 2013, 2015; McLean et al., 2015). Further, the superiority of ERP over risperidone as augmentation to SRI was found to increase with baseline OCD severity (Wheaton, Rosenfield, Foa, & Simpson, 2015). Thus, it can be concluded from available research that the first-line treatment of choice for OCD is specialized CBT and that medication where indicated should be administered in combination with CBT for optimal and sustained results. While further research is required, the studies cited indicate that an update of evidence-based treatment guidelines for OCD (NICE, 2006; APA, 2007) is warranted.

Duration and severity of illness have been reported to impact outcome, highlighting the importance of early intervention (Eisen et al., 2013). Relatively few reports have been published on approaches developed for treatment-resistant samples. Van Dyke and Pollard (2005) underlined the inadequacies of administration of CBT as central to "treatment resistance." In their "St. Louis model," these authors identify and focus on patient-related factors labeled as treatment-interfering behaviors (TIBs) integrated into a comprehensive treatment approach. Inpatient residential treatment that includes ERP of up to three months' duration is indicated for outpatient treatment-resistant cases and has been reported to result in "wellness" status (Yale–Brown Obsessive–Compulsive Scale [YBOCS] ≤ 12) for approximately 25% of admitted patients (Brennan et al., 2014).

The concept of recovery, widely addressed for other mental disorders such as depression, is underexamined in the OCD literature and requires attention (Sookman & Steketee, 2010; Mataix-Cols et al., 2016). Interpretation of treatment outcome depends on response criteria, which are variable across studies. Standardized criteria that include assessment of symptoms, psychosocial functioning, and quality of life would be important for clinical and research purposes (Simpson et al., 2006; Farris, McLean, Van Meter, Simpson, & Foa, 2013; Mataix-Cols, et al., 2016). Sookman and

Steketee (2010, p. 64) described multiple criteria for recovery following specialty CBT for OCD that include no longer meeting diagnostic criteria for OCD, YBOCS ≤ 7, and normalization of salient symptom-related difficulties and psychosocial functioning (duration of gains required for recovery was subsequently updated to one year). In response to specialty treatments involving CBT alone and/or combined treatments, it has been demonstrated that OCD is curable in some cases, using the criterion for recovery of YBOCS ≤ 7 (e.g., Sookman & Pinard, 1999; Sookman, Dalfen, Annable, & Pinard, 2003; Simpson et al., 2006; Belloch, Cabedo, & Carrio, 2008; Rachman et al., 2015). Percentage of recovered patients across studies ranged from 37% to >50% of OCD samples, duration of treatment ranged from three to ten months, with follow-up of six months to two years. Specialized cognitive-behavioral therapy of longer duration and complexity resulted in greater recovery rates. Sookman et al. (2003) examined synchrony of change in beliefs and symptoms with a sample of twenty-five previously CBT-resistant OCD patients. Only patients who were symptomatically recovered in this study (10 out of 25 patients) reported that their dysfunctional beliefs had resolved to within normal limits on self-report cognitive measures of appraisals, assumptions (OCCWG, 2003), and core beliefs (Sookman et al., 2001) characteristic of OCD. It should be noted that research treatment trials are generally time-limited and manualized, and an optimal trial of CBT for OCD often requires longer duration and complexity of specialty interventions. Further research should examine the intervention and individual characteristics of patients who achieve recovery, compared with those who do not, as well as mediators/mechanisms of change in order to validate and refine promising treatment approaches.

CURRENT ISSUES AND INDICATIONS FOR FURTHER RESEARCH

Persistence of OCD symptoms is associated with distress, psychosocial impairment, and susceptibility to symptom exacerbation. Given that our aim is sustained recovery for as many patients as possible, we are still far from our goal for many patients. Despite the progress achieved to date, a substantial number of OCD patients do not respond optimally to CBT combined with pharmacotherapy. This includes patients who refuse to participate fully or drop out of ERP, do not improve, or are relapsed at follow-up. This is in part due to some patients being unable to engage fully with ERP (Simpson et al., 2013; Bloch et al., 2013) and to other patient characteristics, but importantly also to the process and content of CBT administered. A crucial distinction should be made between technical treatment failure when an individual does not improve due to the inadequacy of treatment, and serious treatment failure when an individual does not respond to adequately delivered treatment (Rachman, 1983). In the author's experience, also reported by other OCD experts (e.g., Krebs & Heyman, 2010), the majority of persons with OCD who present as being "treatment resistant" or refractory fall into the technical treatment failure category having received inadequate CBT. Common inadequacies include inaccurate or incomplete psychoeducation; failure to identify and address the patient's misconceptions and fears of initiating or completing CBT (e.g., fear of experiencing strong feelings); insufficient or incorrectly applied cognitive therapy (e.g., oversimplistic conceptualization/intervention such as restricting interventions to "challenging beliefs"); insufficient or incorrectly applied ERP (e.g., partial ERP, solely in the office); conceptual/intervention model of ERP restricted to habituation (anxiety will spontaneously decrease) without adequate consideration of inhibitory learning (formation and retrieval of new nonthreat associations) to optimize corrective learning (Craske et al., 2014); failure to administer treatment that is developmentally adapted or specific to subtype characteristics; therapist unpreparedness to handle therapeutically inevitable distress; sessions of inadequate frequency and/or duration; and premature termination of treatment.

Response rates for responders to specialty treatments for OCD have been reported to range from improved to recovered. However, criteria for treatment response are heterogeneous across studies. A recent study by Mataix-Cols et al. (2016) reported that "lack of agreement was the norm regarding operationalization of these constructs" (abstract). Based on 85.6% consensus among 326 anonymous respondents to a Delphi survey at round two (6.6% response rate; 60% of respondents reported experience with clinical trials of OCD), recovery in this study was defined as follows:

> If a structured diagnostic interview is not feasible, a score of ≤12 on the (C)YBOCS plus CGI rating of 1 (normal, not at all ill) or 2 (borderline mentally ill) lasting for one year." "If a structured interview is feasible, the person no longer meets diagnostic criteria for OCD for at least one year." (p. 19)

It is important to note that some patients in the psychometric category of YBOCS ≤ 12 meet DSM-5 (APA, 2013) diagnostic criteria for OCD, including but not limited to patients with obsessions only. Since standardization of definitions of treatment response has relevance for future randomized controlled trials (RCTs), consistency of interview and psychometric criteria for recovery would increase clarity. Importantly, presence of clinically significant symptoms (YBOCS ≤12) and status of borderline mentally ill may be suitable criteria for "wellness" (Farris, McLean, Van Meter, Simpson, & Foa, 2013) but arguably not for full recovery. This important issue has implications for future outcome studies, as well as for clinical practice, and requires further examination.

Despite general treatment guidelines for this disorder (American Psychiatric Association, 2007; Koran & Simpson, 2013), a mental health crisis characterized by unavailability of specialty treatment spans multiple and diverse international regions. An urgent global issue is the insufficient number of clinicians and clinical sites experienced with assessment and treatment of OCD, resulting in progression to disabling illness for many patients (Dell Osso, Buoli, Hollander, & Altamura, 2010). Early detection and evidence-based treatment improve recovery rates (Hollander et al., 2010). Without timely specialized treatment, remission rates among adults with OCD are low (approximately 20%; Skoog & Skoog, 1999). "Stepped care" has to date not been sufficiently empirically validated for OCD and runs the serious risk of undertreating the disorder (Sookman & Fineberg, 2015). Unfortunately, many individuals with OCD do not receive CBT, and fewer still receive specialized CBT for OCD delivered or supervised by a therapist experienced with this disorder (Stobie, Taylor, Quigley, Ewing, & Salkovskis, 2007; Shafran et al., 2009; Hipol & Deacon, 2013; Fernandez de la Cruz et al., 2015). Research indicates that clinicians report using CBT for OCD and that patients report receiving it, but the content of sessions often does not resemble evidence-based protocols (Stobie et al., 2007). In many regions, there are lengthy waiting lists to access care that may not be evidence-based (e.g., Illing, Davies, & Shlik, 2011; Szymanski, 2012). Prolonged delays in accurate diagnosis, misdiagnosis, and unavailability of specialty treatment are widespread. For example, in a survey of use of specialist services for OCD and BDD in the United Kingdom, patients waited approximately twenty years from first diagnosis to receiving highly specialized treatment, with devastating consequences in terms of illness progression (Drummond, Fineberg, Heyman, Veale, & Jessop, 2013). In a national U.S. survey of office-based practice, only 39% of visits included psychotherapy (Patel et al., 2014). Not receiving CBT is among the variables that predicts poor outcome for OCD patients. Further, perhaps related to the above, there is evidence that prescription practices are not consistent with evidence-based guidelines. For example, in a recent Swedish national study, 67% of a large OCD sample (N = 10,523) had been prescribed anxiolytics/hypnotics (in 75% of cases added to SRIs) or other medications that are not evidence based for OCD (Isomura et al., 2016). Similar findings were reported from a different study of eight international tertiary care sites (Van Ameringen et al., 2014). These results highlight the urgent need for dissemination of expertise in specialty treatments for OCD.

Training in general psychology, psychiatry, and/or CBT is not necessarily sufficient to acquire the clinical skills required for specialized treatment of complex OCD (Sookman & Fineberg, 2015). Additional academic training programs that offer longer-term rotations in the treatment of OCD as an elective would help ensure that the next generation of clinicians is not practicing with inadequate clinical skills, and would serve as well to train sufficient numbers of qualified supervisors. Improvement of existing models of continuing education and training is required to disseminate *advanced* specialty clinical skills in order to optimize illness recovery. Importantly, reliable evaluative methods are required to examine the efficacy of training models.

There is a clear need to define what constitutes evidence-based effective treatment using replicable protocols, specification of measurable core competencies (knowledge and skills) required by clinicians to deliver these, inclusion of multidimensional outcome measures, as well as effective dissemination and evaluative procedures. In order to further examine recovery rates in OCD, RCTs are required that optimize dependent variables and interventions to address inadequacies and to examine innovative new approaches. It is important to report those patients who recover fully (and sustain their recovery) and their characteristics, compared with patients who achieve wellness or clinically meaningful change versus those who do not achieve such gains. The International Accreditation Task Force (ATF) of The Canadian Institute for Obsessive Compulsive Disorders (CIOCD, *www.ciocd.ca*), comprised of seventy-one experts in OCD and related disorders representing fourteen nations, is engaged in an ongoing initiative to achieve transformative change internationally in quality and accessibility of specialized evidence-based treatment for this disorder. During phase 2, at the time of writing, the ATF is establishing specialty knowledge and competency standards recommended for specialized treatments for OCD through the lifespan (specialty CBT and pharmacotherapy), utilizing an evidence-based methodological protocol developed by this task force. ATF phase 3 will involve development and implementation of certification (individual clinicians) and accreditation (clinical sites) criteria and processes based on the established standards. A similar process is planned for OCD-related disorders.

CONCLUSIONS

Treatment for OCD is a specialized field whose aim is recovery of symptoms and restoration of multidimensional quality of life for as many patients as possible. Available outcome studies have reported that this aim is achieved for some cases in response to specialized CBT approaches. Current research underlines the importance of direct access to qualified tertiary care for OCD patients as soon as possible following emergence of symptoms in order to prevent commonly occurring progression of illness. Further research is required to examine new CBT approaches for symptom subtypes and for treatment-resistant samples, using multidimensional and stringent outcome criteria with examination of mediators of sustained change. Randomized controlled outcome trials should optimize treatment characteristics, and should report and characterize those patients who recover fully, those who achieve clinically meaningful improvement or wellness (i.e., into the mild range), and those who do not achieve such benefits. It is important to define treatment resistance as an interaction of intervention factors and patient characteristics *in the context of evidence-based optimally delivered interventions* and to further examine technical treatment failures due to intervention inadequacies. Multisite collaboration is required to improve integration of evidence-based findings from controlled research into clinical practice. There is a well-documented dire insufficiency of clinicians qualified to deliver specialized CBT for OCD. The need to disseminate expertise in this field is urgent. A central issue to be addressed by experts is how to best disseminate expertise available at academic OCD clinics (please see *www.ciocd.ca*).

REFERENCES

Alcolado, G. M., & Radomsky, A. S. (2015). A novel cognitive intervention for compulsive checking: Targeting maladaptive beliefs about memory. *Journal of Behavior Therapy and Experimental Psychiatry, 53,* 75–83.

American Psychiatric Association. (2007). Practice guideline for the treatment of patients with obsessive–compulsive disorder. *American Journal of Psychiatry, 164,* 1–56.

American Psychiatric Association. (2013). *Diagnostic and statistical manual of mental disorders* (5th ed.). Arlington, VA: American Psychiatric Association.

Arntz, A., Rauner, M., & van den Hout, M. A. (1995). "If I feel anxious, there must be a danger": Ex-consequentia reasoning in inferring danger in anxiety disorders. *Behaviour Research and Therapy, 33,* 917–925.

Beck, A. T. (1976). *Cognitive therapy and the emotional disorders.* New York: International Universities Press.

Beck, A. T. (1996). Beyond belief: A theory of modes, personality, and psychopathology. In P. M. Salkovskis (Eds.), *Frontiers of cognitive therapy* (pp. 1–25). New York: Guilford Press.

Beck, A. T., & Clark, D. A. (1997). An information processing model of anxiety: Automatic and strategic processes. *Behavior Research and Therapy, 35,* 49–58.

Beck, A. T., & Haigh, E. P. (2014). Advances in cognitive theory and therapy: The generic cognitive model. *Annual Review of Clinical Psychology, 10,* 1–24.

Belloch, A., Cabedo, E., & Carrio, C. (2008). Cognitive versus behaviour therapy in the individual treatment of obsessive–compulsive disorder: Changes in cognitions and clinically significant outcomes at post-treatment and follow-up. *Behavioural and Cognitive Psychotherapy, 36,* 521–540.

Bloch, M. H., Green, C., Kichuk, S. A., Dombrowski, P. A., Wasylink, S.,

Billingslea, E., . . . Pittenger, C. (2013). Long-term outcome in adults with obsessive–compulsive disorder. *Depression and Anxiety, 30,* 716–722.

Bream, V., Challacombe, F., Palmer, A., & Salkovskis, P. (2017). *Cognitive behaviour therapy for obsessive–compulsive disorder.* New York: Oxford University Press.

Brennan, B. P., Lee, C., Elias, J. A., Crosby, J. M., Mathes, B. M., Andre, M., . . . Hudson, J. I. (2014). Intensive residential treatment for severe obsessive–compulsive disorder: Characterizing treatment course and predictors of response. *Journal of Psychiatric Research, 56,* 98–105.

Bystritsky, A., Liberman, R., Hwang, S., Wallace, C. J., Vapnik, T., Maindment, K., & Saxena, S. (2001). Social functioning and quality of life comparisons between obsessive–compulsive and schizophrenic disorders. *Depression and Anxiety, 14,* 214–218.

Carter, J. D., McIntosh, V. V., Jordan, J., Porter, R. J., Frampton, C. M., & Joyce, P. R. (2013). Psychotherapy for depression: A randomized clinical trial comparing schema therapy and cognitive behavior therapy. *Journal of Affective Disorders, 151,* 500–505.

Craske, M. G., Treanor, M., Conway, C. C., Zbozinek, T., & Vervliet, B. (2014). Maximizing exposure therapy: An inhibitory learning approach. *Behaviour Research and Therapy, 58,* 10–23.

Dell'Osso, B. B., Buoli, M. M., Hollander, E. E., & Altamura, A. C. (2010). Duration of untreated illness as a predictor of treatment response and remission in obsessive–compulsive disorder. *World Journal of Biological Psychiatry, 11,* 59–65.

Denys, D., Tenney, N., van Megen, H. M., de Geus, F., & Westenberg, H. M. (2004). Axis I and II comorbidity in a large sample of patients with obsessive–compulsive disorder. *Journal of Affective Disorders, 80,* 155–162.

Dickhaut, V., & Arntz, A. (2014). Combined group and individual schema therapy for borderline personality disorder: A pilot study. *Journal of Behavior Therapy and Experimental Psychiatry, 45,* 242–251.

Drummond, L. M., Fineberg, N. A., Heyman, I., Veale, D., & Jessop, E. (2013). Use of specialist services for obsessive–compulsive and body dysmorphic disorders across England. *The Psychiatrist, 37,* 135–140.

Eisen, J. L., Sibrava, N. J., Boisseau, C. L., Mancebo, M. C., Stout, R. L., Pinto, A., & Rasmussen, S. A. (2013). Five-year course of obsessive–compulsive disorder: Predictors of remission and relapse. *Journal of Clinical Psychiatry, 74,* 233–239.

Farris, S. G., McLean, C. P., Van Meter, P. E., Simpson, H., & Foa, E. B. (2013). Treatment response, symptom remission, and wellness in obsessive–compulsive disorder. *Journal of Clinical Psychiatry, 74,* 685–690.

Fernandez de la Cruz, L. F., Llorens, M., Jassi, A., Krebs, G., Vidal-Ribas, P., Radua, J., . . . Mataix-Cols, D. (2015). Ethnic inequalities in the use of secondary and tertiary mental health services among patients with obsessive-compulsive disorder. *British Journal of Psychiatry, 207*(6), 530–535.

Foa, E. B., Liebowitz, M. R., Kozak, M. J., Davies, S., Campeas, R., Franklin, M. E., . . . Tu, X. (2005). Randomized, placebo-controlled trial of exposure and ritual prevention, clomipramine, and their combination in the treatment of obsessive–compulsive disorder. *American Journal of Psychiatry, 162,* 151–161.

Foa, E. B., & McNally, R. J. (1996). Mechanisms of change in exposure therapy. In R. M. Rapee (Eds.), *Current controversies in the anxiety disorders* (pp. 329–343). New York: Guilford Press.

Foa, E. B., Simpson, H. B., Liebowitz, M. R., Powers, M. B., Rosenfield, D., Cahill, S. P., . . . Williams, M. T. (2013). Six-month follow-up of a randomized controlled trial augmenting serotonin reuptake inhibitor treatment with exposure and ritual prevention for obsessive–compulsive disorder. *Journal of Clinical Psychiatry, 74*, 464–469.

Foa, E. B., Simpson, H. B., Rosenfield, D., Liebowitz, M. R., Cahill, S. P., Huppert, J. D., . . . Williams, M. (2015). Six-month outcomes from a randomized trial augmenting serotonin reuptake inhibitors with exposure and response prevention or risperidone in adults with obsessive–compulsive disorder. *Journal of Clinical Psychiatry, 76*(4), 440–446.

Freeston, M. H., Ladouceur, R., Gagnon, F., Thibodeau, N., Rheaume, J., & Letarte, H. (1997). Cognitive-behavioral treatment of obsessive thoughts: A controlled study. *Journal of Consulting and Clinical Psychology, 65*, 405–413.

Grisham, J. R., Fullana, M. A., Mataix-Cols, D. D., Moffitt, T. E., Caspi, A. A., & Poulton, R. R. (2011). Risk factors prospectively associated with adult obsessive–compulsive symptom dimensions and obsessive–compulsive disorder. *Psychological Medicine, 41*, 2495–2506.

Guidano, V. F., & Liotti, G. (1985). A constructivist foundation for cognitive therapy. In M. J. Mahoney & A. M. Freeman (Eds.), *Cognitive and psychotherapy* (pp. 101–142). New York: Plenum.

Hipol, L. J., & Deacon, B. J. (2013). Dissemination of evidence-based practices for anxiety disorders in Wyoming: A survey of practicing psychotherapists. *Behavior Modification, 37*(2), 170–188.

Hollander, E., Stein, D., Fineberg, N. A., & Legault, M. (2010). Quality of life outcomes in patients with obsessive-compulsive disorder: Relationship to treatment response and symptom relapse. *Journal of Clinical Psychiatry, 71*, 784–792.

Illing, V., Davies, D., & Shlik, J. (November, 2011). *Champlain District OCD Needs Assessment Survey, Royal Ottawa Health Care Group, University of Ottawa*. Presented at national conference, The Canadian Institute for Obsessive Compulsive Disorders: Mandates and developments, Toronto, Canada.

Isomura, K., Nordsletten, A. E., Rück, C., Ljung, R., Ivarsson, T., Larsson, H., & Mataix-Cols, D. (2016). Pharmacoepidemiology of obsessive–compulsive disorder: A Swedish nationwide cohort study. *European Neuropsychopharmacology, 26*(4), 693–704.

Jacob, M. L., Larson, M. J., & Storch, E. A. (2014). Insight in adults with obsessive–compulsive disorder. *Comprehensive Psychiatry, 55*, 896–903.

Kamath, P., Reddy, Y. C., & Kandavel, T. (2007). Suicidal behaviour in obsessive–compulsive disorder. *Journal of Clinical Psychiatry, 68*, 1741–1750.

Koran, L. M., & Simpson, B. (2013). Guideline watch (March 2013): Practice guideline for the treatment of patients with obsessive-compulsive disorder. *Psychiatryonline*. Retrieved from *http://psychiatryonline.org/content.aspx?bookid=28§ionid=40634994*.

Koran, L. M., Thienemann, M. L., & Davenport, R. (1996). Quality of life for patients with obsessive–compulsive disorder. *American Journal of Psychiatry, 153*, 783–788.

Krebs, G., & Heyman, I. (2010). Treatment-resistant obsessive–compulsive disorder in young people: Assessment and treatment strategies. *Child and Adolescent Mental Health, 15,* 2–1.

Leahy, R. L. (2002). A model of emotional schemas. *Cognitive and Behavioral Practice, 9,* 177–190.

Leahy, R. L., Tirch, D., & Napolitano, L. A. (2011). *Emotion regulation in psychotherapy: A practitioner's guide.* New York: Guilford Press.

Lebowitz, E. R., Panza, K. E., & Bloch, M. H. (2015). Family accommodation in obsessive-compulsive and anxiety disorders: A five-year update. *Expert Review of Neurotherapeutics, 16*(1), 45–53.

Leckman, J. F., Denys, D., Simpson, H., Mataix-Cols, D., Hollander, E., Saxena, S., . . . Stein, D. J. (2010). Obsessive–compulsive disorder: A review of the diagnostic criteria and possible subtypes and dimensional specifiers for DSM-V. *Depression and Anxiety, 27,* 507–527.

Levy, H., & Radomsky, A. S. (2014). Safety behaviour enhances the acceptability of exposure. *Cognitive Behaviour Therapy, 43,* 83–492.

Mataix-Cols, D., Fernández de la Cruz, L., Nordsletten, A. E., Lenhard, F., Isomura, K., & Simpson, H. B. (2016). Towards an international expert consensus for defining treatment response, remission, recovery and relapse in obsessive–compulsive disorder. *World Psychiatry, 15*(1), 80–81.

McLean, C. P., Zandberg, L. J., Van Meter, P. E., Carpenter, J. K., Simpson, H. B., & Foa, E. B. (2015). Exposure and response prevention helps adults with obsessive–compulsive disorder who do not respond to pharmacological augmentation strategies. *Journal of Clinical Psychiatry, 76*(12), 1653–1657.

National Collaborating Centre for Mental Health. (2006). *Obsessive–compulsive disorder and body dysmorphic disorder.* London: British Psychological Society, Royal College of Psychiatrists (National Clinic Practice Guidelines; no. 31).

National Institute for Health and Clinical Excellence (2005). *Obsessive–compulsive disorder: Core interventions in the treatment of obsessive–compulsive disorder and body dysmorphic disorder. Clinical Guideline 31.* London: National Institute for Health and Clinical Excellence. Available at *www.nice.org.uk/nicemedia/pdf/cg031niceguideline.pdf.*

OCCWG. (2003). Psychometric validation of the Obsessive Beliefs Questionnaire and Interpretation of Intrusions Inventory: Part 1. *Behaviour Research and Therapy, 41,* 863–878.

Olatunji, B., Rosenfield, D., Tart, C., Cottraux, J., Powers, & Smits, J. (2013). Behavioral versus cognitive treatment of obsessive–compulsive disorder: An examination of outcome and mediators of change. *Journal of Consulting and Clinical Psychology, 81,* 415–428.

Ost, L. G., Havnen, A., Hansen, B., & Kvale, G. (2015). Cognitive behavioral treatments of obsessive–compulsive disorder: A systematic review and meta-analysis of studies published 1993–2014. *Clinical Psychology Review, 40,* 156–169.

Patel, S. R., Humensky, J. L., Olfson, M., Simpson, H., Myers, R., & Dixon, L. B. (2014). Treatment of obsessive–compulsive disorder in a nationwide survey of office-based physician practice. *Psychiatric Services, 65,* 681–684.

Phillips, K. A. (2000). Quality of life for patients with body dysmorphic disorder. *Journal of Nervous and Mental Disease, 188,* 170–175.

Piaget, J. (1960). *The child's conception of the world* (J. A. Tomilson, Trans.). Totowa, NJ: Littlefield, Adams. (Original work published 1926)

Rachman, S. (1983). Obstacles to the treatment of obsessions. In E. B. Foa & P. M. G. Emmelkamp (Eds.), *Failures in behavior therapy*. New York: Wiley.

Rachman, S. S. (1998). A cognitive theory of obsessions. In E. E. Sanavio (Ed.), *Behavior and cognitive therapy today: Essays in honor of Hans J. Eysenck* (pp. 209–222). Oxford, UK: Oxford University Press.

Rachman, S. (2003). *The treatment of obsessions*. Oxford, UK: Oxford University Press.

Rachman, S. (2006). *Fear of contamination: Assessment and treatment*. Oxford, UK: Oxford University Press.

Rachman, S., Coughtrey, A. E., Shafran, R., & Radomsky, A. (2015). *Oxford guide to the treatment of mental contamination*. Oxford, UK: Oxford University Press.

Radomsky, A. S., Shafran, R., Coughtrey, A. E., & Rachman, S. (2010). Cognitive-behavior therapy for compulsive checking in OCD. *Cognitive and Behavioral Practice, 17*, 119–131.

Romanelli, R. J., Wu, F. M., Gamba, R., Mojtabai, R., & Segal, J. B. (2014). Behavioral therapy and serotonin reuptake inhibitor pharmacotherapy in the treatment of obsessive–compulsive disorder: A systematic review and meta-analysis of head-to-head randomized controlled trials. *Depression and Anxiety, 31*, 641–652.

Rosen, H. (1989). Piagetian theory and cognitive therapy. In A. Freeman, K. M. Simon, L. E. Beutler, & H. Arkowitz (Eds.), *Comprehensive handbook of cognitive therapy* (pp. 189–212). New York: Plenum Press.

Ruscio, A., Stein, D., Chiu, W., & Kessler, R. (2010). The epidemiology of obsessive–compulsive disorder in the National Comorbidity Survey Replication. *Molecular Psychiatry, 15*, 53–63.

Salkovskis, P. M. (1985). Obsessional–compulsive problems: A cognitive-behavioural analysis. *Behaviour Research and Therapy, 23*, 571–583.

Salkovskis, P. M. (1989). Cognitive-behavioural factors and the persistence of intrusive thoughts in obsessional problems. *Behaviour and Research Therapy, 27*, 677–682.

Salkovskis, P. M., & Kobori, O. (2015). Reassuringly calm?: Self-reported patterns of responses to reassurance seeking in obsessive compulsive disorder. *Journal of Behavior Therapy and Experimental Psychiatry, 49*(Part B), 203–208.

Salkovskis, P. M., Shafran, R., Rachman, S., & Freeston, M. H. (1999). Multiple pathways to inflated responsibility beliefs in obsessional problems: Possible origins and implications for theory and research. *Behaviour Research and Therapy, 45*, 2712–2725.

Shafran, R., Clark, D., Fairburn, C., Arntz, A., Barlow, D., Ehlers, A., . . . Ost, L. (2009). Mind the gap: Improving the dissemination of CBT. *Behaviour Research and Therapy, 47*, 902–909.

Shafran, R. R., & Rachman, S. S. (2004). Thought-action fusion: A review. *Journal of Behavior Therapy and Experimental Psychiatry, 35*, 87–107.

Simpson, H. B., Foa, E. B., Liebowitz, M. R., Huppert, J. D., Cahill, S., Maher, M. J., . . . Campeas, R. (2013). Cognitive-behavioral therapy vs. risperidone for augmenting serotonin reuptake inhibitors in obsessive–compulsive disorder: A randomized clinical trial. *JAMA Psychiatry, 70,* 1190–1198.

Simpson, H. B., Huppert, J. D., Petkova, E., Foa, E. B., & Liebowitz, M. R. (2006). Response versus remission in obsessive–compulsive disorder. *Journal of Clinical Psychiatry, 67,* 269–276.

Simpson, H. B., Marcus, S. M., Zuckoff, A., Franklin, M. E., & Foa, E. B. (2012). Patient adherence to cognitive-behavioral therapy predicts long-term outcome in obsessive–compulsive disorder. *Journal of Clinical Psychiatry, 73,* 1265–1266.

Simpson, H. B., & Reddy, J. (2014). Obsessive compulsive disorder for ICD-11: Proposed revisions to the diagnostic guidelines. *Revista Brasileira de Psiquiatria, 36,* 3–13.

Skoog, G., & Skoog, I. (1999). A 40-year follow-up of patients with obsessive–compulsive disorder. *Archives of General Psychiatry, 56,* 121–127.

Solem, S., Håland, Å., Vogel, P. A., Hansen, B., & Wells, A. (2009). Change in metacognitions predicts outcome in obsessive–compulsive disorder patients undergoing treatment with exposure and response prevention. *Behaviour Research and Therapy, 47,* 301–307.

Sookman, D. (2016). *Specialized cognitive behavior therapy for obsessive compulsive disorder: An expert clinician guidebook.* New York: Routledge.

Sookman, D., Abramowitz, J. S., Calamari, J. E., Wilhelm, S., & McKay, D. (2005). Subtypes of obsessive–compulsive disorder: Implications for specialized cognitive behavior therapy. *Behavior Therapy, 36,* 393–400.

Sookman, D., Dalfen, S., Annable, L., & Pinard, G. (2003, March). *Change in dysfunctional beliefs and symptoms during CBT for resistant OCD.* Paper presented at the 23rd annual convention of the Anxiety Disorders Association of America, Toronto, Canada.

Sookman, D., & Fineberg, N. A. (2015). Specialized psychological and pharmacological treatments for obsessive–compulsive disorder throughout the lifespan: A special series by the Accreditation Task Force (ATF) of The Canadian Institute for Obsessive Compulsive Disorders (CIOCD, *www.ciocd.ca*). *Psychiatry Research, 227*(1), 74–77.

Sookman, D., & Pinard, G. (1999). Integrative cognitive therapy for obsessive–compulsive disorder: A focus on multiple schemas. *Cognitive and Behavioral Practice, 6,* 351–362.

Sookman, D., & Pinard, G. (2007). Specialized cognitive behavior therapy for resistant obsessive compulsive disorder: Elaboration of a schema based model. In L. P. Riso, P. L. du Toit, D. L. Stein, & J. E. Young (Eds.), *Cognitive schemas and core beliefs in psychological problems: A scientist-practitioner guide* (pp. 93–109). Washington, DC: American Psychological Association.

Sookman, D., Pinard, G., & Beauchemin, N. (1994). Multidimensional schematic restructuring treatment for obsessions: Theory and practice. *Journal of Cognitive Psychotherapy, 8,* 175–194.

Sookman, D., Pinard, G., & Beck, A. T. (2001). Vulnerability schemas in obsessive–compulsive disorder. *Journal of Cognitive Psychotherapy: An International Quarterly, 15,* 109–130.

Sookman, D., & Steketee, G. (2010). Specialized cognitive behavior therapy for treatment resistant obsessive compulsive disorder. In D. Sookman & R. Leahy

(Eds.), *Treatment resistant anxiety disorders: Resolving impasses to symptom remission* (pp. 31–74). New York: Routledge.

Stewart, S. E., Yu, D. D., Scharf, J. M., Neale, B. M., Fagemess, J. A., Mathews, C. A., . . . Nestadt, G. (2013). Genome-wide association study of obsessive–compulsive disorder: Correction. *Molecular Psychiatry, 18,* 788–798.

Stobie, B., Taylor, T., Quigley, A., Ewing, S., & Salkovskis, P. M. (2007). "Contents may vary": A pilot study of treatment histories of OCD patients. *Behavioural and Cognitive Psychotherapy, 35,* 273–282.

Summerfeldt, L. J. (2007). Treating incompleteness, ordering, and arranging concerns. In M. M. Antony & L. J. Summerfeldt (Eds.), *Psychological treatment of obsessive–compulsive disorder: Fundamentals and beyond* (pp. 187–207). Washington, DC: American Psychological Association.

Szymanski, J., (2012). Using direct-to-consumer marketing strategies with obsessive–compulsive disorder in the nonprofit sector. *Behavior Therapy, 43,* 251–256.

Taylor, S., McKay, D., Miguel, E. C., De Mathis, M. A., Andrade, C., Ahuja, N., Sookman, D., . . . Storch, E. A. (2014). Musical obsessions: A comprehensive review of neglected clinical phenomena. *Journal of Anxiety Disorders, 28,* 580–589.

Thorsen, A., van den Heuvel, O., Hansen, B., & Kvale, G. (2015). *Psychiatry Research: Neuorimaging, 233,* 306–313.

Van Ameringen, M., Simpson, W., Patterson, B., Dell'Osso, B., Fineberg, N., Hollander, E., . . . Zohar, J. (2014). Pharmacological treatment strategies in obsessive compulsive disorder: A cross-sectional view in nine international OCD centers. *Journal of Psychopharmacology, 28*(6), 596–602.

Van Dyke, M. M., & Pollard, C. A. (2005). Treatment of refractory obsessive–compulsive disorder: The St. Louis Model. *Cognitive and Behavioural Practice, 12,* 30–39.

Veale, D., Freeston, M., Krebs, G., Heyman, I., & Salkovskis, P. M. (2009). Risk assessment and management in obsessive–compulsive disorder. *Advances in Psychiatric Treatment, 15,* 332–343.

Veale, D., Page, N., Woodward, E., & Salkovskis, P. (2015). Imagery rescripting for obsessive compulsive disorder: A single case experimental design in 12 cases. *Journal of Behavior Therapy and Experimental Psychiatry, 49*(Pt. B), 230–236.

Wells, A. (2000). *Emotional disorders and metacognition: Innovative cognitive therapy.* Chichester, UK: Wiley.

Wheaton, M. G., Rosenfield, D., Foa, E. B., & Simpson, H. B. (2015). Augmenting serotonin reuptake inhibitors in obsessive–compulsive disorder: What moderates improvement? *Journal of Consulting and Clinical Psychology, 83*(5), 926–937.

Wilhelm, S., Berman, N. C., Keshaviah, A., Schwartz, R. A., & Steketee, G. (2015). Mechanisms of change in cognitive therapy for obsessive compulsive disorder: Role of maladaptive beliefs and schemas. *Behaviour Research and Therapy, 65,* 5–10.

Wilhelm, S., Steketee, G., Fama, J. M., Buhlmann, U., Teachman, B. A., & Golan, E. (2009). Modular cognitive therapy for obsessive–compulsive disorder: A wait-list controlled trial. *Journal of Cognitive Psychotherapy, 23*(4), 294–305.

Williams, M. T., Mugno, B., Franklin, M., & Faber, S. (2013). Symptom dimensions in obsessive–compulsive disorder: Phenomenology and treatment outcomes with exposure and ritual prevention. *Psychopathology, 46,* 365–376.
Wootton, B. M. (2016). Remote cognitive-behavior therapy for obsessive–compulsive symptoms: A meta-analysis. *Clinical Psychology Review, 43*(C), 103–113.
World Health Organization (WHO). (2008). The global burden of disease: 2004 update. Retrieved from *www.who.int/healthinfo/global_burden_disease/2004_report_update/en.*

CHAPTER 20

Cognitive Therapy for Posttraumatic Stress Disorder

Patricia A. Resick

> Let us conjecture, for the moment, that a person's consciousness contains elements that are responsible for the emotional upsets and blurred thinking that lead him to seek help. Moreover, let us suppose that the patient has at his disposal various rational techniques he can use, with proper instruction, to deal with these disturbing elements in his consciousness. If these suppositions are correct, then emotional disorders may be approached from an entirely different route: *Man has the key to understanding and solving his psychological disturbance within the scope of his own awareness.*
>
> —BECK, RUSH, SHAW, AND EMERY (1979, pp. 2–3)

Because, until the *Diagnostic and Statistical Manual* (DSM-5; American Psychiatric Association, 2013), posttraumatic stress disorder (PTSD) was classified as an anxiety disorder, most extant theories of PTSD focused on fear and anxiety. Epidemiology studies (e.g., Kessler, Sonnega, Bromet, Hughes, & Nelson, 1995) made clear that not all traumas have the same effects. Rape and other interpersonal traumas produced greater rates of PTSD than impersonal traumas such as natural disasters and accidents. If PTSD were caused by conditioned reactions to dangerous situations, then the rates of PTSD should be equal across different types of traumas.

Something else must be going on because people who have experienced traumatic events evaluate them relative to their beliefs and prior experiences.

The newest edition of the DSM-5 (APA, 2013) made some major changes influenced by the study of cognitions and emotions with regard to PTSD. With the recognition that fear is not the only emotion involved in PTSD and that PTSD was more closely associated with depression than anxiety (Miller, Resick, & Keane, 2009), the DSM-5 was moved out of the anxiety disorders into a chapter with other event-related disorders. As a result, PTSD has been moved from consideration as an anxiety disorder to consideration as a disorder representing a range of negative emotions, both primary (fear, anger, sadness) and secondary (guilt, shame) and the lack of positive emotions.

Furthermore, cognitions now play a greater role in the diagnosis of PTSD. Erroneous self-blame, or other-blame, overgeneralized beliefs about the effects of the traumatic event (e.g., "no one can be trusted," "I am damaged forever") are now part of a new criterion about cognitions and emotions. Although cognitions have always been studied as part of PTSD, now more than ever, cognitions are acknowledged as important in the development, maintenance, and recovery from PTSD. This chapter will focus on early cognitive theories related to responses to traumatic events as well as more recent theories that correspond more closely to the DSM-5. Clinical applications of cognitive therapy for PTSD by Ehlers and colleagues as well as Resick and colleagues will be described. The final section will present research on cognitive therapy for PTSD.

COGNITIVE MODELS

Cognitive models were proposed even before the diagnosis of PTSD was introduced. As the earliest to focus on the effects of traumatic events, Horowitz (1979) developed an information-processing model that emphasized the role of schemas. He essentially proposed that until the traumatic event is integrated into existing schemas, the trauma will stay in active memory and be repeated. This accounts for the intrusive memories of specific events and a hallmark of PTSD that triggers the strong emotional responses and avoidance or escape behaviors.

McCann and colleagues (McCann & Pearlman, 1990; McCann, Sakheim, & Abrahamson, 1988), developed the constructivist self-development theory regarding traumatic victimization, based on Mahoney and Lyddon's (1988) constructivist perspective in which humans actively create their personal realities, such that new experiences are constrained to determine what "reality" is. McCann et al. proposed a constructivist theory of trauma in which people construct meaning from events. They theorized that aside from frame of reference (the need for a stable and coherent framework for understanding experiences), schemas, mental structures, and needs that are likely to be affected by trauma are those regarding safety, trust, power and control, esteem, and intimacy. McCann and colleagues proposed that adaptation to traumatic events is compromised when previous positive schemas are disrupted or negative schemas are seemingly confirmed. These constructs could be self- or other-directed. Because these constructs appeared so frequently in the discussions with clients, Resick and Schnicke, (1992) included these themes within cognitive processing therapy, but from a cognitive framework of brief therapy.

Although the initial emphasis in the general literature was focused on PTSD as an anxiety disorder and fear conditioning as the predominant model, even the emotional processing models (Lang, 1977; Foa & Kozak, 1986) had a role for meaning elements of threat (e.g., "Blue trucks are dangerous"). They proposed that "fear networks" were composed of stimuli, responses, and meaning elements, which are easily activated. Appraisals of upcoming danger based on prior traumatic events featured prominently in all models of PTSD.

Brewin, Dalgleish, and Joseph (1996) attempted to combine the fear network theories with social learning theories and proposed that there were two types of memory of the traumatic events (dual representation theory). *Autobiographical memory* of the event (verbally accessible memory) is stored in long-term memory as the story of the event, while *situationally accessible memory* is nonconscious, sensory memory of the event that can be triggered by reminders but not deliberately accessed or easily altered. This second type of memory represents images, flashbacks, and other sensory memories that are intrusions. Brewin et al. also proposed two types of emotions: primary emotions such as fear or anger that are conditioned during the trauma, and secondary emotions that result from the person's construction of the meaning of the trauma (e.g., shame, guilt, and erroneous anger).

Ehlers and colleagues (Ehlers & Steil, 1995; Ehlers & Clark, 2000) proposed a cognitive model of PTSD. It, too, was focused on cognitions concerning threat and fear, but Ehlers and Clark recognized the difference between PTSD and the other anxiety disorders with which it was classified. The cognitive models of other anxiety disorders focused on fear appraisals to upcoming dangerous events, while clients with PTSD have problems with their memories of the events that carry into the present as a serious current threat ("nowness").

Their examination of intrusive memories found that they were not thoughts but primarily visual images, not showing the trauma itself, but warning of the impending event (Ehlers, Hackmann, & Michael, 2004; Ehlers et al., 2002). Michael, Halligan, Clark, and Ehlers (2007) found that those with PTSD (versus those with trauma but no PTSD) experienced more distress by intrusions, lack of time perspective (happening now), and lack of context (disconnected from before and afterward). Hackmann, Ehlers, Speckens, and Clark, (2004) classified main intrusions as warning signals 92% of the time. Ehlers and Clark (2000) proposed that when an autobiographical memory is recalled, it includes both specific information about the event and context information. However, in PTSD, the memories are not adequately integrated into their context in time and place and continue to have a "here-and-now" quality. And because of perceptual priming, they have strong memories of what they encountered before and during the trauma. Those with PTSD fail to update their memories with subsequent information ("I did not die"), but instead the reexperiencing symptoms continue to trigger cues that the outcome will happen ("I am going to die").

Not coming from a fear circuitry model, Resick and Schnicke (1992) focused on the full range of emotions. Pitman et al. (1990) found that combat veterans with PTSD who listened to individualized traumatic scripts reported experiencing a range of emotions other than fear. In fact, veterans with PTSD were no more likely to report experiencing fear than other emotions. In a longitudinal investigation of crime victims, Brewin, Andrews, and Rose (2000) also found that, in addition to fear, emotions of helplessness or horror experienced within one month of the crime were predictive of PTSD status six months later. Of the small number who did not report immediate PTSD, but did report PTSD later, they did not report intense fear at the time of the trauma but rather high levels of anger at others or they reported shame. Further, emotions of shame and anger predicted later PTSD status, even after controlling for intense emotions of fear, helplessness, and horror. Similarly, Kaysen, Morris, Rizvi, and Resick (2005) studied peritraumatic emotions and behaviors among female rape and robbery or assault victims. Although 97% of the rape victims and 91% of the robbery/assault victims reported being afraid during the event, 86% of rape and 88% of robbery/assault victims reported being angry and 91% of rape and 69% of robbery/assault victims reported feeling humiliated.

A predominant notion underlying Resick and colleagues' cognitive theory of PTSD (Resick, Monson, & Chard, 2008; Resick, Monson, & Chard, 2017) is that PTSD is a disorder of nonrecovery from a traumatic event. Therefore, PTSD is not a condition that develops over time. Rather, the most severe symptoms of PTSD are experienced during the trauma and in the early days and weeks after exposure to the traumatic event has ended. With time, the majority of people who have been exposed to a traumatic event will experience reduction of PTSD symptoms, or a natural recovery from the trauma, especially if they allow themselves to experience their emotions, seek out social support, and receive corrective information regarding any distorted ideas about their role in the event. However, in a substantial minority of cases, trauma victims will continue to experience symptoms consistent with a diagnosis of PTSD. In other words, for this minority of trauma survivors, natural recovery from the trauma has been blocked in some way.

Cognitive theory of PTSD as presented by Resick et al. (2017) extends beyond informational/emotional processing theories to explain how emotions other than fear develop in PTSD. Some emotions, such as anger, fear, and sadness, that arise as a direct result of the trauma (*natural emotions*) do not need appraisal, whereas other emotions may be the result of the victim's flawed interpretations made (cognitively mediated emotions). For example, if a woman is raped, she may experience fear and anger as a direct result of the danger and abuse that she encountered. However, if she begins to believe that the rape occurred because of something she did (e.g., flirting or walking home alone), she may experience the secondary "manufactured" emotions of guilt or shame. These manufactured emotions are not a direct physiological result of the trauma, but of thoughts and interpretations made about the event. Additionally, though natural emotions tend to decrease over time, manufactured emotions will persist as long as the individual continues to have these interpretations of the event.

Cognitive theory focuses on the content of cognitions and emphasizes the importance of how the traumatic event (new information) integrates with existing schemas. This can happen in several ways. After experiencing a traumatic event, individuals can either assimilate this information into their existing beliefs about themselves and the world, or they can change their beliefs to accommodate information about the trauma—in other words, new learning (Resick & Schnicke, 1992; Resick et al., in press). Accommodation entails altering one's beliefs about self and world just enough to accept the new information that is provided by the event (e.g., "You can be robbed by someone you know"). When PTSD develops, the clients have not been able to accommodate their beliefs about the trauma information. This may be due to discomfort that may arise when they alter their previously held beliefs. People want to believe that they can predict and control their lives and events. For example, if people who held the belief "good things happen to good people, bad things happen to bad people" (*just-world myth*) were the victims of traumatic events, this belief would likely need to be altered. However, accepting the reality that negative events can happen to anyone may lead them to feel more vulnerable to the possibility of future harm, so they may resist changing their belief. As a result, they may engage in assimilation and, rather than accommodating their beliefs to fit with the trauma, they may distort the trauma to keep their beliefs intact. For example, if a combat soldier whose unit is attacked previously believed that his unit would be safe as long as he performed his duties correctly, he may conclude that his actions were to blame for the attack. Another common type of assimilative thinking is hindsight bias, or evaluating the event based on information that is only known after the fact (Fischhoff, 1975).

Alternatively, traumatized individuals may have preexisting negative schemas, usually a result of a history of prior traumatization, emotional abuse, or other negative life events that may include beliefs such as "others cannot be trusted" or they have no control over bad things happening to them. In these cases, traumatic experiences are construed as proof of the preexisting negative schemas. Based on earlier work by McCann and Pearlman (1990), cognitive trauma theory identifies beliefs related to the self and others that are often overaccommodated and contribute to nonrecovery. These beliefs are related to safety, trust, power/control, esteem, and intimacy. A strength of cognitive trauma theory of PTSD is that it accounts for varying preexisting beliefs in each area that may have been positive or negative based on the client's prior trauma history. In cognitive processing therapy (CPT), assimilated and overaccommodated beliefs are labeled "Stuck Points," describing thinking that interferes with natural recovery thereby keeping people "stuck" in PTSD. Stuck Points are targeted in therapy.

Another component of cognitive trauma theory is that instead of accommodating (changing one's beliefs just enough to incorporate this event, this new information, in a balanced and fact-based manner) some people overaccommodate their beliefs from one extreme to the other, as if there are only two categories. This is particularly typical of someone who is traumatized before they have developed more nuanced thinking, after adolescence. A common example of overaccommodation is when a traumatized individual comes to believe, based on his appraisals of his trauma, that the world is a completely unsafe and unpredictable place, when he previously believed that the world was relatively benign, or at least that bad things would not happen to him. Those who overgeneralize or overaccommodate may come to believe, "I must be in control at all times," or "I cannot trust my judgment." These extreme beliefs interfere with the processing of natural emotions produced by the event, such as fear and sadness. Additionally, they may produce manufactured emotions, such as erroneous anger, guilt, and shame.

According to cognitive trauma theory (Resick et al., 2017), clients must allow themselves to experience the natural primary emotions associated with the event that are typically avoided in the case of PTSD. Natural emotions (such as fear or anger accompanying the fight-or-flight response, or sadness from losses) that have been suppressed or avoided contribute to ongoing PTSD symptoms. According to cognitive trauma theory, natural emotions do not perpetuate themselves and thereby, contrary to behavioral theories of PTSD (Foa & Kozak, 1986), do not require systematic exposure to achieve habituation to them. The client is encouraged to approach and feel these natural emotions, which have a rather short course once they are allowed to be experienced.

In contrast, maladaptive misappraisals about the trauma in retrospect (i.e., assimilation), as well as current-day cognitions that have been disrupted (i.e., overaccommodation) are hypothesized to result in secondary, "manufactured" emotions. For example, a drunk driving victim (whose passenger was killed) who believes the crash occurred because she should have been able to swerve in time may feel ongoing guilt and be distrustful of herself. In this way, trauma-related beliefs are manufacturing ongoing negative emotions that will be maintained as long as she continues to make this assumption and will interfere with the natural grief process as well. The key to recovery with regard to manufactured emotions is to foster accommodation of the information about the traumatic event through examining the facts and actual context of the event. In other words, clients are encouraged to alter their thinking enough to account for the event in a realistic manner, without changing their minds too much, resulting in overgeneralized and maladaptive beliefs.

CLINICAL APPLICATIONS

As an extension of these cognitive theories of PTSD, cognitive therapies for PTSD are designed to address cognitive variables as factors that contribute to the development or persistence of PTSD. It is important to note that cognitive therapy is an umbrella term that captures a variety of strategies that are derived from cognitive theory, not simply an added skill included in an otherwise complete treatment. The idea behind these interventions is that an approach that elicits memories of the traumatic event and then directly examines maladaptive beliefs, faulty attributions, and inaccurate expectations may be more direct and effective than exposure therapy alone. While imaginal exposure (IE) activates the memory structure of the traumatic event and facilitates habituation, it does not provide explicit direction in correcting misattributions or other maladaptive beliefs. Therefore, cognitive-behavioral therapies for PTSD often supplement exposure with some type of cognitive intervention, most often cognitive restructuring. The technique of cognitive restructuring involves identifying and challenging thoughts that are maladaptive in specific situations. This type of cognitive restructuring is often more present-centered, focusing on "here-and-now" cognitions that impact mood and functioning. In contrast, other types of cognitive therapy are more likely to address more general trauma-focused themes, rather than challenging only those thoughts that occur in current situations. Cognitive therapy may examine the traumatic event itself, or beliefs about the event. Alternatively, these interventions may address meaning elements of the traumatic events (e.g., tying the event into the meaning of other life events) or underlying themes, and schemas that the trauma represents. Cognitive therapies can also expand the range of emotion states (beyond fear) that can be targeted in treatment.

DESCRIPTION OF COGNITIVE THERAPIES

Cognitive Therapy for PTSD (CT-PTSD)

Ehlers et al. (2004) described a cognitive therapy (CT-PTSD) that is based on their theory of decontextualized trauma memory and sense of serious current threat, either due to excessively negative appraisals of the trauma or its aftermath or a disturbance in the autobiographical memory as described earlier. They suggest that it is necessary for clients to reconstruct exactly what happened during and after the traumatic event. They proposed that this could be done by IE (Foa & Rothbaum, 1998) or by written narratives (Resick & Schnicke, 1993). However, they also suggested that the clients also need to update the event and put it into context by identifying the moments during the traumatic event when they experienced the greatest distress and sense of "nowness" (still occurring and "I am going to die") during recall, The clients also need to identify information through Socratic questioning that updates the information about the traumatic event by identifying the course, circumstances, and outcome of the trauma ("you survived and it is in the past"). Clients are taught to actively update the information into the hotspots, points of the event that elicit the most emotion, using verbal and imagery techniques. In other words, the clients need to learn to discriminate then and now, and to recognize that reexperiencing symptoms are just reminders of the event and not danger cues.

Using the warning signal hypothesis (Ehlers et al., 2002), clients are educated about the associative learning that occurs between some image or sound that occurs just before the trauma that becomes intrusive. They learn that signals that were associated at the time of the trauma do not indicate danger now. Clients may be instructed to bring up the intrusive images in order to practice the discrimination between then and now so that they will update the information. In addition to reconstructing the traumatic event with written or verbal reliving to identify the hotspots that are intrusive and particularly emotional, they may even visit the site of the trauma to both put it into the past and to clarify how the event occurred.

Other components of CT-PTSD include modifying negative appraisals of the trauma and its aftermath through Socratic questioning and behavioral experiments. They are given "reclaiming your life" assignments to reengage in activities or social contacts they have given up since the traumatic event and work to implement behavioral experiments to challenge dysfunctional avoidance behaviors and cognitions (Ehlers et al., 2010; Ehlers, Clark, Hackmann, McManus, & Fennell, 2005).

Cognitive Processing Therapy

CPT focuses primarily on identifying and challenging dysfunctional beliefs that have developed as a result of the traumatic events in order to help clients adopt a more balanced set of beliefs. Treatment traditionally takes twelve sessions and is conducted once or twice a week, with sessions lasting fifty to sixty minutes. Practice assignments are completed in between sessions. There are two versions of CPT, which differ based on whether or not they include a written account of the traumatic event. CPT+A (CPT plus accounts) includes written accounts of the worst event and CPT does not (Resick et al., 2017). CPT can be conducted individually or in groups (or a combination), and the goal, through use of successive worksheets, is to teach clients to analyze and change their own thoughts to become their own therapist—to learn cognitive skills in more balanced evidence-based thinking (as the quote in the beginning of the chapter indicates).

Treatment consists of three phases—moving from education, processing, and then challenging. During the first phase (*education*), clients are educated about symptoms of PTSD, the treatment model, the connection and differences among events (facts), thoughts, and feelings. In order to explore the clients' perceptions about the meaning of the traumatic event, they are assigned a written Impact Statement in which they write about why they think the event occurred and the effects that it has had on their beliefs about themselves, others, and the world. This Impact Statement is used to help the client and the therapist to begin to identify problem areas in their thinking about the event, which are put onto a Stuck Point log for future worksheets. Clients learn to identify Stuck Points and recognize the connections between their thoughts and emotions with the help of A-B-C worksheets. They use these worksheets to identify a situation (column A), a related thought (column B), and a resulting emotion (column C). During this phase of treatment, the therapist begins to use Socratic dialogue to help clients challenge their Stuck Points and demonstrate or learn flexibility in their thinking. Socratic dialogue is a form of questioning that encourages clients to examine and evaluate their own beliefs rather than being told in a directive way.

The second phase of CPT focuses on *processing* the traumatic event. In CPT+A the client is asked to write an account of the index event, including as many sensory details as possible. This account is not intended to serve as an exposure exercise (the goal is not habituation) but to facilitate expression of natural emotions (e.g., fear, anger, sadness) and to gather information to challenge their Stuck Points. In CPT, the trauma account is not used, and the event is explored through Socratic dialogue, with an emphasis on clarifying questions related to the event and how the facts match (or don't match) with the consequent Stuck Points. In both CPT+A and CPT, A-B-C worksheets and Socratic questioning are used to help clients generate alternatives to their assimilated beliefs, with an emphasis on erroneous anger, shame, blame, guilt, and hindsight bias about the event.

In the third phase of treatment (challenging), therapists and clients continue to work together to further examine and challenge Stuck Points about the trauma, as well as overaccommodated beliefs in order to develop more accurate and adaptive beliefs about the event, the self, others, and the world. Several worksheets are introduced, starting with the Challenging Questions Worksheet. Clients use this worksheet to ask themselves questions about their Stuck Points, with the goal of analyzing and challenging their own beliefs. They learn to examine the evidence for and against their beliefs as well as the context in which these beliefs were formed. Next, the Patterns of Problematic Thinking worksheet is introduced to help clients identify maladaptive patterns of thinking that they may be using (e.g., jumping to conclusions, overgeneralizing, or mind reading). This worksheet helps to illustrate how these patterns of thinking contribute to their stuck points and may have preceded the traumatic event. Clients may also become more aware of patterns of problematic thinking that they may be using in their daily lives, with the goal of reducing these types of thinking errors. Finally, the Challenging Beliefs Worksheet is introduced (based on a worksheet from Beck & Emery, 1985). This worksheet combines the material from the A-B-C, Challenging Questions, and Patterns of Problematic Thinking worksheets to help clients to identify Stuck Points and associated emotions, challenge those Stuck Points, and generate more helpful and accurate beliefs and corresponding emotions. This worksheet is then used for the remainder of the treatment. The last five sessions of treatment address themes that are commonly affected by trauma, including safety, trust, power/control, esteem, and intimacy as well as their own unique Stuck Points from the log (which is added to whenever new Stuck Points emerge in therapy). During the esteem and intimacy sessions, clients are given assignments to practice giving and receiving compliments and to do unconditional nice things for themselves each day. Prior to the final session, clients are instructed to write a new impact statement reflecting on their current thoughts about the cause of the traumatic event and beliefs about themselves, others, and the world in the five domains. In the final session, the first and last impact statements are read and compared in order to emphasize changes and progress made during treatment as well as to set future goals.

RESEARCH APPLICATIONS

Randomized Controlled Trials

Two early studies directly compared CT to alternative treatments (Marks, Lovell, Noshirvani, Livanou, & Thrasher, 1998; Tarrier, Pilgrim et al.,

1999). In the first of these studies, four treatments were compared: exposure therapy, cognitive restructuring, exposure combined with cognitive restructuring, and relaxation training (Marks et al., 1998). The participants were eighty men and women who had PTSD from a variety of traumatic stressors. Seventy-seven participants completed treatment, and fifty-two completed the thirty-six-week follow-up. The authors found that, overall, the cognitive, exposure, and combined treatments were more effective than relaxation, but there were no major differences between any of the three treatments. At posttreatment, 35% of the cognitive restructuring group and 37% of the combination exposure/cognitive restructuring group still met the symptom criteria for PTSD. The gains reported in this study were also evident at the six-month follow-up. Marks et al. were the first to suggest that habituation may not be necessary for change but that a change in perspective could be a mechanism of change.

The second study comparing CT with an active alternative treatment included a four-week self-monitoring baseline of symptoms to ensure the persistence of PTSD symptoms (Tarrier, Pilgrim, et al., 1999). Following baseline, seventy-two men and women were assigned to either CT or IE. As with the earlier study, the sample included survivors with PTSD from a variety of traumatic events. The researchers found that both treatment groups improved significantly, but neither form of therapy was superior to the other at posttreatment. At one-year follow-up, the gains from this study were maintained (Tarrier, Sommerfield, Pilgrim, & Humphreys, 1999). This examination demonstrated that relapse was uncommon in the first year following treatment for clients treated with IE or CT. Interestingly, these results changed at five-year follow-up (Tarrier & Sommerfield, 2004), with CT demonstrating superiority. Specifically, including 59% of the originally treated sample, none of the clients in the CT condition had PTSD, whereas 29% of the IE clients had PTSD at five-year follow-up. It is important to note that there was no significant association between type of treatment and attrition in this study. Thus, it appears that the benefits of therapy continue to develop beyond the treatment interval perhaps because of the skills learned in CT.

Bryant, Moulds, R. M., Dang, & Nixon, (2003) compared IE alone and IE with cognitive restructuring (CR) but did not include a condition with CR alone. They found that while both conditions improved, adding CR improved the outcomes better than IE alone for both PTSD and maladaptive coping styles. Ehlers et al. (2003) conducted an RCT of victims of motor vehicle accidents that started with a three-week self-monitoring phase. Those who still had PTSD were randomly assigned to receive CT-PTSD, a self-help booklet based on CT principles, or repeated assessments. At follow-up, only 11% of the CT-PTSD patients had PTSD compared to 61% of those receiving the self-help book. The self-help book was no better than repeated assessments. Ehlers et al. (2014) conducted an RCT of

CT-PTSD with a mixed trauma sample in two CT-PTSD formats, standard weekly and seven-day intensive, along with an emotion-focused supportive therapy or a fourteen-week wait list condition. The results were that 77%, 73%, 43%, and 7%, respectively remitted from their PTSD. This study demonstrated that intensive therapy was as effective as spaced therapy, was well tolerated, and produced faster results.

CPT has been the most widely studied cognitive therapy for PTSD with fourteen published RCTs. The first RCT compared CPT+A with prolonged exposure (PE; Foa, Rothbaum, Riggs, & Murdock, 1991) and a wait list control condition in female rape victims (Resick, Nishith, Weaver, Astin, & Feuer, 2002). Both treatments were highly efficacious in improving PTSD and depression at posttreatment compared with the wait list, with no differences between the active treatments at any assessment. There were a few differences on secondary measures favoring CPT: guilt (Resick et al., 2002), health-related concerns (Galovski, Monson, Bruce, & Resick, 2009), hopelessness (Gallagher & Resick, 2012), and suicidal ideation (Gradus, Suvak, Wisco, Marx, & Resick, 2013). These improvements were sustained at the three-month and nine-month follow-up points.

A long-term follow-up of participants in this study was conducted (Resick, Williams, Suvak, Monson, & Gradus, 2012). Everyone randomized in the study (i.e., intention-to-treat sample) was reached if possible for follow-up assessment five to ten years posttreatment. Of those located (144/171), 88% (N = 126) were reassessed. There were no differences between CPT+A and PE on PTSD and depression outcomes, and they continued to maintain their improvements gained at posttreatment. Moreover, neither further treatment nor subsequent negative life events were significantly associated with the maintained improvements. Gradus et al. (2013) demonstrated differences in suicidal ideation through the long follow-up, with both treatments continuing to improve but for CPT to improve more. Wachen, Jimenez, Smith, and Resick (2014) examined social functioning through treatment and over the long-term follow-up and found large improvements for all forms of functioning and no differences between CPT+A and PE.

Chard (2005), conducted a wait list-controlled trial of CPT with adult survivors of child sexual abuse. She expanded CPT+A to include a combination of group and individual treatment in order to allow not only individual processing of trauma, but also the experience of group cohesion and normalizing of problems that follow child sexual abuse. Aside from differing significantly from wait list, the dropout from treatment rate was quite low, and of those receiving CPT, only 7% met diagnosis for PTSD at posttreatment, 3% at the three-month follow-up and 6% at the one-year follow-up.

Monson et al. (2006) conducted the first CPT+A study with military veterans who were recruited through a U.S. Veterans' Administration Hospital. Sixty veterans (80% of whom were Vietnam veterans) were randomly assigned to CPT+A or treatment as usual. There were significant improvements in PTSD and a range of comorbidities at posttreatment and one-month follow-up for those receiving CPT+A versus wait list. Moreover, service-connected disability status was not associated with treatment outcomes or PTSD diagnostic status. Forbes et al. (2012) conducted a controlled effectiveness trial of CPT+A with veterans served within the Australian veterans' health care system. Like the Monson et al. (2006) study, CPT+A was compared with treatment as usual. They found CPT+A to be superior to usual care with regard to PTSD, anxiety, depression, and social and dyadic relationships, even when delivered by clinicians with varying levels of experience, treatment orientation, and disciplines.

Resick et al. (2008) conducted a dismantling study of CPT+A with 150 female victims of sexual or physical assault. In this study, CPT+A, CPT, and Written Accounts only (WA) were compared, controlling for time spent in the therapy sessions. There was an overall group difference between CPT and WA, but all significantly improved at posttreatment and follow-up periods. The important finding was that the addition of the written accounts slowed the trajectory of change and in the end did not improve the outcomes over cognitive therapy alone.

Galovski, Blain, Mott, Elwood, and Houle (2012) conducted an innovative variable-length study of CPT+A aimed at determining treatment completion based on outcome criteria versus a fixed twelve-session protocol. In this study, an RCT with delayed symptom monitoring control, a treatment completer was not defined as someone who attended all twelve sessions of the CPT+A protocol, but someone who met "good end-state," whether sooner than twelve sessions or up to eighteen sessions. Good end-state was defined as low scores on self-report PTSD and depression scales, agreement between the client and therapist that treatment goals had been reached, and an independent PTSD assessment by a blind evaluator for lack of diagnosis. At the end of session 11, if it was determined that the patient still had higher scores on the self-report PTSD measures, they could receive up to a total of eighteen sessions. They found that the majority were earlier responders (58%), and by the three-month follow-up, only one participant still had PTSD.

Bass et al. (2013) conducted an extraordinary RCT in the Democratic Republic of Congo, which had not only low resources but also high levels of ongoing violence. They randomized participants by village, with women in seven villages receiving group CPT (n = 157) and women in eight villages (n = 248) receiving individual supportive therapy and resources. The therapists had high school education at most, and a majority of the participants were illiterate. They found that CPT was superior to supportive counseling in reducing PTSD, anxiety, and depression and improving functional impairment. At six-month follow-up, only 9% of the CPT participants and 42% of the supportive therapy participants met the criteria for probable PTSD, anxiety, or depression.

Three RCTs examined whether CPT+A was equivalent when conducted in person or by telehealth at a distance (Maieritsch et al., 2016; Morland, Hynes, Mackintosh, Resick, & Chard, 2011; Morland et al., 2015). All three studies, one with male veterans in groups (Morland et al., 2015), one with female veterans or civilians (Morland et al., 2015), and the Maieritsch et al. study with only veterans of the recent wars in Iraq and Afghanistan found both formats of CPT+A to be equivalent.

Recently, Resick and colleagues (2015) compared CPT among U.S. active duty military service members in a group format compared with present-centered therapy (PCT). Both treatments led to improvements in PTSD symptoms, but CPT was superior. Moreover, CPT yielded significant improvements in depression that were maintained at follow-up assessment. An RCT conducted in Germany by Butollo, Karl, Konig, and Rosner (2016) compared CPT with dialogical exposure therapy (DET) based on Gestalt therapy. The trial included 141 male and female clients with PTSD with mixed traumas. Both conditions were variable length with up to twenty-four sessions. The dropout rate was very low for both conditions (12.2% in DET and 14.95 in CPT, including those who never started; 8% of DET and 9% of CPT dropped out after starting therapy). Both types of treatment showed large reductions in PTSD symptoms, but CPT was better at posttreatment and had a larger effect size difference (g = 1.14 for DET and 1.57 for CPT).

CONCLUSIONS

Through theory, therapy, and research on both outcomes and mediators, cognitions play an important role in PTSD treatment. Cognitive therapy has been demonstrated to be an efficacious treatment for PTSD, and change in cognitions is associated with change in PTSD and is not merely a by-product of some other process. Future research needs to examine how we can modify cognitive therapy to make it most efficient and effective for the greatest number of people possible. Civilians appear to show better recovery than veterans or active military, who may have been trained repetitively to think in certain ways that are more resistant to change. Those who served in the military are also more likely to witness killing and other graphic exposures that may be more difficult to process. It was beyond the scope of this chapter to delve into the topics of cross-cultural adaptations or how best to disseminate evidence-based cognitive therapies for PTSD, but both have received recent attention and need more. Because PTSD has more comorbidities and physical ramificactions (e.g., heart problems, immune disorders) than most other psychological disorders, specific attention to comorbidity with PTSD, both psychological and physical, and the effects of treatment will be important for the future.

REFERENCES

American Psychiatric Association. (1980). *Diagnostic and statistical manual of mental disorders* (3rd ed.). Washington, DC: Author.

American Psychiatric Association. (2013). *Diagnostic and statistical manual of mental disorders* (5th ed.). Arlington, VA: Author.

Bass, J. K., Annan, J., McIvor Murray, S., Kaysen, D., Griffiths, S., Cetinoglu, T., . . . Bolton, P. A. (2013). Controlled trial of psychotherapy for Congolese survivors of sexual violence. *New England Journal of Medicine, 368*(23), 2182–2191.

Beck, A. T., & Emery, G. (1985). *Anxiety disorders and phobias: A cognitive perspective.* New York: Basic Books.

Beck, A. T., Rush, A. J., Shaw, B. F., & Emery, G. (1979). *Cognitive therapy of depression.* New York: Guilford Press.

Brewin, C. R., Andrews, B., & Rose, S. (2000). Fear, helplessness, and horror in posttraumatic stress disorder: Investigating DSM-IV criterion A2 in victims of violent crime. *Journal of Traumatic Stress, 13*(3), 499–509.

Brewin, C. R., Dalgleish, T., & Joseph, S. (1996). A dual representation theory of posttraumatic stress disorder. *Psychological Review, 103*(4), 670–686.

Bryant, R. A., Moulds, M. L., Guthrie, R. M., Dang, S. T., & Nixon, R. D. V. (2003). Imaginal exposure alone and imaginal exposure with cognitive restructuring in treatment of posttraumatic stress disorder. *Journal of Consulting and Clinical Psychology, 71*(4), 706–712.

Butollo, W., Karl, R., König, J., & Rosner, R. (2016). A randomized controlled trial of dialogical exposure therapy versus cognitive processing therapy for adult outpatients suffering from PTSD after Type 1 trauma in adulthood. *Psychotherapy and Psychosomatics, 85*, 16–26.

Chard, K. M. (2005). An evaluation of cognitive processing therapy for the treatment of posttraumatic stress disorder related to childhood sexual abuse. *Journal of Consulting and Clinical Psychology, 73*(5), 965–971.

Ehlers, A., & Clark, D. M. (2000). A cognitive model of posttraumatic stress disorder. *Behaviour Research and Therapy, 38*(4), 319–345.

Ehlers, A., Clark, D. M., Hackmann, A., Grey, N., Liness, S., Wild, J., . . . Waddington, L. (2010). Intensive cognitive therapy for PTSD: A feasibility study. *Behavioural and Cognitive Psychotherapy, 38*, 383–398.

Ehlers, A., Clark, D. M., Hackmann, A., McManus, F., & Fennell, M. (2005). Cognitive therapy for post-traumatic stress disorder: Development and evaluation. *Behaviour Research and Therapy, 43*, 413–431.

Ehlers, A., Clark, D. M., Hackmann, A., McManus, F., Fennell, M., Herbert, C., . . . Mayou, R. (2003). A randomized controlled trial of cognitive therapy, a self-help booklet, and repeated assessments as early interventions for posttraumatic stress disorder. *Archives of General Psychiatry, 60*(10), 1024–1032.

Ehlers, A., Hackmann, A., Grey, N., Wild, J., Liness, S., Albert, I., . . . Clark, D. M. (2014). A randomized controlled trial of 7-day intensive and standard weekly cognitive therapy for PTSD and emotion-focused supportive therapy. *American Journal of Psychiatry, 171*, 294–304.

Ehlers, A., Hackmann, A., & Michael, T. (2004). Intrusive re-experiencing in post-traumatic stress disorder: Phenomenology, theory, and therapy. *Memory, 12*(4), 403–415.

Ehlers, A., Hackmann, A., Steil, R., Clohessy, S., Wenninger, K., & Winter, H. (2002). The nature of intrusive memories after trauma: The warning signal hypothesis. *Behaviour Research and Therapy, 40*(9), 995–1002.

Ehlers, A., & Steil, R. (1995). Maintenance of intrusive memories in posttraumatic stress disorder: A cognitive approach. *Behavioural and Cognitive Psychotherapy, 23*(3), 217–249.

Fischhoff, B. (1975). Hindsight is not equal to foresight: The effect of outcome knowledge on judgment under uncertainty. *Journal of Experimental Psychology: Human Perception and Performance, 1,* 288–299.

Foa, E. B., & Kozak, M. J. (1986). Emotional processing of fear: Exposure to corrective information. *Psychological Bulletin, 99,* 20–35.

Foa, E. B., & Rothbaum, B. O. (1998). *Treating the trauma of rape: Cognitive-behavioral therapy for PTSD.* New York: Guilford Press.

Foa, E. B., Rothbaum, B., Riggs, D., & Murdock, T. (1991). Treatment of post-traumatic stress disorder in rape victims: A comparison between cognitive-behavioral procedures and counseling. *Journal of Consulting and Clinical Psychology, 59*(5), 715–723.

Forbes, D., Lloyd, D., Nixon, R. D., Elliott, P., Varker, T., Perry, D., . . . Creamer, M. (2012). A multisite randomized controlled effectiveness trial of cognitive processing therapy for military-related posttraumatic stress disorder. *Journal of Anxiety Disorders, 26*(3), 442–452.

Gallagher, M., & Resick, P. A. (2012). Mechanisms of change in cognitive processing therapy and prolonged exposure therapy for posttraumatic stress disorder: Preliminary evidence for the differential effects of hopelessness and habituation. *Cognitive Therapy and Research, 36*(6), 750–755.

Galovski, T. E., Blain, L. M., Mott, J. M., Elwood, L., & Houle, T. (2012). Manualized therapy for PTSD: Flexing the structure of cognitive processing therapy. *Journal of Consulting and Clinical Psychology, 80,* 968–981.

Galovski, T. E., Monson, C., Bruce, S. E., & Resick, P. A. (2009). Does cognitive-behavioral therapy for PTSD improve perceived health and sleep impairment? *Journal of Traumatic Stress, 22*(3), 197–204.

Gradus, J. L., Suvak, M. K., Wisco, B. E., Marx, B. P., & Resick, P. A. (2013). Treatment of posttraumatic stress disorder reduces suicidal ideation. *Depression and Anxiety, 30,* 1046–1053.

Hackmann, A., Ehlers, A., Speckens, A., & Clark, D. M. (2004). Characteristics and content of intrusive memories in PTSD and their changes with treatment. *Journal of Traumatic Stress, 17,* 231–240.

Horowitz, M. J. (1979). Psychological response to serious life events. In V. Hamilton & D. M. Warburton (Eds.), *Human stress and cognition: An information-processing approach* (pp. 235–263). New York: Wiley.

Kaysen, D., Morris, M., Rizvi, S., & Resick, P. A. (2005). Peritraumatic responses and their relationship to perceptions of threat in female crime victims. *Violence Against Women, 11,* 1515–1535.

Kessler, R. C., Sonnega, A., Bromet, E., Hughes, M., & Nelson, C. B. (1995). Posttraumatic stress disorder in the National Comorbidity Survey. *Archives of General Psychiatry, 52,* 1048–1060.

Lang, P. J. (1977). Imagery in therapy: An information processing analysis of fear. *Behavior Therapy, 8,* 862–886.

Mahoney, M. J., & Lyddon, W. J. (1988). Recent developments in cognitive approaches to counseling and psychotherapy. *Counseling Psychologist, 16*(2), 190–234.

Maieritsch, K. P., Smith, T. L., Hessinger, J. D., Ahearn, E. P., Eickhoff, J. C., & Zhao, Q. (2016). Randomized controlled equivalence trial comparing videoconference and in person delivery of cognitive processing therapy for PTSD. *Journal of Telemedicine and Telecare, 4,* 238–243.

Marks, I., Lovell, K., Noshirvani, H., Livanou, M., & Thrasher, S. (1998). Treatment of posttraumatic stress disorder by exposure and/or cognitive restructuring: A controlled study. *Archives of General Psychiatry, 55*(4), 317–325.

McCann, I. L., & Pearlman, L. A. (1990). *Psychological trauma and the adult survivor: Theory, therapy, and transformation.* New York: Brunner/Mazel.

McCann, I. L., Sakheim, D. K., & Abrahamson, D. J. (1988). Trauma and victimization: A model of psychological adaptation. *Counseling Psychologist, 16,* 531–594.

Michael, T., Halligan, S., Clark, D., & Ehlers, A. (2007). Rumination in posttraumatic stress disorder. *Depression and Anxiety, 24,* 307–317.

Miller, M. W., Resick, P. A., & Keane, T. M. (2009). DSM-V: Should PTSD be in a class of its own? *British Journal of Psychiatry, 194,* 90.

Monson, C. M., Schnurr, P. P., Resick, P. A., Friedman, M. J., Young-Xu, Y., & Stevens, S. P. (2006). Cognitive processing therapy for veterans with military-related posttraumatic stress disorder. *Journal of Consulting and Clinical Psychology, 74*(5), 898–907.

Morland, L. A., Hynes, A. K., Mackintosh, M., Resick, P. A., & Chard, K. M. (2011). Group cognitive processing therapy delivered to veterans via telehealth: A pilot cohort. *Journal of Traumatic Stress, 24*(4), 465–469.

Morland, L. A., Mackintosh, M. A., Rosen, C. S., Willis, E., Resick, P. A., Chard, K. M., . . . Frueh, B. C. (2015). Telemedicine versus in-person delivery of cognitive processing therapy for women with posttraumatic stress disorder: A randomized noninferiority trial. *Depression and Anxiety.* [Epub ahead of print]

Pitman, R. K., Orr, S. P., Forgue, D. F., Altman, B., de Jong, J. B., & Herz, L. R. (1990). Psychophysiologic responses to combat imagery of Vietnam veterans with posttraumatic stress disorder versus other anxiety disorders. *Journal of Abnormal Psychology, 99*(1), 49–54.

Resick, P. A., Galovski, T. E., Uhlmansiek, M. O., Scher, C. D., Clum, G., & Young-Xu, Y. (2008). A randomized clinical trial to dismantle components of cognitive processing therapy for posttraumatic stress disorder in female victims of interpersonal violence. *Journal of Consulting and Clinical Psychology, 76*(2), 243–258.

Resick, P. A., Monson, C. M., & Chard, K. M. (2008). *Cognitive processing therapy veteran/military version: Therapist and patient materials manual.* Washington, DC: Department of Veterans Affairs.

Resick, P. A., Monson, C. M., & Chard, K. M. (2017). *Cognitive processing therapy for PTSD: A comprehensive manual.* New York: Guilford Press.

Resick, P. A., Nishith, P., Weaver, T. L., Astin, M. C., & Feuer, C. A. (2002). A comparison of cognitive processing therapy, prolonged exposure and a waiting condition for the treatment of posttraumatic stress disorder in female rape victims. *Journal of Consulting and Clinical Psychology, 70*(4), 867–879.

Resick, P. A., & Schnicke, M. K. (1992). Cognitive processing therapy for sexual assault victims. *Journal of Consulting and Clinical Psychology, 60*(5), 748–756.

Resick, P. A., & Schnicke, M. K. (1993). *Cognitive processing therapy for rape victims: A treatment manual.* Newbury Park, CA: SAGE.

Resick, P. A., Wachen, J. S., Mintz, J., Young-McCaughan, S., Roache, J. D., Borah, A. M., . . . Peterson, A. L. (2015). A randomized clinical trial of group cognitive processing therapy compared with group present-centered therapy for PTSD among active duty military personnel. *Journal of Consulting and Climical Psychology, 83*(6), 1058–1068.

Resick, P. A., Williams, L. F., Suvak, M. K., Monson, C. M., & Gradus, J. L. (2012). Long-term outcomes of cognitive-behavioral treatments for posttraumatic stress disorder among female rape survivors. *Journal of Consulting and Clinical Psychology, 80*(2), 201–210.

Tarrier, N., Pilgrim, H., Sommerfield, C., Faragher, B., Reynolds, M., Graham, E., . . . Barrowclough, C. (1999). A randomized trial of cognitive therapy and imaginal exposure in the treatment of chronic posttraumatic stress disorder. *Journal of Consulting and Clinical Psychology, 67,* 13–18.

Tarrier, N., & Sommerfield, C. (2004). Treatment of chronic PTSD by cognitive therapy and exposure: 5-year follow-up. *Behavior Therapy, 35,* 231–246.

Tarrier, N., Sommerfield, C., Pilgrim, H., & Humphreys, L. (1999). Cognitive therapy or imaginal exposure in the treatment of posttraumatic stress disorder: Twelve-month follow-up. *British Journal of Psychiatry, 175,* 571–575.

Wachen, J. S., Jimenez, S., Smith, K., & Resick, P. A. (2014). Long-term functional outcomes of women receiving cognitive processing therapy and prolonged exposure. *Psychological Trauma: Theory, Research, Practice and Policy, 27,* 526–534.

CHAPTER 21

Cognitive Therapy for Personality Disorders

Denise D. Davis

It is more important to know what sort of person has the disorder than to know what sort of disorder the person has.
—SIR WILLIAM OSLER

Early adopters of cognitive therapy quickly realized that a substantial number of patients respond in atypical ways, either to their therapist or to standard cognitive interventions (Beck, Davis, & Freeman, 2015). These individuals may present as *exceptionally* anxious, skeptical, confused, cynical, uncooperative, guarded, or perhaps even hostile at the outset. Such responses can make getting an adequate history and setting a basic agenda much more difficult than usual. Some patients may treat the therapist as more of an audience than a helper, while others passively await direction, appear painfully uncomfortable with self-disclosure, or seem suspicious about every question. Under such conditions, it is not surprising that the therapist finds it difficult to connect with the patient, to orient the patient to the treatment model, or to set treatment goals—much less make recognizable progress with a typical treatment plan for anxious or depressive symptoms.

Importantly, the difficulties that often bring these particular patients to treatment are problems that have persisted over time, occur in multiple contexts, and. not infrequently, have expanded well beyond the symptomatic parameters of a single disorder. The patient's personal, work, or community relationships may be fraught with drama, conflict, instability, or estrangement, and personal beliefs about themselves and others are distorted and inflexible. Historically, in the context of other treatment models, these patients have been labeled "neurotic" or "resistant," or are thought to have an irreparably damaged character structure.

These persistent patterns of distorted inner experience and problematic behavior are indicative of personality disorders. As diagnostic systems have evolved, so has conceptualization of a spectrum of disorders where personality functioning is linked with a person's view of self (e.g., identity and self-direction) and view of others (e.g., empathy and intimacy or quality of relationship; APA, 2013). Estimates of personality disorder in the general population suggest that as many as 10% of adults have at least one such disorder (Lensenweger, Lane, Loranger, & Kessler, 2007). Individuals with highly emotional or volatile Cluster B personality disorders (e.g., borderline, antisocial, histrionic, or narcissistic) are most likely to seek treatment (49% for any Cluster B disorder versus 25% for Cluster A and 29% for Cluster C). Surprisingly, the general prevalence of volatile Cluster B disorders is lower (1.5%) than the general prevalence of the odd (Cluster A—paranoid, schizoid, or schizotypal) or anxious (Cluster C—obsessive–compulsive, avoidant, dependent) personality disorders (approximately 6% each; Lensenweger et al., 2007). Further, among those seeking treatment for a symptomatic disorder, the likelihood of a comorbid personality disorder is around 25%, and even higher when the patient presents with two or more symptomatic (Axis I) disorders. According to Lensenweger et al., the most prevalent personality disorders are avoidant (5.2%), followed by schizoid (4.9 %), schizotypal (3.3%), and obsessive–compulsive (2.4%). Although difficulties with emotional instability are associated most often with treatment-seeking, it is important to be alert to the possibility of other prevalent disorders of personality functioning among individuals who inquire about treatment.

Personality disorders have long been recognized as complex conditions that affect a substantial number of individuals and present unique challenges in treatment. Individuals with personality disorders often suffer sustained internal distress, truncated relationships, or troubled, even toxic interactions with the world, and never seek or actively resist the option of seeking help. Research on effective clinical interventions is still in the early stages. Given this clear need, the cognitive model has been adapted as a reasonable and logical treatment option, based on positive results in treating symptomatic disorders and the model's emphasis on personal learning and empowerment (Beck, Freeman, & Associates, 1990; Beck, Freeman, & Davis, 2004; Beck, Davis, & Freeman, 2015).

COGNITIVE MODEL OF PERSONALITY DISORDERS

Personality, whether normal or disordered, consists of predictable individual differences in thoughts, emotional responses, attitudes, preferences, aptitudes, behaviors, and social impressions or impacts. Aristotle's observation, "We are what we repeatedly do. Excellence, then, is not an act, but a habit" (BrainyQuote.com), aptly pinpoints habits as the nucleus of personality. In the cognitive model, personality consists of belief-driven patterns or habitual *modes* of appraisal, emotional coding, and action strategies that in turn comprise a person's sense of self, relation to others, and characteristic navigation of life (Beck, 2015).

In Beck's model, modes are formed from a genetic propensity toward certain normal behaviors, aimed at survival, reproduction, and adaptation to the environment, which in turn are shaped by learning experiences. Various habitual modes form the recognizable features of an individual's personality. As a person navigates through the course of a day, various modes activate and deactivate in a fluid way to meet the person's needs, respond to challenges, to both express and protect the "self." Emotion schemas have an important role in calibrating the movement in and out of modes, which makes them important points of intervention. Optimal personality functioning is flexible and responsive to social cues, yet reflects the unique individual and the individual's cultural context, even in states of high arousal. However, some modes can become hypertrophied or overgrown, while others are underdeveloped, giving rise to the inflexible, pervasive habits that we call personality disorders. Cognitive biases continue to favor these modes, from the point of perception through behavioral response, especially when activated by a highly salient situational challenge or pursuit of a life goal (Beck & Haigh, 2014). The cognitive bias eventually leads to a fusion of the habitual mode and a view of self, to the extent that the individual firmly believes that "this is who I am; this is me," and is apt to resist thinking differently.

The various diagnostic categories of personality disorders can be construed as dysfunctional (overdeveloped) modes such as the obsessive–compulsive mode or the narcissistic mode, each characterized by a specific cognitive profile. For example, in the dysfunctional obsessive–compulsive mode, a particularly strong fear of mistakes, regret, or blame motivates the person to value control or perfection and adopt this as an essential component of their self-image. The patient may say things like, "I'm a perfectionist and I absolutely must strive for high standards." The patient's conditional beliefs often contain "should" or "must," as in "If a person fails to do something right, he should be punished," which reinforces the fear of mistakes. Similarly, a person in a dysfunctional narcissistic mode is preoccupied with verifying his or her self-importance or superiority to others. This individual may hold the conditional belief that "if I have power, that proves my superiority over others and entitlement to special treatment," leading to various efforts to attain power by boasting, dominating, deliberately violating rules, or inflating their status.

The cognitive profile associated with each overdeveloped mode provides the therapist with a roadmap for conceptualization and targeted intervention for the personality difficulties of individual patients (Beck, 2015). Each cognitive profile includes one or more fundamental catastrophic fears about an individual's identity and place in the social world. The individual experiences this fear as both intolerable *and* as something he cannot discount or let go. Therefore, a more superficial compensatory self-image develops as a protective cognitive alternative. This allows the individual to avoid any direct verification of his core fears. At first glance, the compensatory self-image may seem quite adaptive. However, because it functions as a cognitive safety behavior, it is rigid and offers little flexibility in accommodating discrepant information. The individual "must" be able to protect his compensatory self-image, or risk confronting some awful "truth" about his personal competence, lovability, strength, self-determination, normalcy, acceptability, agency, value to others, importance, or worth as a human being.

Table 21.1, which is adapted from Beck (2015), outlines these core fears, compensatory beliefs, key conditional assumptions, and overdeveloped behavioral coping strategies for each personality disorder. For instance, individuals with an avoidant profile greatly fear being perceived as unlikable or inferior to others. Triggers for this fear may be quite diffuse and ever present. Frequent and unpredictable anxious arousal provides the experiential data that underlie their compensatory self-image as emotionally fragile or highly sensitive persons who need to avoid undue stress. This gives rise to conditional assumptions such as "If I reach out and get a negative reaction, I will feel crushed and overwhelmed." Their overdeveloped coping strategy of self-protective avoidance results in persistent sadness, loneliness, and restricted personal growth. Although these modes are recognizable patterns, there is still likely to be considerable variation within the mode with regard to severity, presence of modifying beliefs or skills, overlap and comorbidity with other personality disorders (modes), and environmental factors that impact the person's functioning.

The modes referred to in the Beck model are different from the modes described in Young's schema therapy for personality disorders (Young, 1999; Young, Klosko, & Weishaar, 2003). Although both refer to coping efforts and the predominant state of functioning, the modes are described differently. In Young's model, there are ten schema modes grouped into four descriptive categories: child modes, dysfunctional coping modes, dysfunctional parent modes, and healthy adult modes. In schema therapy, the specific name used for the mode is tailored to fit the feelings and behaviors of the patient, such as "level-headed" mode (healthy adult). Likewise in cognitive therapy, the terms used when discussing modes with patients reflect the primary beliefs, affect, or behavioral habit experienced by the patient, such as "loner," or "detached," modes. The Beck and Young models are quite compatible and can be integrated in the understanding of a specific person. For example, the overcompensating modes of a person with narcissistic personality disorder might include "very important person," mode, and "bully" mode (Behary & Davis, 2015).

For personality disorders, the essential source of difficulty and ultimate targets of intervention are (1) the core fears, (2) compensatory self-image beliefs, and/or (3) the associated overdeveloped and underdeveloped behavioral strategies. The process of altering a person's self-image, view of reality and self-regulating schemas can vary considerably in terms of specific techniques, depending on the individualized case formulation, patient capabilities, and treatment acceptance. Flexibility in using a variety of psychotherapeutic techniques that are adapted for use within the cognitive model is essential, as will be detailed further in the clinical application section below.

CLINICAL APPLICATION

Personality disorders include diverse and potentially overlapping types of functional problems. No single protocol applies to all of the different disorders included in this broad category. Successful treatment will most likely involve an individualized formulation and integration of a range of cognitive, behavioral, experiential, and relational concepts and procedures, with continual and nimble adjustments based on the data of the patient's progress and response to methods used. The following six precepts are offered as a guide to key adaptations needed for ongoing case formulation and dexterous intervention with the various disorders of personality.

Precepts for Cognitive Intervention with Personality Disorders

1. *Listen for Beliefs That Indicate an Inflexible, Compensatory Self-Image, or Negative (Feared) Self-Image.*

It is very important to recognize as early as possible when the patient's difficulties involve maladaptive core beliefs and patterns of coping that underlie their current symptoms. The earliest clinical signs may surface when interactions with a new patient seem notably difficult or unusual in any way. Perhaps the patient is highly guarded, uncooperative, demanding, or brusquely skeptical. This suggests a view of themselves as vulnerable to exploitation and the motivations of others as largely malevolent.

TABLE 21.1. Cognitive Profiles and Overdeveloped Coping Strategies

Personality Disorder	Core Fear	Compensatory Self-Image Beliefs	Key Conditional Assumptions	Overdeveloped Affect/Coping Strategies
Paranoid	"I am a target; vulnerable to personal harm."	"I am intuitive and clever."	"If I stay on guard, I can protect myself."	Fearful, angry, suspicious; Scan for threats; Hide counter-attack
Schizoid	"I am odd, different, or abnormal."	"I am a loner." "I need my space."	"If I am around people, I will have a stressful experience."	Disgust, irritation, nervousness; Refuse social bids; Solitary activity
Schizotypal	"I am weird; a social misfit."	"I am unique; gifted."	"If I appear unusual, others will respect my special gifts."	Anxiety, hostility; Atypical grooming; Endorse magical concepts
Antisocial	"I am deprived; mistreated; a victim."	"I can outsmart the system and get what I want."	"If I see a chance for excitement or advantage, I should take it."	Irritable, proud, contemptuous, restless, bored, thrill-seeking; Exploitative actions
Borderline	"I am damaged; disgusting; a bad person."	"I am a victim; a broken person and cannot help myself."	"If I feel upset, I cannot control myself and must get relief."	Anger, despair; Impulsive decisions and actions
Histrionic	"I am unlovable."	"I am very passionate."	"If I express the depth of my feelings, others will love and validate me."	Anxiety, anger; Intense emotional or sexual display; Tantrums; Somatic complaints
Narcissistic	"I am unimportant."	"I am very special."	"If I have power, that proves I'm superior to others."	Anger, contempt, impatience; Boast; Make demands; Seek power; Dominate others

(*continued*)

TABLE 21.1. (*continued*)

Personality Disorder	Core Fear	Compensatory Self-Image Beliefs	Key Conditional Assumptions	Overdeveloped Affect/Coping Strategies
Avoidant	"I am unlikable; inferior to others."	"I am emotionally fragile."	"If I am very careful, I can prevent humiliation or avoid rejection."	Sadness, loneliness, anxiety; Wishful thinking; Safety behaviors
Dependent	"I am helpless; ineffective; selfish."	"I am a people pleaser."	"If I don't please others, I won't have anyone to lean on."	Anxiety, anger; Complain; Seek help or reassurance; Obligate others
Obsessive–Compulsive	"I am wrong; mistaken; irresponsible."	"I am a perfectionist; I need things done the right way."	"If I find the right way, I can control outcomes and avoid failure, blame, or regret."	Anxiety, anger; Locate and follow rules; Dictate "shoulds"
Passive–Aggressive	"I am trapped; stupid; a loser."	"I am misunderstood; under-appreciated; sensitive to pressure."	"If I do what is expected, I will lose what I want."	Covert anger; Argue; Resist or oppose requests, expectations, or obligations
Depressive	"I am worthless; pathetic, insignificant."	"I am a realist."	"If I don't expect anything, then I won't be disappointed."	Anger, disgust; Cynical, bitter complaints; Avoidance goals; Surrender to frustration

At the other extreme are patients who are notably flattering, ingratiating, or submissive in their behavior. This may stem from the belief that they are helpless or unworthy and must make a special effort to please or avoid displeasing the therapist to merit any treatment. In general, the likelihood of personality disorder is greater when the patient presents symptomatic problems that are complex, comorbid, and long-standing.

Because compensatory beliefs have a more positive tone, it may be easier to inquire directly about characteristics such as perfectionism, exceptional intelligence, social superiority, strong passion, and an ability to outsmart "the system." These indications are not sufficient for diagnosing psychopathology per se, but they can aid in early conceptualization. Personality disorder is based on evidence of pervasiveness and inflexibility that leads to clinically significant internal distress or functional impairment in relating to the world. There may be a lack of synchrony between internal and external problems, as the perfectionist may suffer inwardly and yet receive approbation in the world, while the con artist is smug or proud of exploiting or aggravating others and callous to the impact of their actions.

Core fears are more likely to be accessible when an individual is experiencing some triggering stress. Typical triggers can include new developmental demands, relationship changes or conflicts, real-world consequences of the overcompensating or undercompensating behavior, or simply the difficulty of managing recurrent negative affect such as pervasive loneliness, severe anxiety, or chronic resentment. In any case, the compensatory self-image is somehow rattled, and the individual needs a new way to cope. Some patients will openly share a struggle they are having with a recurring belief that they are bad, worthless, or inferior. Others may vehemently deny any such concern, although they identify the fear as emotionally relevant to them. For example, a young man was despondent over failing to receive a significant performance award at work because he believed his special talents deserved more recognition. He concurred that one of his strongest fears was being ignored or treated as unimportant, even though he most certainly did not believe himself to be unimportant.

Guided discovery can be used to explore beliefs that the patients endorse as descriptive of who they are and how they usually behave, to collaboratively conceptualize personality related beliefs. To separate core beliefs from more transient mood-driven reactions, therapists can ask about duration and cross-situation evidence of these beliefs. When rapport is strong enough and there is sufficient time to respond with support, the therapist might ask the patients if there is anything that they have often feared might be true about them. A follow-up question might be to ask what the patients wish could be true about them as persons. The patients' thoughts about the therapist or what the therapist might be thinking about them are also another important source of information. These thoughts are typically most accessible when the patient shows an affective shift in the session; this is an opportune time to make an inquiry.

Discussion of core beliefs requires a degree of self-reflection that is difficult or uncomfortable for some patients, especially early in therapy. Thus, it may be useful to offer brief psychoeducation on the value of discussing self-schemas as a means of improving self-esteem, self-direction, and self-care (well-being), and creating calmer, more satisfying relationships with others, while also being sensitive to the patient's emotional reactions to the topic of "self." As a technical concept, self-schemas might be likened to an inner set of personal instructions or adopted roles that provide a key to understanding why certain personal scenarios recur. For example, a dependent patient complained of feeling overwhelmed and of being unable to say "no" to others. This was because she saw herself as "the one who is always there for others." If she didn't enact this role of constant supporter, she feared that she would be cast as "the selfish one." Again and again, she would stay up too late, take on too much, listen too long, and feel cranky, resentful, and overwhelmed. When she examined the implications of selfishness, she recognized that she feared rejection because she viewed herself as helpless on her own. Recognizing the beliefs connected to her habitual self-sacrifices helped her to add more flexibility to her valued position of caring for herself and others, and to evaluate her view of her own competence. Specifically, she was able to state her desired role as "one who supports others in mutually healthy ways," rather than being a constant "people pleaser" as a constant hedge against helplessness.

Self-reflection can be framed as an essential skill that provides the basis for effective self-understanding and direction, and it can be gradually developed through guided practice with the therapist. The amount of time spent on these specific discussions will depend on patient acceptance and emotional tolerance, as some patients will collaborate readily while others need more time to develop trust and reduce their guardedness in the therapeutic interaction.

2. *Review Personal Beliefs about the Feasibility of Personality Change and Possible Mechanisms of Change.*

Personality is often likened to a hardened "structure" that is relatively predetermined and intractable to further change once it is set in place. Based on this assumption of a determined and set construction, therapists and patients alike may believe that personality change is not possible, or at least not likely for the individual in question. Biological concepts often ground this perspective, with genetic inheritance and nervous system wiring as the immutable building blocks. The presence of a complex family history of problems is then interpreted as evidence of a biological substrate that cannot be altered, with an inevitable life trajectory. A related belief is that early negative experiences add structural damage and decrease any potential for adaptive plasticity. This essential view of set personality is very important because of the implication that personality cannot change. This last point is very significant because the idea that personality cannot change is more prediction than established fact.

Although the model of personality structure as concretized by biology and very early experience has been extremely influential in popular and clinical contexts, a more differentiated perspective has emerged from the last two decades of scientific study. Looking first at normal personality development, Roberts, Walton, and Viechtbauer (2006) have summarized compelling longitudinal and cross-sectional evidence that personality changes occur across the lifespan, well into old age, albeit with young adulthood as the period of most intense change. The normal direction of change is usually positive, with increases in emotional stability, agreeability, conscientiousness, and greater confidence and independence in social contexts, while social energy and desire for new experiences may drop off somewhat during middle to later years. Individual differences in these patterns are also evident over the lifespan, as well as cohort effects that reflect variations in cultural values during certain historical periods. Considering what factors prompt personality changes, Roberts and colleagues propose that "most personality change occurs through the press of contingencies found in age graded social roles" (2006, p. 18). Role expectations serve as guides for coping, and role opportunities provide catalyzing experiences that foster personality change. Thus, there is ample evidence that personality can and does change and that life experiences and life lessons play a larger role than genetic factors in shaping personality development (Roberts et al., 2006).

But what evidence is there to support an expectation of change among persons with disordered personality? This is a more complicated question from an empirical standpoint. The presumption of stability has been examined in four longitudinal studies of the course of personality disorders and summarized by Morey and Hopwood (2013). Although Morey and Hopwood caution against any single conclusion due to significant methodological issues, they note that the diagnostic remission rates found in longitudinal studies of personality disorders exceed expectations based on clinical assumptions and that remission rates are increased by treatment, whether or not it is specific to the personality disorder.

For example, among a sample of inpatients with borderline personality disorder (BPD) who were reassessed every two years posttreatment, 39% achieved remission within the first two years, and 88% achieved remission of the BPD diagnosis by the ten-year follow-up (Zanarini, Frankenburg, Hennen, Reich, & Silk, 2006). At the sixteen-year follow-up (Zanarini, Frankenburg, Reich, & Fitzmaurice, 2012), the cumulative rate of a remission (less than two criteria for diagnosis over the duration of two years) was 99%, although some had experienced relapse and levels of functional impairment were not as dramatically improved. A smaller comparison sample of patients with other personality disorders demonstrated similar rates of remission that were achieved in shorter time periods and had low recurrence rates. The BPD recurrence rates ranged from 10 to 36%, while the comparison PDs were under 10%, with recurrence less likely the longer that remission was maintained. Similar longitudinal data from a different study were reported by Gunderson et al. (2011), where 85% of outpatients with BPD achieved remission at ten-year follow-up, had a 12% relapse rate, and experienced minimally slower progress compared to a group of patients with cluster C (anxious) personality disorders.

These studies provide important information on the instability of personality disorder diagnosis, yet they do not delineate the mechanisms of how disordered personality characteristics can be changed. As Morey and Hopwood note (2013), the rates of maladaptive core personality traits and functional difficulties tend to be more stable and enduring than symptoms across various studies. They propose that core personality traits are slowly evolving constellations and functional impairments are compromised attempts to cope or compensate for these traits.

Evidence to support the role of beliefs as a potential mechanism for altering personality traits and behaviors is provided by the work of Dweck (2008). For example, when individuals believe that their basic qualities can be changed by their own actions, they demonstrate much greater persistence and ability to self-regulate (Blackwell, Trzesniewski, & Dweck, 2007; Dweck, 1999). Dweck has termed this the *malleable* self-theory, as contrasted with a *fixed* theory of the traits and abilities of self and others. Malleable theory can be taught, and when it is, the result is greater motivation and better response to challenges. Dweck makes the important point that praising an individual's process or effort facilitates adoption of a malleable theory, while praising specific traits (e.g., intelligence) will reinforce fixed theory beliefs (Mueller & Dweck, 1998). In either case, beliefs are the bridge or mechanism for altering personality traits (e.g., conscientiousness), and even small interventions that increase the malleability of core beliefs can produce a large impact on how well a person functions in her life (Dweck, 2008).

This evidence is consistent with the cognitive model of personality functioning (Beck, 2015), where cognitive control schemas are thought to play a crucial role in self-image and self-regulation (Beck, 2015). These schemas organize the processes of self-direction and regulation, derived from the underlying self-concepts and a medley of rules acquired from life lessons. Thus, it is important for therapists to help their patients to consider the malleable self-theory and to understand that what people believe about themselves and their place in reality is an ongoing construction that can change with new experience. Change-blocking beliefs such as "It runs in the family," or "My history of abuse caused irreparable damage," or "I have to be who I have *always* been," might be framed as true or partially true statements but do not provide sufficient rationale for continuing maladaptive actions (overdeveloped strategies).

3. *Use Your Personality Strengths to Facilitate New Learning.*

The person-to-person interaction takes on special significance as a *therapeutic* component in treatment of personality disorders. One of the first things therapists often notice among patients with personality difficulties is the patient's heightened sensitivity to interpersonal interactions. This may be confined to certain people or groups of people (e.g., authority figures; significant others), or it may reflect a generalized sensitivity in interacting with the world. How the patient reacts to the therapist can provide a valuable window into how the patient interacts with others and what sorts of impacts their behavior may have on others. Interactions with the therapist also provide an essential opportunity to gain new information that can help to de-activate overdeveloped coping strategies and encourage potentially helpful but underdeveloped strategies.

Rather than attempting to adopt a very neutral stance in service of "transference," the CBT therapist deliberately behaves in ways that exemplify the adaptive poles of major personality traits (see APA, 2013, pp. 779–781, for details on maladaptive domains and features). These traits include presenting themselves as emotionally stable (vs. moody, negative, or unpredictable); friendly and engaged (vs. judgmental, condescending or detached); agreeable and considerate (vs. critical or insensitive); conscientious (vs. careless or impulsive); and clear and understandable (vs. disorganized and obscure). The actions that exemplify these traits can be thought of as the micro-skills that therapists use to effectively set patients at ease and prompt their involvement in therapeutic collaboration. Because patients with personality disorders often have notable difficulty engaging and collaborating, it is especially important for therapists to deliberately employ behaviors that model and prompt the desired responses from the patients.

Therapists can use these basic interpersonal skills as foundational efforts or, more simply, as what to do all the time, and as what they can *always* do when they are unsure of the best way to proceed. For example, they can smile, relax their posture, practice self-calming, and show the patient how to remain emotionally steady by their own example. They can demonstrate the skill of accepting feedback by inviting it and responding with appreciation rather than defensiveness or anger. Taking time to express genuine interest in the patient's life, showing warmth and appreciation for the patient's efforts, and empathy for the patient's struggles are all important features of a truly therapeutic interaction.

Perhaps even more important is the process of respectfully drawing the patient into decision making about what problems to address, how to approach them, and what homework might be helpful. The therapist avoids controlling the agenda without input, lecturing, giving advice without being asked, imposing his or her opinion as expert, moving too quickly without checking with the patient, or pushing for certain outcomes or timetables without patient agreement. Instead, the therapist guides the session flow and invites the patient's participation without dominating or being too passive. The therapist keeps his own attention focused and filters personal impulses. Therapists avoid confusing or upsetting terms, and endeavor to make the therapeutic goals and methods transparent and understandable to the patient. With permission or when invited to do so, they share their train of thought and invite the patients to verify, correct, extend, or redirect their thoughts. Last, but certainly not least, therapists model congruence between verbal and nonverbal messages, and check for the possibility of any confusion or misinterpretation. This gives the patient a chance to identify his or her perceptions and check them out directly, and thereby strengthen and normalize an underdeveloped strategy. All of this may require the therapist to adjust his internal timeline for progress, as much more time may be needed to focus on these more subtle therapeutic interactions. How the patient and therapist interact matters just as much as, if not more than, what topic they specifically address on the agenda and how far they get with that topic.

Because many patients with personality disorders are (1) sensitive to interpersonal threats, (2) prone to exhibit maladaptive traits, and (3) cope by avoidance or interpersonal dominance, therapists can prepare to spot these patterns, resist taking the behavior personally, and deploy specific therapeutic responses that gently evoke more adaptive patient responses. In this way, they can foster trust, provide the patient with a healthy example, and create opportunities for practicing cognitive and interpersonal flexibility. Of note in schema-focused cognitive therapy (e.g., Arntz, 2015), the therapist strategically acts in ways that target the patient's unmet childhood emotional needs, such as warm acceptance or consistent limits, to facilitate development of the patient's healthy adult mode.

4. *Stay Grounded in the Cognitive Model to Guide the Focus, Pace, and Methods of Change.*

Hopefully, it is clear that the general goal of cognitive therapy for personality disorders is to help individuals develop a malleable self-theory and flexible core beliefs that support adaptive personality functioning. Such adaptive personality functioning can include (1) the ability to consider multiple perspectives on a situation; (2) tolerance of new or different experiences; (3) appreciation of a range of emotions in living; (4) identification and pursuit of personal goals; (5) expression of compassion or kindness to self and others; (6) respect and reciprocation in relationships; and (7) low tendency to exaggerate strengths or hide vulnerabilities (or vice versa; Fulton & Siegel, 2013).

Specific objectives for individual patients will depend on the features of their cognitive profile and case formulation as well as their basic values and desires for a productive and satisfying life. For example, Clark and Hilchey note that key treatment goals for an individual with depressive personality disorder would likely include correcting negative future expectancies, reducing solicitation of negative feedback, and altering behavioral self-handicapping patterns (2015, pp. 233–234). These are key skills relevant to recognizing multiple perspectives on a situation and the pursuit of personal goals. With avoidant individuals, Padesky and Beck target cognitive and emotional avoidance and work on skills of self-reflection and interpersonal self-expression (2015, pp. 183–184), to assist these individuals in appreciating their range of emotions, achieving a desired level of intimacy and reciprocation with others, and decreasing their tendency to anxiously hide vulnerabilities.

Change generally takes place much more slowly in the treatment of personality disorders, as compared to uncomplicated mood or anxiety disorders (Beck, Freeman, & Davis, 2015). This, however, is not necessarily verification of the idea that personality cannot change or that it requires Herculean effort. The pace of change can be affected by many variables and will likely include bursts of progress or lulls when it may seem that little change is happening. A persistence of functional difficulties is to be expected and is not interpreted to mean that the cognitive model is inappropriate, ineffective, or should be discarded. The therapist can use ongoing case formulation, including developmental history, core beliefs, assumptions, and coping strategies that are over- and underdeveloped, and apply a variety of evidence-based methods to prompt the patient's initiative toward greater adaptive functioning.

Patients with personality difficulties often present in a state of general distress, or at least distress over their predicaments, but this does not necessarily indicate a readiness to change. Their personality modes may leave them chronically distressed, but the targets for change are vague. They may feel confused about who they really are or what they want out of life, and lack consistent or enjoyable relationships with others. They may be surprised or distressed by external pressures and resent others for confronting them or expecting them to change. The displeasure of others may be triggering resistance to change such that the patients are less open to self-reflection, less receptive to suggestions, and more concerned with protecting their compensatory self-image. Furthermore, the patients may be frustrated by a long history of conflicts with others, being pushed toward therapy, or participating in previous therapies that seemed to have little impact. Thus, therapists will do well to address such ambivalence with effective methods such as motivational interviewing (Miller & Rollnick, 2012). Skillful use of motivational interviewing can help the therapist draw out the patient's own interests in and reasons for change, noting the thoughts that argue against change and facilitating the shift into considering personal reasons for change and possible ways to make it happen (Mitchell, Tafrate, & Freeman, 2015).

Typically, the patient's most pressing functional problems provide the initial as well as ongoing focus for consideration of change. Patients who do not endorse any pressing problems or distress, who are angry and want others to change (or at least stop pestering them), or who are highly suspicious or overcontrolled may be among the most difficult to engage. In these kinds of interactions, the therapist might feel pressured, puzzled, anxious, or doubtful about using the cognitive model, or at a loss in terms of direction. Despite the images popularized in entertainment media, using "get tough" confrontation is seldom very effective (Mitchell et al., 2015). Rather than abandoning the cognitive model or deeming the patient unsuitable, the therapist can conceptualize such problems through the lens of readiness for change. When the patients do not identify any personal problems despite evidence to the contrary, they are said to be in a state of pre-contemplation. This state of pre-contemplation must be addressed for therapy to effectively continue. Adequate resolution of this state will lead into the subsequent states of thinking constructively about change, preparing for action, taking action, and maintaining change.

The mainstay of collaborative strategies for moving from pre-contemplation into contemplation of change is Socratic questions and guided discovery, framed in the nonexpert stance of a motivational interviewer. Because the patients' beliefs and behavior function as protection against any experience that might risk confirming their core fear, it is important to invest due diligence in helping such patients identify a problem that they are willing to tackle so that they are oriented to therapy as a process of considering and enacting change. For example, an antisocial patient who abuses substances may only be willing to work on job interviewing skills early in therapy because the substance use is associated with seeing himself as shrewd and powerful. Confronting the substance use as a problem will challenge these compensatory core beliefs. Patients who believe that they are vulnerable to exploitation or being manipulated will likely lean toward negative views of therapy, unless the therapist can help them become aware of the advantages of therapeutic discussions (Renton & Mankiewicz, 2015). Patients who fail to perceive a down side to their current way of coping might benefit from empathic relational feedback or therapist self-disclosure (Arntz, 2015; Behary & Davis, 2015; Sungur & Gündüz, 2015) or from assisted self-appraisal of lifestyle (Mitchell et al., 2015). Patients who fear the emotional arousal of self-disclosure will be more likely to engage in constructive contemplation of self-change when they can trust that the interpersonal process will be supportive and reinforcing, not critical and punitive. Signaling safety through friendly, respectful actions such as explaining the cognitive model, involving the patient in setting the agenda, providing positive reinforcement for emotional disclosures, and seeking the patient's feedback all help patients tolerate the stress of considering change (Brauer & Reinecke, 2015; Fusco, 2015; Padesky & Beck, 2015; Simon, 2015). Some patients may respond best to a blend of these various methods (Clark & Hilchey, 2015). Finally, it is not unusual for people to become disengaged from their motivation to change during treatment, necessitating a return to these considerations.

The cognitive model for treatment of personality disorders specifically emphasizes a collaborative, individual conceptualization based on the patient's view of current life problems, their developmental history and information gathered from interaction with the therapist (Beck et al., 2015). Given the developmental nature of personality disorders, it is valuable to use a tripartite approach to examine beliefs and supporting experiences in these three spheres: (1) current concerns, (2) personal history or life narrative, and (3) therapeutic interaction (Brauer & Reinecke, 2015). Thus, intervention is more person-focused than symptom-focused. The selection of specific therapy techniques is tailored to the individual based on a collaborative formulation, and a range of cognitive, behavioral, psychoeducational, and experiential methods is used in the service of increasing cognitive flexibility and skill in regulating thoughts, emotions, and behavior. With increased cognitive flexibility, the individuals' underdeveloped coping strategies become accessible options, core self-image fears have lower valence, self-esteem is more stable and less contingent on projecting their compensatory self-image, and their relationships are more fluid and growth-oriented rather than being stressful or unsatisfying to self and others.

Table 21.2 provides a selected overview of some underdeveloped cognitive coping strategies that correspond to typical vulnerabilities associated with each of the different personality disorders.

Based on individual patient needs, any or all of the following interventions may be appropriate.

- Predict the long-term implications of making no changes.
- Identify which areas of adaptive functioning are strengths and which areas need further attention (see Precept 4 for a list of adaptive functions).
- Reduce self-handicapping habits such as physical or financial self-harm, procrastination, passivity, seeking negative feedback; dominating, manipulating, or purposely frustrating others, acting on unfiltered impulses, and avoiding constructive feedback or reasonable personal responsibility.
- Practice mindfulness skills to heighten present-moment engagement and reduce brooding, distraction, or stress.
- Use acceptance strategies as a response to distressing thoughts or emotions.
- Identify values that support more emotionally secure relationships with self and others.
- Practice making decisions and setting goals that are consistent with chosen values.
- Identify personal history relevant to core self-image and integrate new information into a personal narrative.

TABLE 21.2. Underdeveloped Cognitive Coping Strategies

Personality Disorder	Selected Cognitive Coping Strategies to Strengthen
Paranoid	Test hypotheses about threats and consider benign and positive possibilities. Ask direct questions instead of covertly searching for clues to confirm suspicions. Consider potential benefits of social involvements.
Schizoid	List positive aspects of other people and shared experiences. Scale perceived demands from others, situation by situation.
Schizotypal	Evaluate the loss to benefit aspects of nonconforming choices in appearance, ideas, or social participation. Practice thinking about the logic of thoughts (metacognition).
Antisocial	Filter cognitions for dangerous, exploitive, or criminogenic ideas. Identify prosocial values and align with personal strengths or skillful choices.
Borderline	Observe and describe emotional states, behavioral urges, and potential consequences of impulses. Label action as a conscious choice. Rehearse images of constructive alternative actions and evoke positive emotions. Assess reasons for trust or mistrust of others and rate intensity.
Histrionic	Expand emotional vocabulary and metacognition about options for emotional expression.
Narcissistic	Evaluate potential loss to benefit ratio of validating others. Trace the implications of trumpeting strengths and avoiding vulnerability. Predict and test the possible benefits of compassion for others and social give and take.
Avoidant	Identify long-term consequences of emotional avoidance. Rate difficult emotions on a scale of intensity to build tolerance. Practice self-encouragement and self-direction to pursue goals, solve problems, and increase social initiative.
Dependent	Direct and sustain attention to planning, goal setting, decision making, task initiation, and accurate self-appraisal of strengths and potential.
Obsessive–Compulsive	Identify ambiguity and practice cognitive acceptance of uncertainty. List benefits of relaxation, release of tension, and compassion for self and others.
Passive–Aggressive	Compare the benefits of persistence (stubbornness) versus flexibility, cooperation or compromise. Identify reflexive opposition and detect social and personal costs. Direct attention to goal setting, task initiation, and decision-making.
Depressive	Appraise personal strengths and positive experiences. Construct positive emotional experiences with attention to planning, goal-directed persistence and awareness of valence between negative and positive appraisals.

Many patients will also benefit from reviewing pivotal events from their personal history, usually when memories are particularly salient such as at anniversaries or when old conflicts are stirred up in current situations. These reflections can provide insight or increased understanding of how certain self-schemas and behavior patterns "make sense" as part of a person's life story. They also provide an opportunity to test the validity of core beliefs in a past-versus-present context. Developmental insight is helpful for increasing cognitive distance and self-acceptance, and it can be combined with experiential exercises to reduce emotional pain, increase mastery, reconceptualize assumptions about reality, and mark the transition to a new "chapter" in the personal narrative. However, not everyone wants or needs to engage in a developmental review to successfully build a more flexible self-mode. Patients who have extensively explored their past in previous therapy may want to focus more on the here-and-now and need not be pushed to look back yet again. Therapists can support and affirm the work the patients have already done and help them to link their knowledge to the relevant self-schemas and coping modes that are the focus of current therapy. Therapists will want to monitor the usefulness of any developmental review, not pushing or dismissing these efforts, and discerning when it is helpful rethinking and when it is unhelpful ruminating about negative core beliefs.

The dysfunctional personality mode is also the patient's default mode. This means that it will take time, persistence, and some measure of ingenuity to craft and activate a more adaptive mode. Both patient and therapist need to understand that they are actually constructing a "new normal" mode of personality function and that they need to temper their expectations for how quickly and easily this should be attained. Patients may think that they have tried everything, even cognitive therapy, and may have periods of discouragement about its value. Therapists may face similar worrisome thoughts such as "maybe they really can't change," or "I can't get them to engage in cognitive therapy." Therapists may feel anxious about the range of techniques or the length of time needed to make substantial progress because this does not fit their image of a cognitive therapy protocol. Because the patient's core beliefs are embedded in primal schemas related to basic survival, health, identity, and attachments to others (Beck & Haigh, 2014), more effort, patience, and creativity are needed to significantly impact the patient's self-image and view of reality, and to stabilize a functional shift. Even when patients know their perceptions are skewed and they very much want to acquire new skills, it takes repetition across domains to build new strengths-based schemas, to make new coping strategies into habits, and to weaken the predominance of default modes.

For example, the first year of Meg's therapy focused on overcoming depressed mood, making decisions about her marriage, and coping with work stress. However, she was still vulnerable to significant mood swings and impulses toward self-harm because of her difficulties in coping with strong emotions and because of her persistent beliefs that she was a bad person who could not meet the expectations of others. When Meg felt criticized by others or disappointed in herself, which was often, her "hate mode" would activate, with screaming tirades, alcohol binges, and self-attacking rages that included vivid images of harming herself. Her therapist asked her to rehearse and use replacement images of self-care, and modeled calm persistence in helping her to develop skills in cognitive and behavioral redirection. Although Meg made diligent efforts, she had considerable difficulty expressing compassion to herself and altering some of her self-harming behaviors. Her feelings of guilt and discomfort in offering warm support to herself provided a memory bridge back to negative experiences from childhood and early adulthood when she experienced similar feelings. Over the course of several such emotional history reviews, Meg recognized unacknowledged sexual trauma as well as a family dynamic of rage, ridicule, and emotional aggression. These insights helped her to understand the origins of her assumption that she should attack and negatively judge herself, and to see the lack of support or nurturance as an unmet emotional need.

On several occasions, Meg's therapist guided her in imagery rescripting, which is an experiential exercise for using imagery to reprocess certain emotionally pivotal interactions from the past (Arntz, 2015; Sunger & Gündüz, 2015). The objective is to embed an image of how negative experiences might have been resolved more successfully, so that dysfunctional beliefs about the self can be challenged (e.g., "I'm bad"; "I don't deserve help"), and the patient can evoke feelings of empowerment and protection in a way that strengthens healthy adult skills. During one of these exercises, Meg recalled an experience of being ridiculed by her mother, and then imagined her adult self entering the scene and assertively redirecting the mother toward more effective problem solving, and comforting her frightened younger self. This helped Meg to link the past with her present schema of herself as an inadequate, bad person. It also helped to diminish the intrusiveness of the negative memories of her mother, and to increase her mastery and confidence in self-soothing skills. As therapy progressed, her marital relationship improved, she communicated her feelings more calmly and directly, she altered her pattern of alcohol use; she initiated more social activities for pleasure, and her self-harm urges and behaviors diminished.

5. *Infuse Homework with a Sense of Shared Curiosity and Potential Reward.*

Much of the art of engaging any patient resides in the therapist's ability to communicate a sense of adventure, personal caring, and the realistic hope for improved well-being. More than an outcome carrot at the end of the stick, the process of discovery itself needs to be intriguing, positive, interpersonally warm, and safe from punitive or discouraging messages. However, even the most skillful therapist can face significant challenges in attempting to provide this positive structure with this patient population. This can be particularly evident when it comes to the tasks of planning and following through on homework. Sometimes relabeling homework in various ways, such as self-coaching, personal practice, or terms the patient prefers can make the effort more appealing and valuable. However, strategic choice of words is only the beginning of engaging the personality-disordered patient in change efforts that extend beyond the session.

The therapist's task with homework is to assist patients in planning what to do between sessions to maximize their progress. Therapist effectiveness in this task has been linked to outcome improvements in symptoms and personality functioning among personality-disordered patients (Ryum, Stiles, Svartberg, & McCullough, 2010). Effectiveness with homework, as noted by Ryum and colleagues, has more to do with quality and strategy than with just adhering to a protocol or generating quantity. To maximize homework productivity, the therapist can (1) custom tailor it to the patient's interest and current energy; (2) articulate reasons why it might be helpful or rewarding; (3) elicit reactions to the idea and anticipated difficulties; (4) provide encouragement and guidance; (5) debrief the effort at the next session, link to progress and value; and (6) exchange feedback on the homework process.

The more a patient is involved in choosing specific homework activities, the more likely it is that he or she will value the effort and follow through. However, some personality-disordered patients either lack the skills or are too emotionally distracted to collaborate in generating homework ideas. So therapists may have to take the lead and generate suggestions or offer ideas as potential options. To reduce the risk of immediate resistance or avoidance, the therapist can draw a possible link between effort and reward in the form of a question. For example, one might ask a dependent patient, "Do you think it could be any fun at all to spend an afternoon by yourself, working on a project of your choosing?" "Could this possibly boost your self-confidence?" When the therapist poses a question about the link between homework and its potential benefits, the patient's curiosity will hopefully be aroused and her interest in testing the idea will increase. The notion of focusing on fun should not trivialize the homework, but rather emphasize the constructive, rewarding aims. This applies even when activities involve some discomfort. For example, exposures to feared situations provide the building blocks of self-confidence, which is desirable to most people. True collaboration involves adapting homework so that the plan is acceptable to the patient, and asking if they are willing to test the idea for its usefulness.

When patients are reluctant to try any homework, it may useful to observe that they are already doing something between sessions, and to ask them if there are any particular reasons for not trying something different. At the same time, it is also important to communicate emotional support for the patient's self-determination and to downplay any potential pressure to do a specific activity that the patient finds averse, or to produce a specific result. Particularly with guarded and fearful patients, it is crucial to communicate support for their autonomy and to avoid triggering fears of interpersonal control or manipulation. For example, the therapist might say, "I really want you to get the most from your therapy, and your thoughts about homework activities will help us both to know what might work best for you." In a very basic sense, homework is simply the pursuit of maximum rewards, with curiosity leading the way, at a pace that is tolerable and effective for the individual patient.

6. *Sustain Your Self.*

As the saying goes, "You can't pour from an empty cup." The complexities of treating personality disorders can tax a therapist's emotional and intellectual resources more than working with problems that are straightforward and amenable to basic protocols. Substantial energy may be needed to stay positively invested in the therapeutic relationship, to draw the patient into collaboration, to select, adapt, and implement treatment interventions, and to sustain productivity along the way. It is not unusual for therapists to be concerned about what they might be missing or disheartened by slow progress or difficult rapport. Stress level is more likely to escalate quickly when the patient encounters a crisis, as he or she may hold a higher risk of extreme or impulsive actions. Patients with personality disorders tend to elicit strong, often difficult emotions in others, including therapists. Emotional reactions such as feeling unusually anxious, frustrated, bored, or puzzled, or feeling particularly excited, interested, or elated are signs of what is often called "countertransference" or emotional responses to the patient's problems. Therapists may specifically worry that their technical skills are insufficient to the task of treating these challenging problems, or that someone else would have much greater success. While that may be true, the cultivation of a calm presence will contribute a great deal to one's ability to respond to emotionally charged interactions or intractable problems with creative perspective and functional professional objectivity. The therapist's emotion-regulating skills are important not only in session but beyond it as well.

Consulting regularly with colleagues can be invaluable for testing out thoughts about one's treatment approach and generating fresh options. Colleagues can also provide encouragement and support when a therapist is unsure about treatment continuation or referral. Therapists can assess whether they are accurately estimating their progress or objectivity with the patient, as these are common questions when dealing with personality problems. In addition to colleague consultation, a personal routine of relaxation and self-care activities can promote emotional distance and energy renewal needed to maintain a therapeutic balance of objectivity and involvement. It can also reduce the risk of unproductive, therapy-interfering thoughts, attitudes, and actions that put the therapist at risk of burnout. Sustaining oneself as a therapist is essential for remaining hopeful and persistent in adapting cognitive therapy for disorders of personality.

RESEARCH

Cognitive-behavioral interventions, including cognitive therapy (CT), schema therapy (ST), dialectical behavior therapy (DBT), acceptance and commitment therapy (ACT), and rational emotive behavior therapy (REBT), are the most investigated and supported forms of treatment for personality disorders (David & Freeman, 2015). Borderline personality disorder has been investigated most often, while schizoid and schizotypal personality disorders have received scant investigation. In treatment studies of symptomatic disorders where patients with various comorbid personality disorders were included, treatment gains were obtained for obsessive–compulsive disorder (McKay, Neziroglu, Todaro, & Yaryura-Tobias, 1996), panic (Black et al., 1996), social phobia (Hope, Herbert, & White, 1995), generalized anxiety (Sanderson, Beck, & McGinn, 1994), or depression (Kuyken, Kurzer, DeRubeis, Beck, & Brown, 2001; Lynch et al., 2007), with some concomitant improvement in personality traits. Although treatment dropout rates for patients with personality disorders are problematic in general, maladaptive avoidant and paranoid beliefs have been linked with poorer participation. This suggests that these particular types of beliefs exert a greater influence on outcome of symptomatic treatment than personality disorder diagnosis per se (Kuyken et al., 2001).

Investigations of cognitive interventions specifically targeted to personality disorders are promising, though limited in number and scope. In a randomized controlled trial for brief treatment of avoidant personality disorder, 91% of the patients who received CBT (twenty sessions) no longer met criteria for the disorder and maintained gains at the six-month follow-up (Emmelkamp et al., 2006). Another randomized controlled trial involving a mixed group of patients with Cluster C (avoidant, dependent, obsessive–compulsive), passive–aggressive, self-defeating, or comorbid personality disorders found that forty weekly sessions of cognitive therapy produced significant gains that continued to accrue over time. At a two-year follow-up, 42% were recovered on measures of symptoms, and 40% showed improvements in interpersonal and personality functioning

(Svartberg, Stiles, & Seltzer, 2004). In a large-scale, multicenter, randomized controlled trial that compared schema therapy to treatment as usual as well as a clarification-oriented therapy for patients with Cluster C, paranoid, narcissistic, and histrionic personality disorders, Bamelis and colleagues (2014) found that fifty sessions of schema therapy proved superior to the other treatments, with an 80% recovery rate at the three-year follow-up, including improvement of life function. These investigators highlight the following as distinctive aspects of schema therapy: (1) directiveness and psychoeducation; (2) treatment relationship interactions geared toward the patient's unmet (childhood) emotional needs; (3) focus on childhood experiences of trauma or neglect; (4) behavioral pattern breaking; and (5) integration of cognitive, behavioral, interpersonal, and experiential techniques.

Investigations of cognitive interventions with borderline personality disorder (BPD) are also encouraging. In a long-term follow-up of patients with BPD who were treated in a randomized controlled trial with one year of cognitive therapy, 50% had remitted six years posttreatment and had fewer inpatient days or suicidal acts than patients treated as usual (Davidson, Tyrer, Norrie, Palmer, & Tyrer, 2010). In an open clinical trial of cognitive therapy for BPD where patients were offered fifty weeks of treatment, 55% were remitted at the one-month follow-up, and overall dysfunctional beliefs improved (Brown, Newman, Charlesworth, Crits-Cristoph, & Beck, 2004). Giesen-Bloo and colleagues (2006) found intensive schema therapy (three years of sessions twice per week) to be more effective than similarly intensive transference-focused psychotherapy in treatment of BPD, although all patients improved in terms of symptoms, personality, and life function.

Lastly, a small-scale feasibility study of a community sample of violent men with antisocial personality disorder randomized participants into treatment as usual (TAU) or TAU plus up to thirty sessions of CBT (Davidson et al., 2009). The failure to find any significant effects of CBT on relevant measures in this study may have been due to low literacy levels as well as a high dropout rate either before CBT started or after one session. Among those who did participate, the trend was toward more positive personality beliefs, less harmful alcohol use, and better social functioning. The results of this study point toward the importance of conceptualizing the cognitive profile that is specific to the personality disorder. The patterns of aggressive and criminogenic cognitions and beliefs among persons with antisocial personality disorder (ASPD) are highly divergent from the patterns observed among persons with other personality disorders. Antisocial beliefs can even be a mirror opposite of the kinds of beliefs usually encountered among persons presenting with depression or anxiety problems. This can be quite confusing to many clinicians (Mitchell et al., 2015).

CONCLUSIONS

The cognitive model conceptualizes personality disorders as overdeveloped modes of potentially adaptive functioning in need of balance and flexibility, particularly with regard to self-concepts and cognitive control schema. Individualized treatment seeks to alter the cognitive profile by strengthening skills for coping with the fears associated with core negative self-schemas, testing perceptions of reality, exploring the theory of a malleable self, and reducing overreliance on compensatory self-schemas. Cognitive therapy helps the individual develop a new normal mode of functioning as an alternative to the maladaptive default mode that maintains their identity and way of relating to others. This process takes patience, persistence, creativity, and strong conceptual and interpersonal skills, and challenges the therapist to practice good personal stress management. Access to adequate treatment is often limited by negative beliefs about the potential for personality change, or perceptions that treatment is too difficult, too slow, or too weak for personality disorders. Given that personality disorders are common in the general population and prevalent among clinical populations, more research on treatment refinement and training of clinicians is needed. Although human tendencies and traits most certainly pass from one generation to the next, personality is still an ongoing, lifelong construction.

REFERENCES

American Psychiatric Association. (2013). *Diagnostic and statistical manual of mental disorders* (5th ed.). Arlington, VA: Author.

Arntz, A. (2015). Borderline personality disorder. In A. Beck, D. Davis, & A. Freeman (Eds.), *Cognitive therapy of personality disorders* (3rd ed., pp. 366–390). New York: Guilford Press.

Bamelis, L. L. M., Evers, S. M. A. A., Spinhoven, P., & Arntz, A. (2014). Results of a multicenter randomized controlled trials of the clinical effectiveness of schema therapy for personality disorders. *American Journal of Psychiatry, 171*, 305–322.

Beck, A. T. (2015). Theory of personality disorders. In A. Beck, D. Davis, & A. Freeman (Eds.), *Cognitive therapy of personality disorders* (3rd ed., pp. 19–62). New York: Guilford Press.

Beck, A., Davis, D., & Freeman, A. (2015). *Cognitive therapy of personality disorders* (3rd ed.). New York: Guilford Press.

Beck, A. T., Freeman, A., & Associates. (1990). *Cognitive therapy of personality disorders*. New York: Guilford Press.

Beck, A., Freeman, A., & Davis, D. B. (2004). *Cognitive therapy of personality disorders* (2nd ed.). New York: Guilford Press.

Beck, A. T., & Haigh, E. (2014). Advances in cognitive theory and therapy: The generic cognitive model. *Annual Review of Clinical Psychology, 10*, 1–24.

Behary, W., & Davis, D. (2015). Narcissistic personality disorder. In A. Beck, D.

Davis, & A. Freeman (Eds.), *Cognitive therapy of personality disorders* (3rd ed., pp. 299–324). New York: Guilford Press.

Black, D. W., Monahan, P., Wesner, R., Gabel, J., & Bowers, W. (1996). The effect of fluvoxamine, cognitive therapy, and placebo on abnormal personality traits in 44 patients with panic disorder. *Journal of Personality Disorders, 10*(2), 185–194.

Blackwell, L., Trzesniewski, K., & Dweck, C. S. (2007). Implicit theories of intelligence predict achievement across an adolescent transition: A longitudinal study and an intervention. *Child Development, 78*, 246–263.

Brauer, L., & Reinecke, M. (2015). Dependent personality disorder. In A. Beck, D. Davis, & A. Freeman (Eds.), *Cognitive therapy of personality disorders* (3rd ed., pp. 155–173). New York: Guilford Press.

Brown, G. K., Newman, C. F., Charlesworth, S., Crits-Cristoph, P., & Beck, A. T. (2004). An open clinical trial of cognitive therapy for borderline personality disorder. *Journal of Personality Disorders, 18*(3), 257–271.

Clark, D. A., & Hilchey, C. A. (2015). Depressive personality disorder. In A. Beck, D. Davis, & A. Freeman (Eds.), *Cognitive therapy of personality disorders* (3rd ed., pp. 223–243). New York: Guilford Press.

David, D. O., & Freeman, A. (2015). Overview of cognitive behavioral therapy of personality disorders. In A. T. Beck, D. D. Davis, & A. Freeman (Eds.), *Cognitive therapy of personality disorders* (3rd ed., pp. 3–18). New York: Guilford Press.

Davidson, K. M., Tyrer, P., Norrie, J., Palmer, S., & Tyrer, H. (2010). Cognitive therapy v. usual treatment for borderline personality disorder: Prospective 6-year follow-up. *British Journal of Psychiatry, 197*, 456–462.

Davidson, K. M., Tyrer, P., Tata, P., Cooke, D., Gumley, A., Ford, I., . . . Crawford, M. J. (2009). Cognitive behaviour therapy for violent men with antisocial personality disorder in the community: An exploratory randomized controlled trial. *Psychological Medicine, 39*, 569–577.

Dweck, C. S. (1999). *Self-theories: Their role in motivation, personality and development.* Philadelphia: Taylor and Francis/Psychology Press.

Dweck, C. S. (2008). Can personality be changed? *Current Directions in Psychological Science, 17*(6), 391–394.

Emmelkamp, P. M. G., Benner, A., Kuipers, A., Feiertag, G. A., Koster, H. C., & van Apeldoorn, F. J. (2006). Comparison of brief dynamic and cognitive-behavioral therapies in avoidant personality disorder. *British Journal of Psychiatry, 189*, 60–64.

Fulton, P. R., & Siegel, R. D. (2013). Buddhist and western psychology: Seeking common ground. In C. K. Germer, R. D. Siegel, & P. R. Fulton (Eds.), *Mindfulness and psychotherapy* (2nd ed., p. 48). New York: Guilford Press.

Fusco, G. (2015). Passive–aggressive personality disorder (negativistic personality disorder). In A. Beck, D. Davis, & A. Freeman (Eds.), *Cognitive therapy of personality disorders* (3rd ed., pp. 276–298). New York: Guilford Press.

Giesen-Bloo, J., van Dyck, R., Spinhoven, P., van Tilburg, W., Dirksen, C., van Asselt, T., . . . Arntz, A. (2006). Outpatient psychotherapy for borderline personality disorder, randomized trial of schema-focused therapy vs transference-focused psychotherapy. *Archives of General Psychiatry, 63*, 649–658.

Gunderson, J. G., Stout, R. L., McGlashan, T. H., Shea, M. T., Morey, L. C., &

Zanarini, M. C. (2011). Ten-year course of borderline personality disorder: Psychopathology and function from the Collaborative Longitudinal Personality Disorders Study. *Archives of General Psychiatry, 68,* 827–837.

Hope, D., Herbert, J., & White, C. (1995). Diagnostic subtype, avoidant personality disorder, and efficacy of cognitive-behavioral group therapy for social phobia. *Cognitive Therapy and Research, 19,* 399–417.

Kuyken, W., Kurzer, N., DeRubeis, R. J., Beck, A. T., & Brown, G. K. (2001). Response to cognitive therapy in depression: The role of maladaptive beliefs and personality disorders. *Journal of Consulting and Clinical Psychology, 69*(3), 560–566.

Lenzenweger, M. F., Lane, M. C., Loranger, A. W., & Kessler, R. C. (2007). DSM-IV personality disorders in the National Comorbidity Survey Replication. *Biological Psychiatry, 62*(6), 553–564.

Lynch, T. R., Cheavens, J. S., Cukrowicz, K. C., Thorp, S. R., Bronner, L., & Beyer, J. (2007). Treatment of older adults with co-morbid personality disorder and depression: A dialectical behavior therapy approach. *International Journal of Geriatric Psychiatry, 22*(2), 31–143.

McKay, D., Neziroglu, F., Todaro, J., & Yaryura-Tobias, J. A. (1996). Changes in personality disorders following behavior therapy for obsessive–compulsive disorder. *Journal of Anxiety Disorders, 10*(1), 47–57.

Miller, W. R., & Rollnick, S. (2012). *Motivational interviewing: Helping people change* (3rd ed.). New York: Guilford Press.

Mitchell, D., Tafrate, R. C., & Freeman, A. (2015). Antisocial personality disorder. In A. Beck, D. Davis, & A. Freeman (Eds.), *Cognitive therapy of personality disorders* (3rd ed., pp. 346–365). New York: Guilford Press.

Morey, L., & Hopwood, C. (2013). Stability and change in personality disorders. *Annual Review of Clinical Psychology, 9,* 499–528.

Mueller, C. M., & Dweck, C. S. (1998). Intelligence praise can undermine motivation and performance. *Journal of Personality and Social Psychology, 75,* 33–52.

Padesky, C., & Beck, J. (2015). Avoidant personality disorder. In A. Beck, D. Davis, & A. Freeman (Eds.), *Cognitive therapy of personality disorders* (3rd ed., pp. 174–202). New York: Guilford Press.

Renton, J., & Mankiewicz, P. (2015). Paranoid, schizotypal, and schizoid personality disorders. In A. Beck, D. Davis, & A. Freeman (Eds.), *Cognitive therapy of personality disorders* (3rd ed., pp. 244–275). New York: Guilford Press.

Roberts, B. W., Walton, K. E., & Viechtbauer, W. (2006). Patterns of mean-level change in personality traits across the life course: A meta-analysis of longitudinal studies. *Psychological Bulletin, 132,* 1–25.

Ryum, T., Stiles, T., Svartberg, M., & McCullough, L. (2010). The effects of therapist competence in assigning homework in cognitive therapy with Cluster C personality disorders: Results from a randomized controlled trial. *Cognitive and Behavioral Practice, 17,* 283–289.

Sanderson, W. C., Beck, A. T. & McGinn, L. K. (1994). Cognitive therapy for generalized anxiety disorder: Significance of co-morbid personality disorders. *Journal of Cognitive Psychotherapy: An International Quarterly, 8,* 13–18.

Simon, K. (2015). Obsessive–compulsive personality disorder. In A. Beck, D. Davis, & A. Freeman (Eds.), *Cognitive therapy of personality disorders* (3rd ed., pp. 203–222). New York: Guilford Press.

Sungur, M., & Gündüz, A. (2015). Histrionic personality disorder. In A. Beck, D. Davis, & A. Freeman (Eds.), *Cognitive therapy of personality disorders* (3rd ed., pp. 325–345). New York: Guilford Press.

Svartberg, M., Stiles, T. C., & Seltzer, M. H. (2004). Randomized, controlled trial of the effectiveness of short-term dynamic psychotherapy and cognitive therapy for cluster C personality disorders. *American Journal of Psychiatry, 161,* 810–817.

Young, J. E. (1999). *Cognitive therapy for personality disorders: A schema-focused approach* (3rd ed.). Sarasota, FL: Professional Resource Press/Professional Resource Exchange.

Young, J. E., Klosko, J., & Weishaar, M. E. (2003). *Schema therapy: A practitioner's guide.* New York: Guilford Press.

Zanarini, M. C., Frankenburg, F. R., Hennen, J., Reich, D. B., & Silk, K. R. (2006). Prediction of the 10-year course of borderline personality disorder. *American Journal of Psychiatry, 163,* 827–832.

Zanarini, M. C., Frankenburg, F. R., Reich, D. B., & Fitzmaurice, G. (2012). Attainment and stability of sustained symptomatic remission and recovery among patients with borderline personality disorder and Axis II comparison subjects: A 16-year prospective follow-up study. *American Journal of Psychiatry, 169,* 476–483.

CHAPTER 22

Concluding Thoughts

Robert L. Leahy

When I first met Aaron Beck in December 1981 at the Center for Cognitive Therapy at the University of Pennsylvania Medical School, it seemed that cognitive therapy was just beginning to gain some recognition. It was the "new kid on the block," and there was considerable excitement that we were part of a revolution in the field of psychotherapy. From 1982 to 1983 when I was associated with them, the Center had a number of future stars—Arthur Freeman, Jeff Young, Norm Epstein, John Riskind, and others—but we all felt that we were learning from a singular giant whose soft-spoken demeanor deceptively hid the brilliant and even provocative ideas that were the foundation of cognitive therapy. Beck held the "Anxiety Seminar" every week, where many of us might have felt anxious—but the topic was how we could apply the cognitive model to the treatment of anxiety. This was before the DSM had become dominant, often clouding the thinking of clinicians about the underlying processes. Beck would run the seminar like a Socratic dialogue asking participants about patients and then why the thought or situation would bother the patient. Each question was an attempt to find the underlying meaning of sensations, situational triggers, thoughts, and assumptions. Beck shared with us his curiosity about how patients thought and reacted—rather than focusing on psychodynamics or contingencies that were important in other theories. I had previously been involved in research in developmental psychology where Piaget's constructivist model was influential. Beck's clinical inquiry with patients seemed like it could have been a branch of Piagetian theory—perhaps, "The patient's construction of threat, loss, and hopelessness." Beck's model was nothing less than a description of the patient's theory of the world.

At that time, in the early 1980s, the cognitive model only had empirical support from the early research on depression. Beck avoided making any grandiose claims about proven efficacy of cognitive therapy for anything other than depression. The data just were not there yet—the studies had not been done. Beck wanted to proceed cautiously, basing his work on scientific findings, not overreaching.

As this volume reflects, the field has expanded immensely in the last thirty-five years—far more than I think Beck or any of us thought it would. As the research reviews indicate, we now have evidence that cognitive therapy—or CBT—is effective in the treatment of major depressive disorder, dysthymia, bipolar disorder, borderline personality, social anxiety disorder, generalized anxiety disorder, PTSD, panic disorder, and agoraphobia, obsessive–compulsive disorder, schizophrenia, couples issues, family problems, child and adolescent disorders, and eating disorders. The field of behavioral medicine has also benefited from CBT models in the treatment of irritable bowel syndrome, headaches, pain management, traumatic brain injury, weight management, and other problems.

The cognitive approach provides a sophisticated and complex model of how different forms of psychopathology may arise, how these problems are maintained or exacerbated, and how they are treated. This may sound rather simplistic—but it's not, in my view. By identifying the evolutionary, socialization, neurobiological, and cognitive elements of a disorder—such as panic disorder with agoraphobia—the clinician can elaborate a case conceptualization that can be used with the patient. The "cognitive architecture" that underpins panic disorder (or any of the other disorders) allows the clinician to identify idiosyncratic automatic thoughts, maladaptive assumptions, and core beliefs, which are driven by confirmation bias and by selective memory and evaluation of negative information. These different levels of cognitive processing can also be targeted for intervention, behavioral experiments can be developed with the patient, and the credibility of these levels of thought can be modified. Unhelpful safety behaviors (such as reassurance seeking, reliance on others, specific habits of walking or breathing, avoidance of anxiety-provoking situations) can be relinquished, and the underlying catastrophic predictions can be tested. Thus, models of etiology, activation, and maintenance are directly related to specific intervention strategies.

Now this is different from the psychodynamic model that CBT has largely surpassed in influence. I recall a story told by Ed Zigler at Yale in my undergraduate course in "Abnormal Psychology" many years ago. Ed was working in a hospital, and a psychoanalytic colleague was describing the Oedipal Complex of one of the patients on the ward. Ed kept asking, "How do you know this is true," and the analyst kept pointing to the conceptualization of parental conflict and "underlying motivations." Ed said, "Make a prediction that we can test." So the analyst said, "When the orderly asks him to help out on the ward, the patient will rebel because he will see the orderly as a father figure—and this will make him rebel." The next week the orderly was called into the meeting, and the analyst asked him how the patient responded to him. The orderly said, "He was one of the most helpful patients I have seen here. He asked how he could help out and thanked me for asking him." The analyst then dismissed the orderly. Ed said, "You said he would rebel but he was cooperative." The analyst turned to Zigler and said, "Don't you see? It was reaction formation!"

I will never forget that story because it illustrates one of the main reasons that Beck felt the need to develop a testable model. Beck did not want to get caught in circular fictional conceptualizations that would have little relevance to effective treatment. As Rachel Rosner's fascinating chapter in this volume illustrates, Beck had hoped that his new cognitive model would become an extension of the ego psychology current at that time. He wanted to improve on the psychodynamic model. But the analysts would not have anything to do with him. He was voted off the island, as they say. As a result, the cognitive model—and the CBT models in general—went their own way, building conceptualizations that could be tested out—making clinical psychology into an empirical field rather than a closed system.

Our colleague David Clark at Oxford University has been instrumental in disseminating CBT in the National Health Service in the United Kingdom. The government-run program—The Initiative for Accessible Psychological Treatments—is the largest program to disseminate effective psychological treatment ever conducted anywhere in the world. It is telling that Clark collaborated with Richard Layard, an economist at the London School of Economics, to "sell" this program—first to Tony Blair's Labour government and then to David Cameron's Conservative/Liberal coalition administration. One would like to think that the selling point was the compassion and humanity in providing effective treatment for depression. But politics being what it is, we know that the main selling point was that psychological treatment is cost effective. The government—and, therefore the taxpayer—will save money if people are able to get back to work, get off government aid, and require fewer health care services. And that is exactly what has happened. The psychological treatments are largely CBT—and it is reassuring to know that it works.

The chapters in this volume do not cover every aspect of CBT—a book that did would be extremely long. But I hope that the reader has been able to get a clear idea of the current state of much of the field that has been influenced by the cognitive model. There are other CBT models that are valuable and effective—such as dialectical behavior therapy, behavioral activation, and acceptance and commitment therapy—and it is a reflection of the richness of the field that we, as clinicians, have such a plethora of techniques and strategies that we can use. After all, it all comes down to helping people who are suffering, whose lives are transfixed by fear and hopelessness, who have lost any shred of meaning in their lives. The contributors to this volume have helped in our shared effort to provide a path out of misery, to empower clinicians—throughout the world—with new tools and strategies that seem to proliferate daily. Somewhere someone's mother or father, sister or brother, son or daughter—or friend—will follow that path out of the darkness. They will not know, of course, all the years of work by other clinicians and researchers who have made that path possible.

And, for that and for so much more, I am grateful to the contributors to this volume.

Index

Note. *f* or *t* following a page number indicates a figure or a table.

H

I

J

L

M

N

O

P